# Challenging Concepts in Interventional Radiology and Endovascular Procedures

## Published and forthcoming titles in the Challenging Concepts in series

**Anaesthesia** (Edited by Dr Phoebe Syme, Dr Robert Jackson, and Professor Tim Cook)

**Cardiovascular Medicine** (Edited by Dr Aung Myat, Dr Shouvik Haldar, and Professor Simon Redwood)

**Emergency Medicine** (Edited by Dr Sam Thenabadu, Dr Fleur Cantle, and Dr Chris Lacy)

**Infectious Disease and Clinical Microbiology** (Edited by Dr Amber Arnold and Professor George Griffin)

**Interventional Radiology and Endovascular Procedures** (Edited by Dr Miltiadis Krokidis, Dr Irfan Ahmed, and Dr Tarun Sabharwal)

**Neurology** (Edited by Dr Krishna Chinthapalli, Dr Nadia Magdalinou, and Professor Nicholas Wood)

**Neurosurgery** (Edited by Mr Robin Bhatia and Mr Ian Sabin)

**Obstetrics and Gynaecology** (Edited by Dr Natasha Hezelgrave, Dr Danielle Abbott, and Professor Andrew Shennan)

**Oncology** (Edited by Dr Madhumita Bhattacharyya, Dr Sarah Payne, and Professor Iain McNeish)

**Oral and Maxillofacial Surgery** (Edited by Mr Matthew Idle and Dr Andrew Monaghan)

**Respiratory Medicine** (Edited by Dr Lucy Schomberg and Dr Elizabeth Sage)

# Challenging Concepts in Interventional Radiology and Endovascular Procedures

## *Cases with Expert Commentary*


*Edited by*

Miltiadis Krokidis
Consultant Vascular and Interventional Radiologist,
Department of Radiology, Cambridge University Hospitals
NHS Foundation Trust, Cambridge, UK

Irfan Ahmed
Consultant Vascular and Interventional Radiologist,
Department of Radiology, Guy's and St Thomas'
NHS Foundation Trust, London, UK

Tarun Sabharwal
Consultant Vascular and Interventional Radiologist,
Department of Radiology, Guy's and St Thomas'
NHS Foundation Trust, London, UK

*Series editors*

Dr Aung Myat BSc (Hons) MBBS MRCP
BHF Clinical Research Training Fellow, King's College London British Heart Foundation
Centre of Research Excellence, Cardiovascular Division, St Thomas' Hospital, London, UK

Dr Shouvik Haldar MBBS MRCP
Electrophysiology Research Fellow & Cardiology SpR, Heart Rhythm Centre, NIHR Cardiovascular
Biomedical Research Unit, Royal Brompton & Harefield NHS Foundation Trust, Imperial College
London, London, UK

Professor Simon Redwood MD FRCP
Professor of Interventional Cardiology and Honorary Consultant Cardiologist, King's College London
British Heart Foundation Centre of Research Excellence, Cardiovascular Division and Guy's and
St Thomas' NHS Foundation Trust, Dr Thomas' Hospital, London, UK



OXFORD
UNIVERSITY PRESS

**OXFORD**
**UNIVERSITY PRESS**

Great Clarendon Street, Oxford, OX2 6DP,
United Kingdom

Oxford University Press is a department of the University of Oxford. It furthers the University's objective of excellence in research, scholarship, and education by publishing worldwide. Oxford is a registered trade mark of Oxford University Press in the UK and in certain other countries



Impression: 1



Published in the United States of America by Oxford University Press
198 Madison Avenue, New York, NY 10016, United States of America

British Library Cataloguing in Publication Data
Data available

Library of Congress Control Number: 2015934018

ISBN 978–0–19–966438–2

Printed in Great Britain by
Ashford Colour Press Ltd, Gosport, Hampshire

# FOREWORD

Interventional radiology has come of age, and has an established place in modern medical care. Its techniques have been shown to be clinically effective, safe, and less expensive than most equivalent open surgical procedures. There are now several excellent textbooks of interventional radiology which deal with all aspects of the discipline. The Cardiovascular and Interventional Radiological Society of Europe has created a robust examination, which is rapidly setting training standards in this discipline within Europe and beyond.

This book does not aim to provide systematic instruction in the techniques of interventional radiology at either a basic or at an advanced level. Instead, the editors, Miltos Krokidis, Irfan Ahmed, and Tarun Sabharwal, have adopted an innovative and fresh approach—they have focused on important current issues in interventional radiology. In each case, instead of an exhaustive review of the literature and a series of vague statements presenting all views on an individual topic, they have chosen to deal with each issue with clarity and confidence, and have tried to offer a clear opinion on each subject.

The book contains 31 cases. The emphasis is on endovascular procedures, but important nonvascular topics, mainly in interventional oncology, are also included. Each case has been written by either an interventional radiologist in training or a young staff radiologist. There are clear descriptions of techniques, examples of challenging cases, learning points, and a focus on these points by experts in the subject. The layout is clear, colourful, and easy to navigate. This approach has resulted in a fresh and topical volume, and a 'no-nonsense' practical approach. There is no attempt to cover each subject in a comprehensive fashion, or to present the latest research on each topic. But the trainee, or the young staff radiologist seeking guidance on some of the most important issues in this discipline, will enjoy reading this excellent and refreshing book, and will want to keep a copy within easy reach.

Andreas Adam CBE, MB, BS(Hons),
PhD, FRCP, FRCR, FRCS, FFRRCSI(Hon),
FRANZCR(Hon), FACR(Hon), FMedSci
Professor of Interventional Radiology,
King's College London

# CONTENTS

# EXPERTS

**Professor Andreas Adam**
Professor of Interventional Radiology
King's College London
Department of Radiology
Guy's and St Thomas' NHS Foundation Trust
London
UK

**Dr Irfan Ahmed**
Consultant Vascular and Interventional Radiologist
Department of Radiology
Guy's and St Thomas' NHS Foundation Trust
London
UK

**Professor Anna-Maria Belli**
Professor of Interventional Radiology
St Georges Medical School
Department of Radiology
St George's University Hospitals NHS Foundation Trust
London
UK

**Professor Elias Brountzos**
Professor of Interventional Radiology
Athens University Medical School
Second Department of Radiology
Attikon University Hospital
Athens
Greece

**Dr Fabrizio Fanelli**
Vascular and Interventional Radiologist
Vascular and Interventional Radiology Unit
Department of Radiological Sciences
Sapienza University Hospital
Rome
Italy

**Professor Afshin Gangi**
Professor of Diagnostic and Interventional Radiology
University of Louis Pasteur
Department of Radiology
University Hospital of Strasbourg
Strasbourg
France

**Dr Panos Gkoutzios**
Consultant Vascular and Interventional Radiologist
Department of Radiology
Guy's and St Thomas' NHS Foundation Trust,
London
UK

**Dr Mo Hamady**
Consultant Interventional Radiologist
Honorary Senior Lecturer
Department of Surgery and Cancer
Imperial College
London
UK

**Ass. Prof Adam Hatzidakis**
Assistant Professor of Radiology
University of Crete Medical School
Department of Medical Imaging
University Hospital of Heraklion
Heraklion
Greece

**Dr Hanno Hoppe**
Vascular and Interventional Radiologist
Linderhof Hospital
Bern
Switzerland

**Professor Vittorio Iaccarino**
Professor of Interventional Radiology
University of Naples Medical School
Department of Cardiovascular and Interventional Radiology
University Hospital Federico II
Naples
Italy

**Ass Prof Dimitrios Karnabatidis**
Associate Professor of Radiology
University of Patras Medical School
Department of Interventional Radiology
Patras University Hospital
Rio
Greece

**Dr Narayan Karunanithy**
Consultant Vascular and Interventional Radiologist
Department of Radiology
Guy's and St Thomas' NHS Foundation Trust
London
UK

**Dr Konstantinos Katsanos**
Consultant Vascular and Interventional Radiologist
Department of Radiology
Guy's and St Thomas' NHS Foundation Trust
London
UK

**Dr Philip Kwok**
Consultant Radiologist
Department of Radiology and Imaging
Queen Elizabeth Hospital
Kowloon
Hong Kong

**Professor Michael J Lee**
Consultant Interventional Radiologist
Beaumont Hospital
Professor of Radiology
Royal College of Surgeons in Ireland
Department of Radiology
Beaumont Hospital
Dublin
Ireland

**Dr Robert Morgan**
Consultant Vascular and Interventional Radiologist
Department of Radiology
St George's University Hospitals NHS Foundation Trust
London
UK

**Dr Praveen Peddu**
Consultant Interventional Radiologist
Department of Radiology
King's College Hospital NHS Foundation Trust
London
UK

**Dr Iain Robertson**
Consultant Interventional Radiologist
Department of Interventional Radiology
Gartnavel General Hospital
Glasgow
UK

**Ass Prof Michele Rossi**
Associate Professor of Radiology
Department of Radiological, Oncological and Pathological Sciences
Sapienza University of Rome
Italy

**Dr Tarun Sabharwal**
Consultant Vascular and Interventional Radiologist
Department of Radiology
Guy's and St Thomas' NHS Foundation Trust
London
UK

**Professor Dimitrios Siablis**
Professor of Interventional Radiology
University of Patras Medical School
Department of Interventional Radiology
Patras University Hospital
Rio
Greece

**Professor Małgorzata Szczerbo-Trojanowska**
Professor of Interventional Radiology
Department of Interventional Radiology and Neuroradiology
Medical University of Lublin
Lublin
Poland

**Professor Peter Taylor**
Professor of Vascular Surgery
King's College London
Department of Vascular Surgery
Guy's and St Thomas' NHS Foundation Trust
London
UK

**Professor Anthony Watkinson**
Professor of Interventional Radiology
The Peninsular Medical School
Department of Radiology
Royal Devon and Exeter Hospital NHS Foundation Trust
Exeter
UK

**Dr Andrew Winterbottom**
Consultant Vascular and Interventional Radiologist
Department of Radiology
Cambridge University Hospitals NHS Foundation Trust
Cambridge
UK

# CONTRIBUTORS

**Dr Ali Alsafi**
Specialist Registrar in Clinical Radiology
Imperial College Healthcare NHS Trust
London
UK

**Dr Christopher Burke**
Fellow in Interventional Radiology
Department of Radiology
Guys' and St Thomas' NHS Foundation Trust
London
UK

**Dr Alessandro Cannavale**
Specialist Registrar in Radiology
Vascular and Interventional Radiology Unit
Department of Radiological Sciences
Sapienza University Hospital
Rome
Italy

**Dr Andrew Christie**
Consultant Interventional Radiologist
Department of Interventional Radiology
Gartnavel General Hospital
Glasgow
UK

**Dr Raymond Chung**
Fellow in Interventional Radiology
Department of Radiology
St George's University Hospitals NHS Foundation Trust
London
UK

**Mrs Rachel Clough**
Vascular and Endovascular Fellow
Department of Vascular Surgery
Guy's and St Thomas' NHS Foundation Trust
London
UK

**Dr Raj Das**
Consultant Interventional Radiologist
Department of Radiology
St George's University Hospitals NHS Foundation Trust
London
UK

**Dr Athanasios Diamantopoulos**
Consultant Vascular and Interventional Radiologist
Department of Radiology
Guy's and St Thomas' NHS Foundation Trust
London
UK

**Dr Nicos Fotiadis**
Consultant Interventional Radiologist
Department of Radiology
The Royal Marsden NHS Foundation Trust
London
UK

**Dr Angie Galea**
Specialist Registrar in Clinical Radiology
Peninsula Radiology Academy
Plymouth
UK

**Dr Bhaskar Ganai**
Lecturer in Interventional Radiology
Royal College of Surgeons in Ireland
Department of Radiology
Beaumont Hospital
Dublin
Ireland

**Dr Richard Guinness**
Consultant Radiologist
Royal Devon and Exeter Hospital NHS Foundation Trust
Exeter
UK

**Dr Venus Hedayati**
Consultant Radiologist
Department of Radiology
King's College Hospital NHS Foundation Trust,
London
UK

**Dr Riccardo Inchingolo**
Interventional Radiologist
Diagnostic and Interventional Radiology Unit
"Madonna delle Grazie" Hospital
Matera
Italy

**Dr Magdalena Jarząbek**
Fellow in Interventional Radiology,
Department of Interventional Radiology and
Neuroradiology
Lublin University Hospital
Lublin
Poland

**Dr Panagiotis Kitrou**
Vascular and Interventional Radiologist
Department of Interventional Radiology
Patras University Hospital
Rio
Greece

**Dr Miltiadis Krokidis**
Consultant Vascular and Interventional Radiologist
Department of Radiology
Cambridge University Hospitals NHS Foundation Trust
Cambridge
UK

**Mr Christos Lioupis**
Vascular and Endovascular Fellow
Department of Vascular Surgery
Guy's and St Thomas' NHS Foundation Trust
London
UK

**Dr Leto Maili**
Consultant Vascular and Interventional
Radiologist
Department of Radiology
St George's University Hospitals NHS Foundation
Trust
London
UK

**Dr Peter Mezes**
Consultant Interventional Radiologist
North Bristol NHS Trust
Bristol
UK

**Dr Gianluigi Orgera**
Interventional Radiologist
Department of Radiological
Oncological and Pathological Sciences
Sapienza University of Rome
Rome
Italy

**Dr Aneeta Parthipun**
Fellow in Interventional Radiology
Department of Radiology
Guys' and St Thomas' NHS Foundation Trust
London
UK

**Dr Vyzantios Pavlidis**
Specialist Registrar in Radiology
Second Department of Radiology
Attikon University Hospital
Athens University Medical School
Athens

**Mr Shirish Prabhudesai**
Specialist Registrar in Surgery
Department of Biosurgery and Surgical Technology
Imperial College
St Mary's Hospital
London
UK

**Dr Nadeem Shaida**
Consultant Vascular and Interventional
Radiologist
Department of Radiology
Cambridge University Hospitals NHS Foundation
Trust
Cambridge
UK

**Dr Aidan Shaw**
Fellow in Interventional Radiology
Department of Radiology
Guy's and St Thomas' NHS Foundation Trust
London
UK

**Dr Stavros Spiliopoulos**
Vascular and Interventional Radiologist
Department of Interventional Radiology
Patras University Hospital
Rio
Greece

**Dr Victoria St Noble**
Specialist Registrar in Clinical Radiology
Department of Radiology
Royal Brompton Hospital
London
UK

**Dr Kendrick Tang**
Specialist Registrar in Radiology
Department of Radiology
Pamela Youde Nethersole Eastern Hospital
Chai Wan
Hong Kong

**Dr Piotr Trojanowski**
ENT Surgeon,
ENT Department
Lublin University Hospital
Lublin
Poland

**Dr Georgia Tsoumakidou**
Interventional Radiologist
Department of Radiology
University Hospital of Strasbourg
Strasbourg
France

**Dr Piero Venetucci**
Vascular and Interventional Radiologist,
Department of Cardiovascular and Interventional Radiology
University Hospital Federico II
Naples
Italy

# ABBREVIATIONS

| | |
|---|---|
| A&E | Accident and Emergency |
| AAA | abdominal aortic aneurysm |
| ABC | aneurysmal bone cyst |
| ABF | aorto-bifemoral |
| ABI | ankle–brachial pressure index |
| ABPI | ankle–brachial pressure index |
| ACCF | American College of Cardiology Foundation |
| ACT | activated clotting time |
| ADHF | acute decompensated heart failure |
| AFP | alpha-fetoprotein |
| AHA | American Heart Association |
| ALI | acute limb ischaemia |
| ALP | alkaline phosphatase |
| AP | anteroposterior |
| aPTT | activated partial thromboplastin time |
| ASA | American Society of Anesthesiologists |
| AST | aspartate aminotransferase |
| ATA | anterior tibial artery |
| AV | arteriovenous |
| AVM | arteriovenous malformation |
| BAE | bronchial artery embolization |
| BCLC pathway | Barcelona Clinic Liver Cancer pathway |
| BCS | Budd–Chiari syndrome |
| BMS | bare metal stent |
| BPH | benign prostate hypertrophy |
| BTK | below the knee |
| CAS | carotid artery stenting |
| CCA | common carotid artery |
| CCT | controlled clinical trial |
| CDT | catheter-directed thrombolysis |
| CDU | clinical decision unit, colour Doppler ultrasound |
| CEA | carotid endarterecomy |
| ce-CT | contrast-enhanced computed tomography |
| CEMRA | contrast-enhanced magnetic resonance angiography |
| CFA | common femoral artery |
| CI | confidence interval |
| CIA | common iliac artery |
| CKD | chronic kidney disease |
| CLI | critical limb ischaemia |
| COPD | chronic obstructive pulmonary disease |
| CPR | cardiopulmonary resuscitation |
| Cr | creatinine |
| CSS | cancer-specific survival |
| CT | computed tomography |
| CTA | CT angiography |
| CTO | chronic total occlusion |
| CXR | chest X-ray |
| DEB | drug-eluting balloon |
| DFS | disease-free survival |
| DIC | disseminated intravascular coagulopathy |
| DIPS | direct intrahepatic portocaval shunt |
| DLco | diffusing capacity of lung for carbon monoxide |
| DMSO | dimethyl sulphoxide |
| DP | dorsalis pedis |
| DPA | descending palatine artery, dorsalis pedalis artery |
| DSA | digital subtraction angiography |
| DU | Doppler ultrasound |
| DVT | deep vein thrombosis |
| ECA | external carotid artery |
| ECG | electrocardiogram |
| ECOG | Eastern Cooperative Oncology Group |
| EDV | end diastolic velocity |
| eGFR | estimated glomerular filtration rate |
| EIA | external iliac artery |
| EL | endoleak |
| ePTFE | expanded polytetrafluoroethylene |
| ESC | European Society of Cardiology |
| ET | essential thrombocythemia |
| EVAR | endovascular aortic repair |
| FA | facial artery |

| | |
|---|---|
| FAST | focused abdominal ultrasonography |
| FDG | fludeoxyglucose |
| $FEV_1$ | forced expiratory volume in 1 second |
| FEVAR | fenestrated endovascular aortic repair |
| $FiO_2$ | fraction of inspired oxygen |
| FNA | fine-needle aspiration |
| FVC | forced vital capacity |
| GA | general anaesthetic |
| GCS | Glasgow coma scale |
| GFR | glomerular filtration rate |
| GGT | gamma glutamyl transferase |
| GI | gastrointestinal |
| GP | general practitioner |
| GTN | glyceryl trinitrate |
| Hb | haemoglobin |
| HCC | hepatocellular carcinoma |
| HE | hepatic encephalopathy |
| HFDU | high-frequency duplex ultrasound |
| HHT | hereditary haemorrhagic telangiectasia |
| HoLAP | holmium laser ablation of the prostate |
| HR | hazard ratio |
| HTC | haematocrit |
| HU | Hounsfield unit |
| ICA | internal carotid artery |
| ICBT | intercostal bronchial trunk |
| ICER | incremental cost-effectiveness ratio |
| ICU | intensive care unit |
| IIAOB | internal iliac artery occlusion balloon |
| IM | intramuscular |
| IMA | internal mammary artery, internal maxillary artery |
| INR | international normalized ratio |
| IPSS | International Prostate Symptom Score |
| ISR | in-stent re-stenosis |
| ISV | internal spermatic vein |
| IVC | inferior vena cava |
| IVUS | intravascular ultrasound |
| JRA | juxtarenal aneurysm |
| LAD | left anterior descending artery |
| LAO | lateral anterior oblique |
| LCA | lateral calcaneal artery |
| LPA | lateral plantar artery |
| LSA | left subclavian artery |
| LUTS | lower urinary tract symptoms |
| MAI | mycobacterium avium-intracellulare |
| MCA | medial calcaneal artery |
| MDCTA | multidetector computed tomography angiography |
| MDT | multidisciplinary team |
| MELD | Model for End-Stage Liver Disease |
| MFS | metastasis-free survival |
| MI | myocardial infarction |
| MIP | multiple intensity projection |
| MPA | medial plantar artery |
| MPR | multiplanar reconstruction |
| MRA | magnetic resonance angiography |
| MRI | magnetic resonance imaging |
| NAFLD | non-alcoholic fatty liver disease |
| NBCA | n-butyl cyanoacrylate |
| NIHSS | National Institutes of Health Stroke Scale |
| NSCLC | non-small-cell lung cancer |
| NTT | number needed to treat |
| od | once daily |
| OLT | orthotopic liver transplantation |
| OS | overall survival |
| OSR | open surgical repair |
| PA | peroneal artery |
| $PaCO_2$ | partial pressure of carbon dioxide in arterial blood |
| PAD | peripheral arterial disease |
| PAE | pelvic arterial embolization, prostate artery embolization |
| $PaO_2$ | partial pressure of oxygen in arterial blood |
| PAOD | peripheral arterial occlusive disease |
| PCA | patient-controlled anaesthesia |
| PCD | phlegmasia cerulea dolens |
| PE | pulmonary embolism |
| PEI | percutaneous ethanol injection |
| PET | positron emission tomography |
| PMMA | polymethylmethacrylate |
| PMT | pharmacomechanical thrombectomy |
| PN | partial nephrectomy |
| PP | pampiniform plexus |

| | |
|---|---|
| PR | per rectum |
| PSA | prostate-specific antigen |
| PSV | peak systolic velocity |
| PT | posterior tibia, prothrombin time |
| PTA | percutaneous transluminal angioplasty, posterior tibial artery |
| PTFE | polytetrafluoroethylene |
| PTS | post thrombotic syndrome |
| PTT | partial thromboplastin time |
| PV | percutaneous vertebroplasty |
| PVA | polyvinyl alcohol |
| PVD | peripheral vascular disease |
| RAS | renal artery stenosis |
| RCC | renal cell carcinoma |
| RCT | randomized controlled trial |
| RFS | recurrence-free survival |
| r-tPA | recombinant tissue plasminogen activator |
| SAFARI | subintimal arterial flossing with antegrade–retrograde intervention |
| SEMS | self-expanding metallic stent |
| SFA | superficial femoral artery |
| SIA | sub-intimal angioplasty |
| SIRT | selective internal radiation treatment |
| SLA | superior labial artery |
| SMA | superior mesenteric artery |
| SPA | sphenopalatine artery |
| SUV | standard uptake value |
| SVC | superior vena cava |
| SVS | Society for Vascular Surgery |
| TAA | thoracic aortic aneurysm |
| TACE | transarterial chemoembolization |
| TAD | thoracic aortic dissection |
| TASC | Transatlantic Inter-Society Consensus |
| TEVAR | thoracic endovascular aortic repair |
| TIA | transient ischaemic attack |
| TIPS | transjugular intrahepatic portosystemic shunt |
| TLC | total lung capacity |
| TLR | target-lesion revascularization |
| TOE | transoesophageal echocardiography |
| tPA | tissue plasminogen activator |
| TUEVP | transurethral electrovaporization of the prostate |
| TUR | transurethral resection |
| TURP | transurethral resection of the prostate |
| UCSD | ultrasound colour Doppler |
| UFE | uterine fibroid embolization |
| US | ultrasound |
| UTI | urinary tract infection |
| VA | alveolar volume |
| VAS | visual analogue score |
| VC | vital capacity |
| VCF | vertebral compression fracture |
| VRT | volume rendering technique |
| VTE | venous thromboembolism |
| WIT | warm ischaemia time |

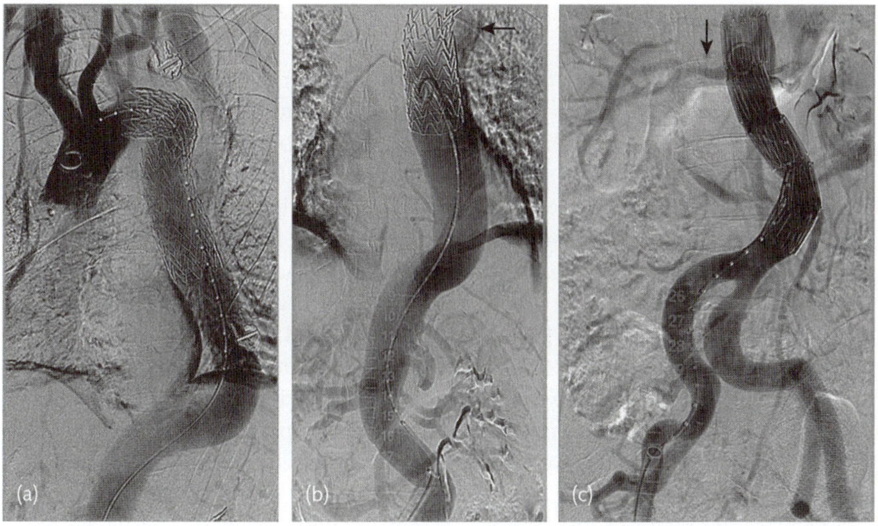


**Figure 1.2** (a) The stent graft has prevented antegrade flow into the false lumen by covering the entry tear. (b) Retrograde flow is seen at the lower end of the device within the false lumen (arrow). (c) Good flow is seen in the right renal artery (arrow) and right common iliac artery after deployment of two bare metal stents

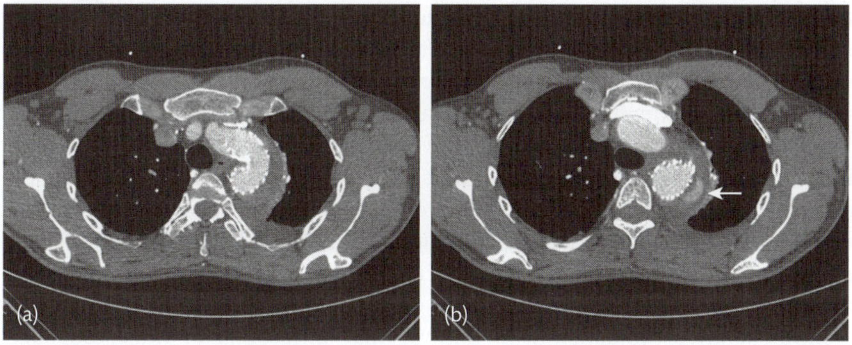


**Figure 1.3** (a) The stent graft has opened the stenosis in the true lumen. (b) Contrast enhancement of the false lumen at the lower portion of the stent graft (arrow)

with resolution of the chest pain and sensory deficit of the right leg. The chest pain returned on the third post-operative day and CT angiography showed some filling of the false lumen in the proximal descending thoracic aorta at the distal section of the cTAG stent graft (Figure 1.3). The true lumen in the region of the proximal TXD device had fully expanded and the false lumen could not be seen. There was contrast within the false lumen at the level of the second TXD device in the lower descending aorta, and the right renal and right common iliac arteries were patent although there was still some delay apparent in the right nephrogram. No further procedure was deemed necessary because the primary entry tear had been covered proximally and therefore the patient was treated with analgesia and hypotensive medication.

However, later that day the patient suffered a cardiac arrest and died despite cardiopulmonary resuscitation. Post-mortem examination showed that the false lumen had ruptured at the level of the primary entry tear in the proximal descending thoracic aorta.

## Discussion

The goals of thoracic endovascular aortic repair (TEVAR) for acute aortic type B dissection include coverage of the proximal entry tear, expansion of the true lumen with restoration of flow to the visceral vessels, and obliteration of false lumen flow with subsequent thrombosis [1–5]. When these goals of endovascular therapy are successfully achieved, aortic remodelling should occur with subsequent prevention of future aneurysmal degeneration of the outer wall of the false lumen. The EuroSTAR (European Collaborators on Stent/Graft Techniques for Aortic Aneurysm Repair) and UK Registry report is the largest group of patients treated with stent grafts to date: 131 patients with aortic dissection (5% proximal, 81% distal, 144% not classified) were treated with stent grafts and 57% had symptoms of rupture, aortic expansion, or side branch occlusion. Although no long-term data are available, primary technical success was achieved in 89%, 30-day mortality was 8.4%, paraplegia occurred in 0.8% of those treated, and survival at one year was reported in 90% of the patients who completed follow-up [6].

Endovascular repair of aortic disease associated with connective tissue disease is controversial, although it can be justified in emergencies with careful pre-operative planning [7]. Care should be taken in elective cases as the long-term durability of devices relying on oversizing may be compromised by a dilating aortopathy.

> **Expert comment**
> The presence of a subclavian artery aneurysm with aortic dissection and the sudden death of a young first-degree relative suggest connective tissue disorder as the primary pathology in this case. Genetic screening of first-degree relatives should be performed.

Stent-graft sizing is very important in treating patients with type B dissections. Most of the emphasis on treating complicated type B aortic dissection with stent grafts has been about the proximal sizing of the device. Too much can cause retrograde type A dissection and device collapse [8]. It is recommended that oversizing a stent graft relative to the proximal undissected aorta should be much less in aortic dissection than for degenerative aneurysm; 5–10% oversizing is considered adequate for dissections whereas aneurysms should be oversized by 15–30%. Balloon dilation is to be avoided in dissection because of the risk of retrograde dissection. The aortic lumen may not be the same diameter along its length and, as in this case, this can result in inadequate sealing of the distal end, allowing retrograde entry of blood into the false lumen.

> **Expert comment**
> This patient may have died because the distal end of the stent graft did not adequately seal the true lumen, allowing flow to pressurize the false lumen. If the stent graft was longer, a distal seal would have been achieved because the whole aortic diameter decreased distally. However, longer devices are associated with an increased risk of paraplegia so the risks have to be carefully evaluated.

Intra-operative evaluation with intravascular ultrasound or transoesophageal echocardiography might have shown retrograde flow into the false lumen around the distal end of the stent graft. The findings of retrograde flow around the device on digital subtraction angiography were subtle, and the significance of these was not appreciated at the time of implantation. Only careful inspection after the death of the patient showed the real cause of the problem. Unfortunately, intravascular ultrasound is expensive and is not used in our hospital, and echocardiography is not used routinely for endovascular thoracic repair of acute aortic dissections.

A bare stent may be used to increase the size of the true lumen and it has been suggested as a way of overcoming branch vessel compromise. In this case the right renal and right common iliac arteries, which were compromised even with stent graft in place, were opened.

> **Expert comment**
> The bare stents, by completely occluding the false lumen in the distal thoracic aorta, may have played a part in the patient's death. The continued perfusion of the false lumen (retrogradely alongside the distal portion of the device) through the primary entry tear and the distal occlusion of the false lumen by the TXD stents may have pressurized the false lumen and ultimately led to aortic rupture.

Continued or recurrent pain following endovascular treatment of an acute type B aortic dissection is a sinister sign which should prompt further investigation. The CT angiographic findings of continued perfusion of the false lumen at the level of the device, with no false lumen filling distally at the level of the proximal bare stent, may represent an unsatisfactory post-operative imaging finding. Use of further stent grafts rather than TXD devices might have excluded flow from the false lumen and prevented this fatal complication.

### Learning points

- Endovascular repair in connective tissue disease is not recommended except in cases of emergency.
- Accurate placement of both the proximal and distal ends of the stent graft is important to prevent continued filling of the false lumen.
- Careful intra-operative evaluation following stent-graft placement should be performed (with two X-ray views or rotational angiography, intravascular ultrasound, or transoesophageal echocardiography) to exclude retrograde flow alongside the device with continued perfusion of the false lumen through the primary tear.
- The use of bare stents distal to the covered stent has been recommended as a means of improving outcome, however, in the presence of continued false lumen perfusion, occlusion of the false lumen outflow may cause pressurization resulting in aortic rupture and death.
- Continuing or recurrent pain after endovascular repair of acute type B aortic dissection is a sinister sign which should prompt further investigation.

### Clinical tip Evaluation of type B dissection with CT angiography

CT angiography provides useful anatomical correlates for endovascular therapy with imaging of the true and false lumens and entry tear sites.

- In most cases, the true lumen may be localized by its continuity with the undissected segment of the aorta.
- The presence of intraluminal thrombus is a good marker of the false lumen, though in patients with concomitant degenerative aneurysms thrombus may be present in the true lumen.
- In the descending thoracic aorta, the false lumen is larger than the true lumen in more than 90% of cases [9].
- The orientation and mobility of the dissection flap can be assessed with CTA. If the dissection flap is concave toward the false lumen, a true lumen pressure deficit can be predicted [10].

Marked compression of the true lumen (true lumen collapse) is evidence of dynamic aortic obstruction and should raise the index of suspicion for malperfusion syndrome.

### Clinical tip Endovascular treatment of malperfusion syndrome

The endovascular management of an acute type B aortic dissection complicated with malperfusion syndrome involves the following.

- True lumen access from either a brachial or a femoral approach. Typically, because the type B dissection is distal to the left subclavian artery, rapid true lumen access is easily obtained through a right transbrachial approach.
- Recognition of the entry tear and the proximal zone of fixation.
- Visualization of all aortic branches before intervention, since changes in flap mobility secondary to relief of obstruction may alter perfusion of other aortic side branches.
- Wire access into the distal true lumen of compromised aortic side branches should be secured if the origin of the branch is uncovered by the dissection
- If stenting of the proximal descending thoracic aorta and coverage of the entry tear does not restore flow to the compromised aortic side-branches, uncovered dissection stents can be deployed in the aorta. If these fail to restore patency, placement of self-expanding stents into the aortic branches should be performed

### Learning point Indications for left subclavian artery (LSA) revascularization

In patients who need urgent TEVAR for acute aortic syndromes it is suggested that revascularization should be individualized. In selected patients whose anatomy compromises perfusion to critical organs, routine pre-operative LSA revascularization is strongly recommended. Such configurations include:

- presence of a patent left internal mammary artery to coronary artery bypass graft
- termination of the left vertebral artery at the posterior inferior cerebellar artery or other discontinuity of the vertebrobasilar collaterals

(continued)

- absent, diminutive, or occluded right vertebral artery
- a functioning arteriovenous shunt in the left arm
- prior infrarenal aortic repair
- planned long-segment (>20cm) coverage of the descending thoracic aorta where critical intercostal arteries originate
- internal iliac artery occlusion.

**Evidence base** Prospective multicenter clinical trial (STABLE) on the endovascular treatment of complicated type B aortic dissection using a composite device design [11]

- Prospective single-arm multicentre study.
- Patients with complicated type B aortic dissection were treated with an endovascular system consisting of a proximal TX2 thoracic stent graft and distal bare metal dissection stents (Zenith Dissection Endovascular System; Cook Medical, Bloomington, IN).
- Indications for enrolment were branch vessel malperfusion, impending rupture, aortic diameter ≥40mm, rapid aortic expansion, and persistent pain or hypertension despite maximum medical therapy.
- One-year follow-up results, including clinical and radiographic (CT and X-ray) evaluation, were available for this study.
- Forty patients were enrolled in this study.
- The onset of symptoms was acute (≤14 days) in 24 patients (60%).
- A majority of patients (77.5%; 31 of 40 patients) presented with impending aortic rupture (indicated by peri-aortic effusion/haematoma) or branch vessel malperfusion.
- The 30-day mortality rate was 5% and the one-year survival rate was 90%. Two deaths were secondary to aortic rupture.
- Morbidity occurring within 30 days included stroke (7.5%), transient ischaemic attack (2.5%), paraplegia (2.5%), retrograde progression of dissection (5%), and renal failure (12.5%). Additional morbidity after 30 days included one case of retrograde progression of dissection and one case of renal failure.
- Favourable aortic remodelling was observed during the course of follow-up.
- Initial data with a composite TEVAR construct have demonstrated favourable clinical and anatomical results.

## References


1. Trimarchi S, Nienaber CA, Rampoldi V, et al. Role and results of surgery in acute type B aortic dissection: insights from the International Registry of Acute Aortic Dissection (IRAD). *Circulation* 2006; 114(1 Suppl): I357–64.
2. Eggebrecht H, Nienaber CA, Neuhauser M, et al. Endovascular stent-graft placement in aortic dissection: a meta-analysis. *Eur Heart J* 2006; 27(4): 489–98.
3. Fattori R, Tsai TT, Myrmel T, et al. Complicated acute type B dissection: is surgery still the best option? A report from the International Registry of Acute Aortic Dissection. *JACC Cardiovasc Interv* 2008; 1(4): 395–402.
4. Tsai TT, Trimarchi S, Nienaber CA. Acute aortic dissection: perspectives from the International Registry of Acute Aortic Dissection (IRAD). *Eur J Vasc Endovasc Surg*. 2009; 37(2): 149–59
5. Coady MA, Ikonomidis JS, Cheung AT, et al. Surgical management of descending thoracic aortic disease: open and endovascular approaches. A scientific statement from the American Heart Association. *Circulation* 2010; 121(25): 2780–804.
6. Leurs LJ, Bell R, Degrieck Y, et al. Endovascular treatment of thoracic aortic diseases: combined experience from the EUROSTAR and United Kingdom Thoracic Endograft registries. *J Vasc Surg* 2004; 40(4): 670–80.

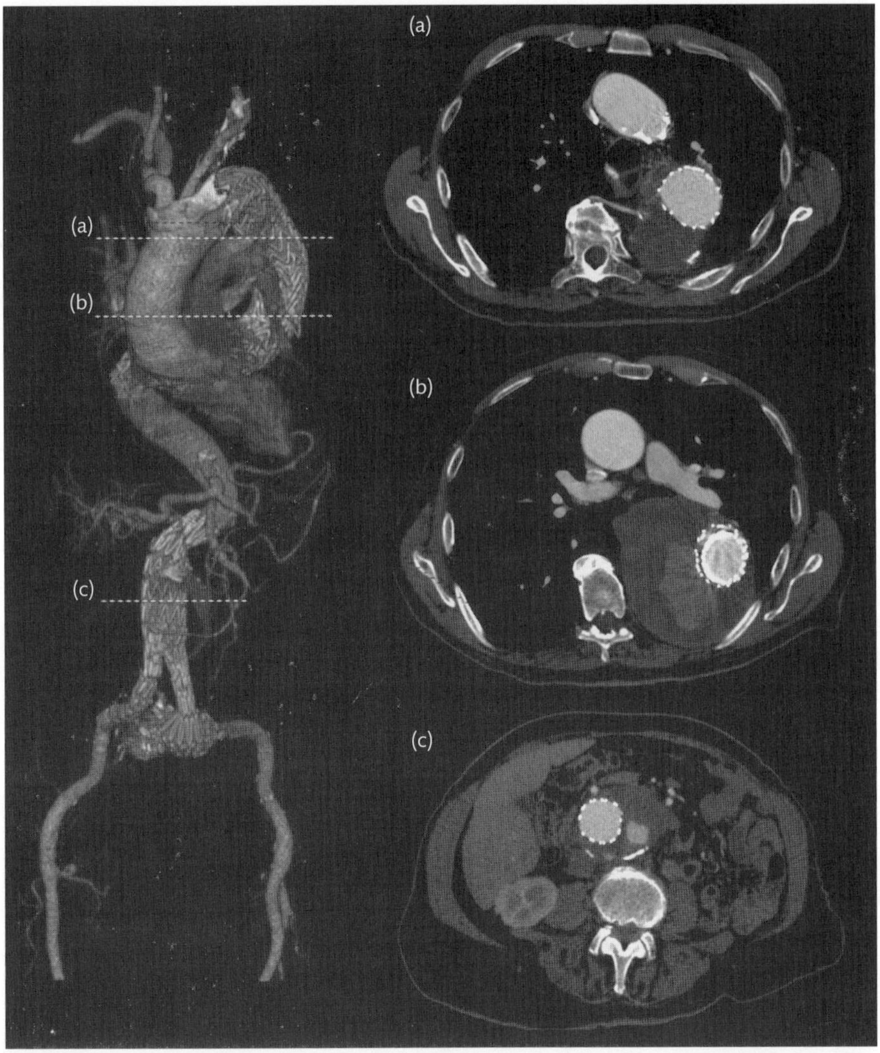


**Figure 2.2** 3D volume render from the admission CT angiogram with axial images demonstrating the thoracic and abdominal endoleaks: (a) intercostal vessels feeding the TAA sac (type II endoleak); (b) TAA endograft with contrast in the TAA sac; (c) AAA endograft with contrast in the enlarged aneurysm sac.

tributaries (Figure 2.3). A CT two days later showed persistent opacification of the aneurysm sac from intercostal arteries. A second attempt at embolizing the feeder vessels again via a right brachial artery approach was abandoned due to challenging anatomy.

Following further MDT discussion, the TAA sac, which occupied most of the left hemithorax, was directly punctured under ultrasound and 3D rotational fluoroscopy guidance, where a 6Fr catheter was inserted, permitting selective catheterization of the two feeding branches, followed by embolization using Onyx. The outflow vessels were also embolized and the aneurysm sac filled with embolic material and thrombin (Figure 2.4). A follow-up CT three months later showed a reduction in TAA size to 10cm with resolution of the type II endoleak (Figure 2.5).

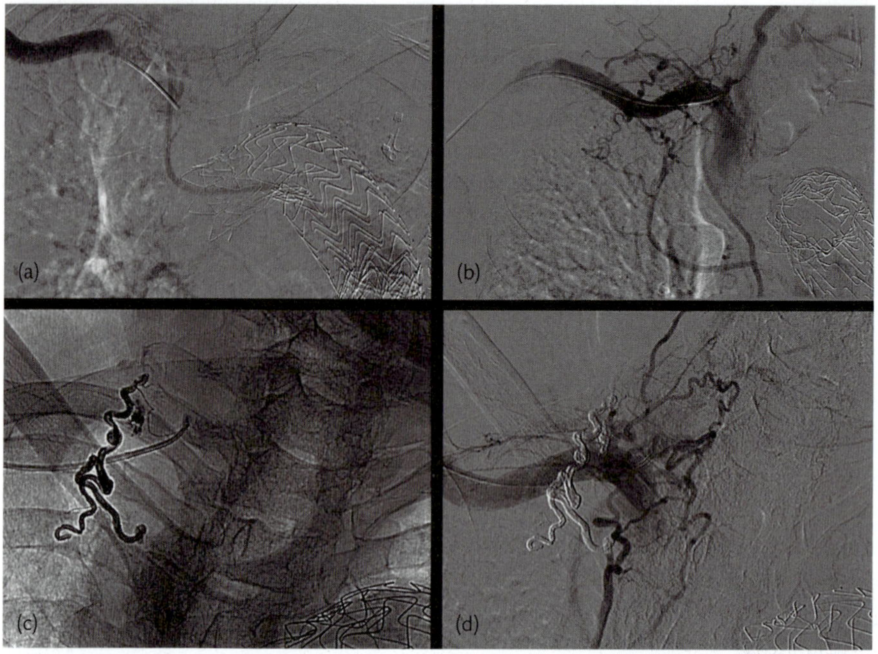


**Figure 2.3** Angiography images following a right brachial artery puncture demonstrating (a) contrast in the TAA sac, (b) origin of the feeder vessel from the thyrocervical trunk, and (c, d) persistent filling of the TAA sac feeder vessels following embolization of several thyrocervical trunk branches.

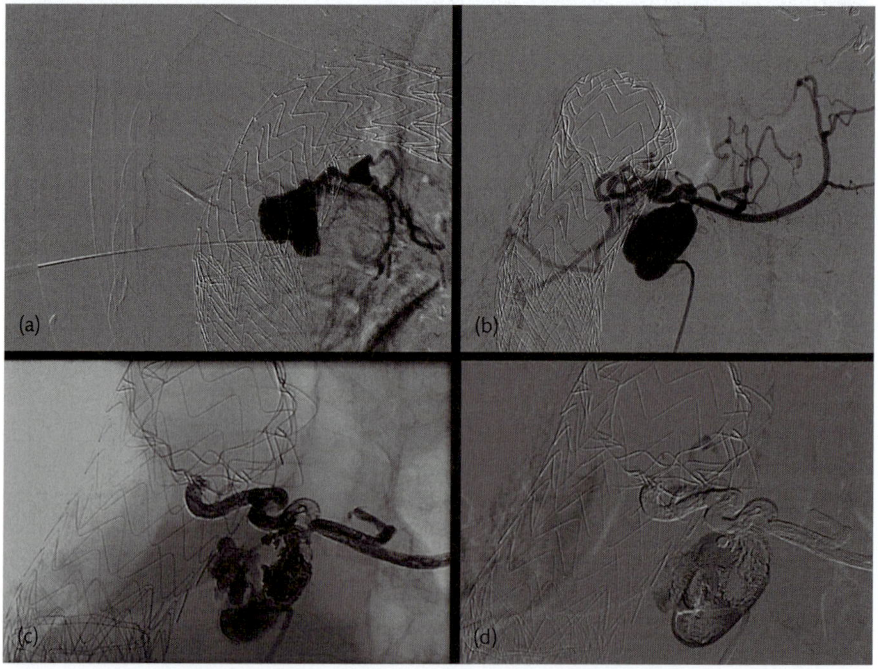


**Figure 2.4** DSA of the TAA aneurysm sac after direct puncture: (a, b) contrast in the aneurysm sac and feeder vessels; (c) Onyx in the TAA sac, feeder, and draining vessel; (d) aneurysm sac after embolization demonstrating minimal contrast opacification.

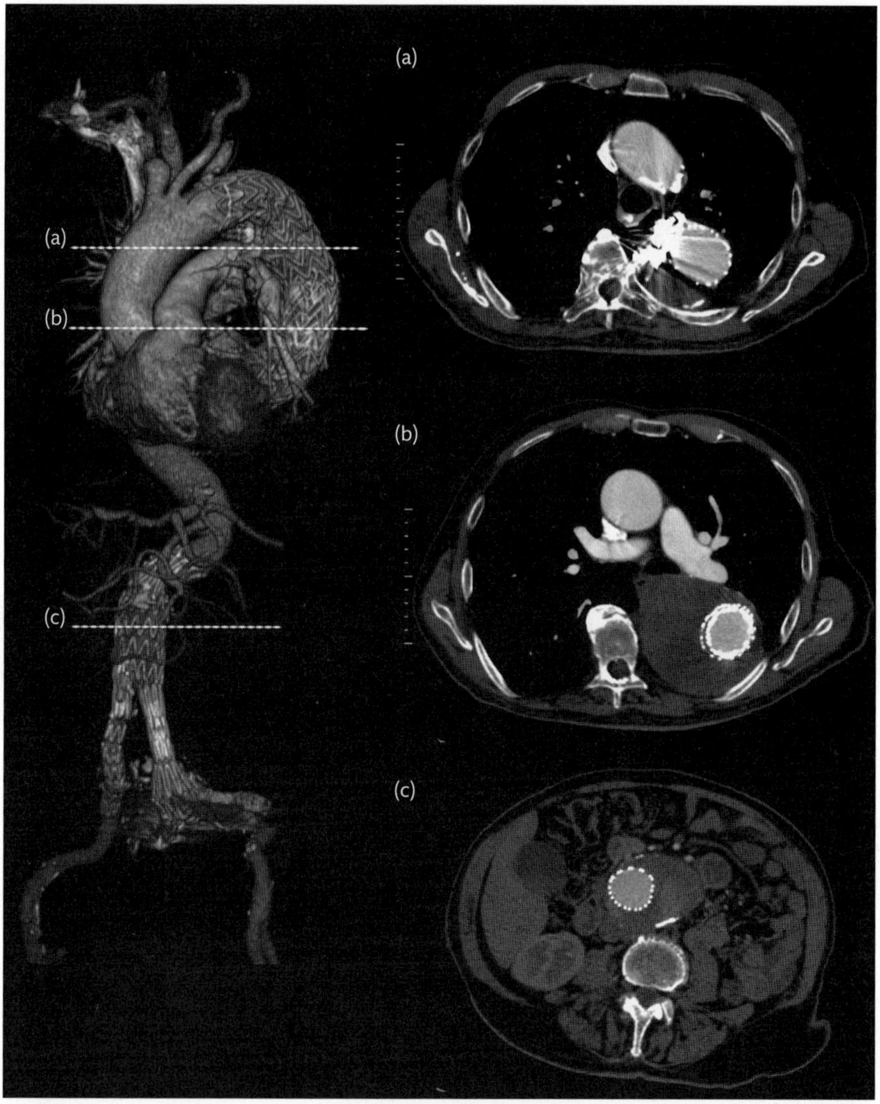


**Figure 2.5** 3D volume render from a CT angiogram following embolization: (a) high density embolic material (Onyx) in the feeder vessels and TAA sac; (b) TAA sac has reduced in size; (c) AAA sac with minimal residual contrast secondary to a residual type II endoleak.

The abdominal type Ib endoleak was treated with staged bilateral internal iliac artery embolization and extension of the stent grafts into the external iliac arteries. Enough time (two weeks) was allowed for collaterals to develop between the procedures. The inferior mesenteric artery, supplied by a branch of the superior mesenteric artery (SMA), was identified as the main feeder vessel of the abdominal aneurysm sac. With a selective catheter at the SMA, a microcatheter was introduced coaxially through the feeder vessel and into the aneurysm sac. The sac was then embolized using liquid embolic material (Onyx) with a good angiographic result. A follow-up CT demonstrated stable sac size and no residual endoleak.

## Discussion

TAAs affect 10.4 in 100,000 people per year, with up to 25% being associated with a concomitant AAA (6, 7). The estimated incidences of TAA rupture and dissection are both 3.5 per 100,000 per year [7], with a high (90%) mortality rate in cases of acute rupture [6]. The aim of TAA treatment is to reduce the risk of rupture and death.

### TEVAR as a viable alternative to open surgical aortic repair

Open surgical repair of type B thoracic aortic aneurysms is associated with significant mortality (5–22%) and morbidity even in the elective setting [8–11]. As such, TEVAR has become a viable, acceptable, and in many cases preferred alternative to open surgical repair (OSR) for the treatment of thoracic aortic disease [12–14].

### Endovascular treatment

Since Dake et al. published the first case series detailing their experience of TEVAR in 1994 [12], multiple further studies have confirmed its safety and efficacy for follow-up periods of up to six years, but no long-term data are available at present [13–16]. There is a suggestion from a recent study that TEVAR may be associated with lower long-term survival rates; however, patients undergoing TEVAR have a higher comorbid burden, with TEVAR becoming the treatment of choice for poor surgical candidates [17].

TEVAR has emerged as the treatment modality of choice in complicated thoracic aortic dissection (TAD), i.e. for those with persistent or recurrent pain, uncontrolled hypertension despite full medical treatment, malperfusion, and rupture. In uncomplicated type B dissection, medical management remains the treatment of choice [18–20].

TEVAR has also become the treatment of choice in aortic injuries, which may be either immediate, in the case of acute transection or delayed otherwise [21–23]. Connective tissue disorders remain one of the main relative contraindications to TEVAR, except acutely as an interim measure or in cases of previous surgical repair where the stent graft will lie completely within the surgical graft [24,25].

### Endoleak rates in TEVAR trials

**Evidence base** Five-year follow-up of the VALOR trial [26]

A prospective non-randomized trial which followed up 195 patients who had TEVAR for fusiform TAA using the Medtronic Vascular Talent Thoracic Stent Graft System over a five-year period.

- 32 (16%) patients had type I endoleaks over the study period, and 44% of these had a significant increase in the size of the aneurysm sac.
- 49 (35%) type II and 11 (5.6%) type III endoleaks, all of which were junctional, were reported.
- 87% of the additional interventions performed were to treat endoleaks.

**Evidence base** VALOR II trial [27]

A prospective non-randomized trial assessing the Medtronic Valiant Thoracic Stent Graft System in the treatment of TAA: 160 patients were recruited and TEVAR was successfully performed in 154. The overall rate of endoleaks was 15.8% at one month and 13.0% at one year. Most of the endoleaks at one year were type II (7%), followed by type I (3%), and type III (1%). Compared with the VALOR patients, VALOR II patients required fewer secondary interventions for type I and III endoleaks.

**Learning point** Onyx®

Onyx is a liquid embolic agent—ethylene vinyl alcohol copolymer dissolved in dimethyl sulphoxide. It solidifies upon contact with blood, blocking flow distal to its deployment site. Onyx is approved in the USA for use in neurointervention as a temporary embolic agent for arteriovenous malformations [2]. Increasingly, Onyx has been used in a variety of new settings including the treatment of endoleaks after endovascular aortic repair.

**Clinical tip**

Exposure of Onyx to diathermy during surgical procedures is potentially hazardous, resulting in spark formation and combustion [3,4]. Bipolar diathermy is safer in this context, although ignition has been observed at higher energy settings [5].

**Evidence base** GORE TAG trial [14]

Multicentre prospective non-randomized phase II trial, which recruited surgical candidates with descending non-dissecting TAA: 140 patients who had TEVAR with the GORE TAG device, 137 successfully, were followed up for five years.

- Endoleaks occurred in 10.6% of cases, mostly type I, with 3.5% of patients requiring further intervention related to these.
- No type II endoleaks required treatment.

Some of the discrepancies in the rates of endoleaks between the different trials are probably due to differences in reporting endoleaks.

## Complications

A meta-analysis in 2010, which analysed 42 non-randomized comparative studies with a total of 5,888 patients, showed lower mortality and morbidity for patients undergoing TEVAR at 30 days and at one year compared with those who had OSR, but no clear difference over five years [29]. Both TEVAR and OSR were associated with a similar risk of stroke. However, patients undergoing TEVAR had a lower risk of paraplegia and paraparesis with shorter intensive care unit (ICU) and hospital stay [29].

## Endoleaks

Endoleaks have been described as the 'Achilles' heel' of endovascular aortic repair. Ricotta et al. [30] assessed 19 studies with a total of 3,002 patients who had TEVAR and estimated the average rate of endoleaks as 10.4% at 30 days and 9.5% at one year, with an overall rate of 18% (ranging from 9% to 38%). The majority of endoleaks were type I (8.4%); 4% were type III and 2% type II. Almost half the endoleaks were actively treated, with 85% technical success and a low rate of conversion to OSR (3.6%).

Some anatomical and technical factors need to be considered to minimize the incidence of endoleaks, namely the contour and tortuosity of the thoracic aorta as well as the extent of the proximal and distal landing zones. Small degrees of graft migration during endograft deployment may result in an incomplete aneurysm seal, leading to systemic pressurization and sac enlargement. This results in type I endoleaks, which require early/immediate treatment.

Type II endoleaks are the result of retrograde aneurysm sac filling, often from intercostal, bronchial, or a covered left subclavian artery. These feeder vessels have a lower pressure than systemic circulation, do not result in significant aneurysm sac enlargement, and often do not require treatment as they tend to thrombose spontaneously. However, the case discussed here illustrates significant enlargement of the aneurysm sac that did require aggressive treatment, highlighting the importance of close surveillance post-TEVAR. A recent conference abstract suggests that volumetric assessment of endoleak cavity may be a good predictor of aneurysm sac enlargement (post-EVAR) and may become a risk stratification tool for early identification of patients who will need re-intervention prior to significant sac enlargement [31].

### Evidence base

Shah et al. recently published a prospective cohort study detailing the outcomes of 332 patients who underwent 297 TEVARs at a single centre over a six-year period [28].

- 12% of procedures required re-intervention at a mean of 8 ± 14 months, most commonly for type I endoleaks (5%). This reduced over time, perhaps due to an initial learning curve.
- Survival was similar in patients requiring re-intervention and those who did not ($p = 0.26$).

### Clinical tip Imaging of endoleaks

Digital subtraction angiography is the gold standard for diagnosing endoleaks. CT angiography has become the mainstay for diagnosis with a high sensitivity and specificity, with the added advantage of assessing aneurysm sac size [32]. Once the presence of an endoleak is determined and treatment is contemplated, conventional angiography is performed to better define the anatomy with a view to intervention.

For a full assessment of the endograft, the aneurysm sac, and the presence and nature of endoleaks, a pre-contrast CT followed by an arterial phase and then a delayed-phase study are recommended, with endoleaks best appreciated on the delayed-phase imaging [33]. Contrast within the aneurysm sac indicates the presence of an endoleak.

Triphasic contrast-enhanced MRI of the aorta has been shown to have higher sensitivity for detection of endoleaks post-EVAR and may have a role in follow-up post-TEVAR when the endograft used does not contain a stainless steel skeleton [34].

Intra-procedure transoesophageal echocardiography (TOE) can identify primary (type I) endoleaks as well as guide endograft placement [35,36].

## Management of endoleaks

Type I endoleaks are treated by securing the attachment sites, initially by balloon angioplasty to fully expand the endograft and to create an adequate seal. If this fails, a bare metal stent can be deployed if the endograft coverage is adequate albeit with poor aortic wall apposition; otherwise extension of the endograft may be required. Visceral debranching may be necessary to extend the landing zone in cases where endograft extension is contemplated. If interventional treatment fails, OSR is recommended as type I endoleaks are associated with rapid sac enlargement and an increased risk of aortic rupture.

Most type II endoleaks will resolve spontaneously, but intervention may be necessary if they persist, if the aneurysm sac expands, or in symptomatic patients. Embolization of the feeder vessels is the mainstay of treatment, which may be either transarterial or transthoracic as in the case discussed herein. Ultrasound or CT-guided aneurysm sac puncture may be necessary.

As with type I endoleaks, type III endoleaks require aggressive treatment, usually by deployment of an additional endograft to seal the defect. As stent-graft technology improves, these are becoming less common.

Type IV endoleaks almost invariably resolve after anticoagulation is reversed and are increasingly of historical value as endograft technology improves and porosity reduces.

## A final word from the expert

TAA affects 10.4 in 100,000 people per year, with increasing risk of rupture as aneurysm size increases. The diameters for ascending and descending TAA for which the risk of rupture is thought to outweigh the risk of intervention are 5.5cm and 6.0cm, respectively.

TEVAR has become a viable treatment for thoracic aortic disease, but this relatively novel procedure has created a new set of challenges and complications which were not previously seen with open surgical treatment. As such, it is imperative that patients undergo regular follow-up imaging post TEVAR to detect problems early. One such complication is endoleaks, whereby there is continual blood flow into the aneurysm sac, causing it to enlarge. Five types of endoleaks have been described, and these can be divided into two broad categories. 'High pressure endoleaks', where blood flow into the aneurysm sac is under systemic arterial pressure (types I and III), are associated with significant sac enlargement and warrant prompt treatment. On the other hand, 'low pressure endoleaks' (type II), such as in cases of backflow from covered left subclavian, intercostal, or bronchial arteries, are usually less problematic and often spontaneously resolve. They do require close follow-up however, in order to identify sac enlargement and may occasionally require aggressive treatment, rarely necessitating direct puncture of the aneurysm sac to embolize the feeder vessels.

It is important to note that there are no robust guidelines on how endoleaks should be treated. Management is often based on case series and reports and is largely guided by local expertise with some extrapolation from prior EVAR experience, but must always be tailored to the individual patient. Therefore careful planning and discussion within an expert MDT are paramount.

## References

1. White GH, Yu W, May J. Endoleak—a proposed new terminology to describe incomplete aneurysm exclusion by an endoluminal graft. *J Endovasc Surg* 1996; 3(1): 124–5.
2. Ayad M, Eskioglu E, Mericle RA. Onyx: a unique neuroembolic agent. *Expert Rev Med Devices* 2006; 3(6): 705–15.
3. Smith SJ, Thomas A, Ashpole RD. Intra-operative combustion of Onyx embolic material. *Br J Neurosurg* 2009; 23(1): 76–8.
4. Mull A, Marshallek F, Tejada J, Flores RL. A cautionary report: creation of intraoperative sparks and embers from Onyx embolic material during surgical resection of arterio-venous malformations. *Plast Reconstr Surg* 2012; 129(2): 401e–2e
5. Schirmer CM, Zerris V, Malek AM. Electrocautery-induced ignition of spark showers and self-sustained combustion of Onyx ethylene-vinyl alcohol copolymer. *Neurosurgery* 2006; 59(4 Suppl 2): ON S413–18.
6. Bickerstaff LK, Pairolero PC, Hollier LH, et al. Thoracic aortic aneurysms: a population-based study. *Surgery* 1982; 92(6): 1103–8.
7. Clouse WD, Hallett JW Jr, Schaff HV, et al. Acute aortic dissection: population-based incidence compared with degenerative aortic aneurysm rupture. *Mayo Clin Proc* 2004; 79(2): 176–80.
8. Coselli JS, LeMaire SA, Conklin LD, Adams GJ. Left heart bypass during descending thoracic aortic aneurysm repair does not reduce the incidence of paraplegia. *Ann Thorac Surg* 2004; 77(4): 1298–303.
9. Estrera AL, Rubenstein FS, Miller CC, III, et al. Descending thoracic aortic aneurysm: surgical approach and treatment using the adjuncts cerebrospinal fluid drainage and distal aortic perfusion. *Ann Thorac Surg* 2001; 72(2): 481–6.
10. Rigberg DA, McGory ML, Zingmond DS, et al. Thirty-day mortality statistics underestimate the risk of repair of thoracoabdominal aortic aneurysms: a statewide experience. *J Vasc Surg* 2006; 43(2): 217–23.
11. Cowan JA, Jr, Dimick JB, Henke PK, et al. Surgical treatment of intact thoracoabdominal aortic aneurysms in the United States: hospital and surgeon volume-related outcomes. *J Vasc Surg* 2003; 37(6): 1169–74.
12. Dake MD, Miller DC, Semba CP, et al. Transluminal placement of endovascular stent-grafts for the treatment of descending thoracic aortic aneurysms. *N Engl J Med* 1994; 331(26): 1729–34.
13. Fairman RM, Criado F, Farber M, et al. Pivotal results of the Medtronic Vascular Talent Thoracic Stent Graft System: the VALOR Trial. *J Vasc Surg* 2008; 48(3): 546–54.e2.
14. Makaroun MS, Dillavou ED, Wheatley GH, Cambria RP. Five-year results of endovascular treatment with the Gore TAG device compared with open repair of thoracic aortic aneurysms. *J Vasc Surg* 2008; 47(5): 912–18.
15. Dake MD, Kato N, Mitchell RS, et al. Endovascular stent-graft placement for the treatment of acute aortic dissection. *N Engl J Med* 1999; 340(20): 1546–52.
16. Fairman RM, Tuchek JM, Lee WA, et al. Pivotal results for the Medtronic Valiant Thoracic Stent Graft System in the VALOR II trial. *J Vasc Surg* 2012; 56(5): 1222–31
17. Goodney PP, Travis L, Lucas FL, et al. Survival after open versus endovascular thoracic aortic aneurysm repair in an observational study of the Medicare population. *Circulation* 2011; 124(24): 2661–9.
18. Szeto WY, McGarvey M, Pochettino A, et al. Results of a new surgical paradigm: endovascular repair for acute complicated type B aortic dissection. *Ann Thorac Surg* 2008; 86(1): 87–94.
19. Nienaber CA, Kische S, Ince H, Fattori R. Thoracic endovascular aneurysm repair for complicated type B aortic dissection. *J Vasc Surg* 2011; 54(5): 1529–33.
20. Lombardi JV, Cambria RP, Nienaber CA, et al. Prospective multicenter clinical trial (STABLE) on the endovascular treatment of complicated type B aortic dissection using a composite device design. *J Vasc Surg* 2012; 55(3): 629–L40e2.

21. Fattori R, Napoli G, Lovato L, et al. Indications for, timing of, and results of catheter-based treatment of traumatic injury to the aorta. *AJR Am J Roentgenol* 2002; 179(3): 603–9.
22. Scheinert D, Krankenberg H, Schmidt A, et al. Endoluminal stent graft placement for acute rupture of the descending thoracic aorta. *Eur Heart J* 2004; 25(8): 694–700.
23. Dake MD, White RA, Diethrich EB, et al. Report on endograft management of traumatic thoracic aortic transections at 30 days and 1 year from a multidisciplinary subcommittee of the Society for Vascular Surgery Outcomes Committee. *J Vasc Surg* 2011; 53(4): 1091–6.
24. Cooper DG, Walsh SR, Sadat U, et al. Treating the thoracic aorta in Marfan syndrome: surgery or TEVAR? *J Endovasc Ther* 2009; 16(1): 60–70.
25. Ince H, Rehders TC, Petzsch M, et al. Stent-grafts in patients with Marfan syndrome. *J Endovasc Ther* 2005; 12(1): 82–8.
26. Foley PJ, Criado FJ, Farber MA, et al. Results with the Talent thoracic stent graft in the VALOR trial. *J Vasc Surg* 2012; 56(5): 1214–21e1.
27. Fairman RM, Tuchek JM, Lee WA, et al. Pivotal results for the Medtronic Valiant Thoracic Stent Graft System in the VALOR II trial. *J Vasc Surg* 2012; 56(5): 1222–31.
28. Shah AA, Barfield ME, Andersen ND, et al. Results of thoracic endovascular aortic repair 6 years after United States Food and Drug Administration approval. *Ann Thorac Surg* 2012; 94(5): 1394–9.
29. Cheng D, Martin J, Shennib H, et al. Endovascular aortic repair versus open surgical repair for descending thoracic aortic disease: a systematic review and meta-analysis of comparative studies. *J Am Coll Cardiol* 2010; 55(10): 986–1001.
30. Ricotta JJ 2nd. Endoleak management and postoperative surveillance following endovascular repair of thoracic aortic aneurysms. *J Vasc Surg* 2010; 52(4 Suppl): 91S–9S.
31. Demehri S, Signorelli J, Wake N, et al. Volumetric quantification of type II endoleak cavity: a predictor for aneurysm sac enlargement following endovascular abdominal aortic repair. Presented at Radiological Society of North America Annual Meeting, November 2012.
32. Stavropoulos SW, Clark TW, Carpenter JP, et al. Use of CT angiography to classify endoleaks after endovascular repair of abdominal aortic aneurysms. *J Vasc Interv Radiol* 2005; 16(5): 663–7.
33. Rozenblit AM, Patlas M, Rosenbaum AT, et al. Detection of endoleaks after endovascular repair of abdominal aortic aneurysm: value of unenhanced and delayed helical CT acquisitions. *Radiology* 2003; 227(2): 426–33.
34. Alerci M, Oberson M, Fogliata A, et al. Prospective, intraindividual comparison of MRI versus MDCT for endoleak detection after endovascular repair of abdominal aortic aneurysms. *Eur Radiol* 2009; 19(5): 1223–31.
35. Swaminathan M, Lineberger CK, McCann RL, Mathew JP. The importance of intraoperative transesophageal echocardiography in endovascular repair of thoracic aortic aneurysms. *Anesth Analg* 2003; 97(6): 1566–72.
36. Rocchi G, Lofiego C, Biagini E, et al. Transesophageal echocardiography-guided algorithm for stent-graft implantation in aortic dissection. *J Vasc Surg* 2004; 40(5): 880–5.

CASE

# 3 Juxtarenal abdominal aortic aneurysms: fenestrations versus chimneys


Nadeem Shaida

Expert commentary Andrew Winterbottom


## Case history

A 75-year-old asymptomatic man underwent ultrasound (US) screening for abdominal aortic aneurysm (AAA). He had a past medical history of hypertension, hypercholesterolaemia, and ischaemic heart disease and had previously had a coronary artery stent placed. He was taking clopidogrel, aspirin, ramipril, bisoprolol, and atorvostatin. Pre-operative blood results showed a creatinine level of 86μmol/l and haemoglobin of 15.2g/dl. Screening US demonstrated an AAA and he was subsequently referred for a CT examination for further evaluation. CT demonstrated a Crawford type IV thoraco-abdominal aneurysm (TAA) extending from the level of the coeliac artery origin to just above the aortic bifurcation (Figures 3.1 and 3.2).

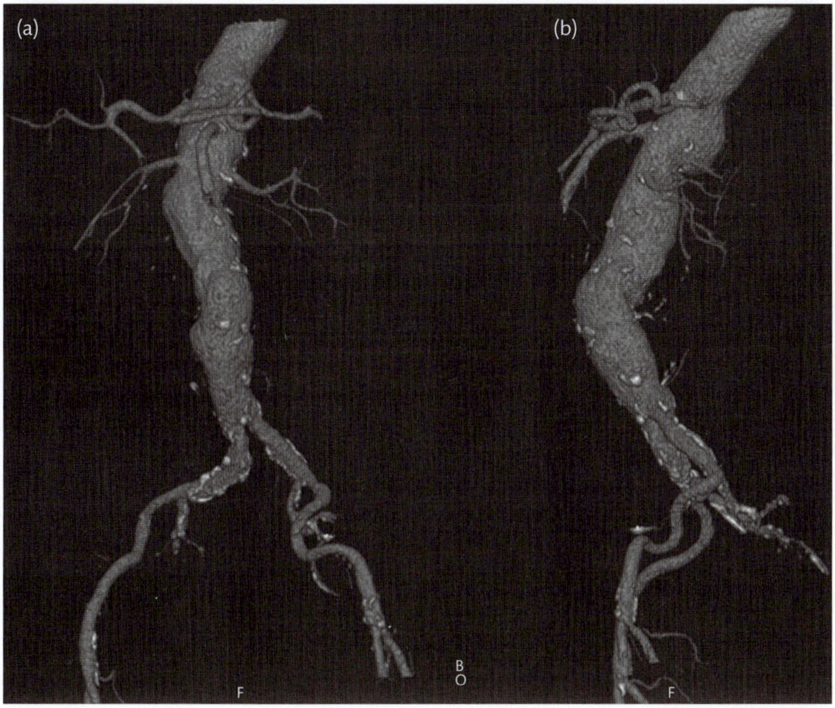


**Figure 3.1** VRT reconstruction demonstrating AAA extending above the renal arteries to the level of the coeliac artery in (a) AP and (b) lateral planes.

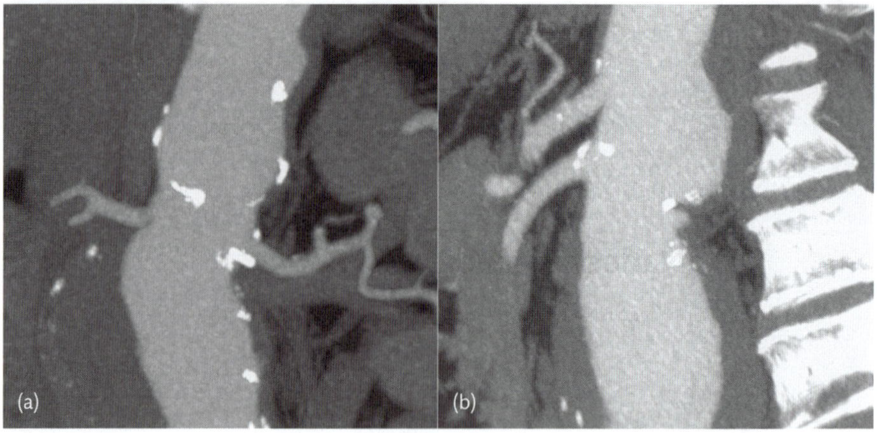


**Figure 3.2** CT MIP of the visceral artery branches in (a) AP and (b) lateral planes.

**Learning point** The Crawford classification (Figure 3.3)

- Type I begins in the proximal descending thoracic aorta and extends to the level of the coeliac artery.
- Type II is more extensive and involves the whole of the abdominal aorta and descending thoracic aorta.
- Type III is defined by its superior extent, which is not above the level of the T6 vertebra or inferior pulmonary vein and involves a variable amount of abdominal aorta.
- Type IV begins at the level of the coeliac artery and extends into the infrarenal aorta.
- Type V: a later modification of this classification [1] added a further type that extends from the mid descending thoracic aorta to the level of the renal arteries.

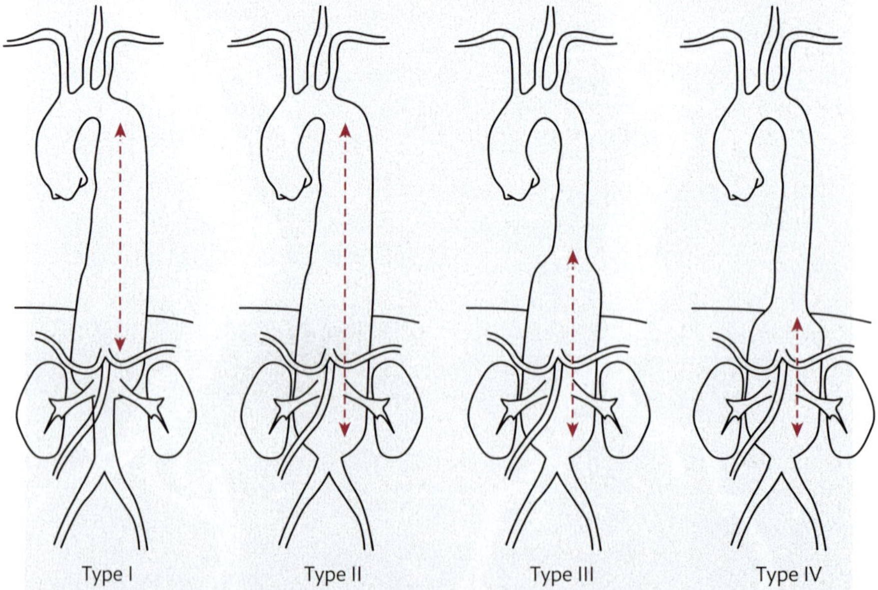


**Figure 3.3** Schematic representation of the Crawford classification of thoraco-abdominal aneurysms (TAAs).

Reproduced from Huynh TT, Miller CC 3rd, Estrera AL, et al. Determinants of hospital length of stay after thoracoabdominal aortic aneurysm repair. *J Vasc Surg* 2002; 35(4): 648–53 with permission from Elsevier.

**Learning point** Juxtarenal aneurysms

There is some variation within the literature in terms of the definition of juxtarenal aneurysm (JRA). Traditionally, the definition has been based on the principle of surgical repair with a JRA defined as one in which the surgeon was unable to safely place an infrarenal clamp. Typically this occurs with an infrarenal neck length less than 5mm.

In the case shown in Figure 3.4 there is a 'true' juxtarenal AAA with a short proximal neck of less than 5mm. This patient was treated with a two-vessel fenestrated endovascular aortic repair (FEVAR). With the advent of more advanced endovascular techniques this definition is no longer so clear cut and, with no universal classification system in place, outcome data following FEVAR should be interpreted with some caution.

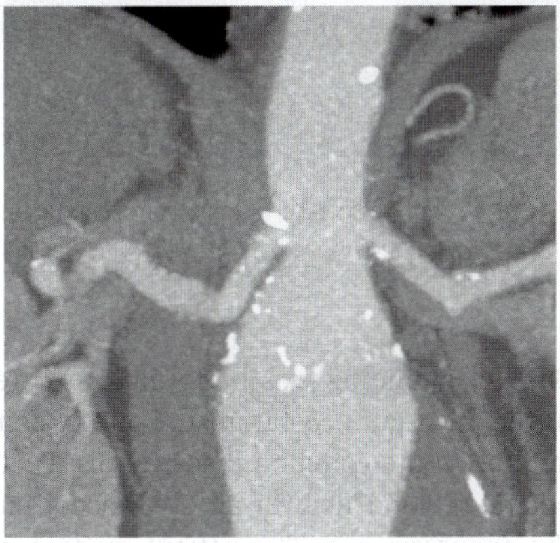

**Figure 3.4** A 'true' juxtarenal abdominal aortic aneurysm.

## Procedure

Following MDT discussion, the decision was made to proceed to insertion of a four-vessel fenestrated endovascular aortic stent graft. The procedure was performed under general anaesthetic in the angiography suite. Bilateral surgical groin cut-downs were performed. The fenestrated body of the stent graft was positioned such that the markers around each fenestration aligned with the visceral artery origins (Figure 3.5). Each visceral artery was then cannulated in turn and stent grafts placed into each one (Figure 3.6). The visceral artery stent grafts were then deployed.

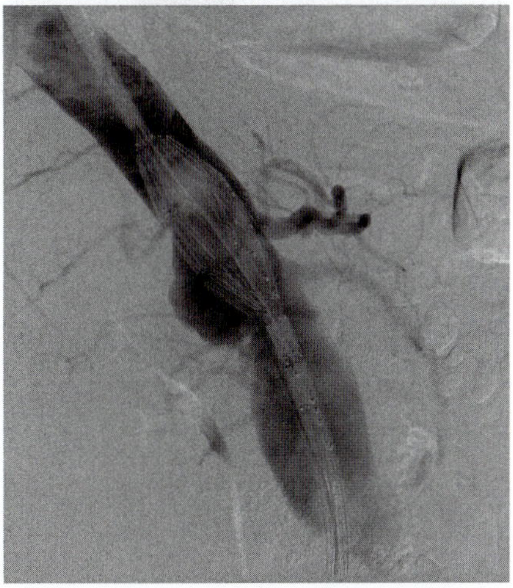

**Figure 3.5** Lateral aortogram showing alignment of the fenestrated graft adjacent to the coeliac trunk and superior mesenteric artery (SMA).

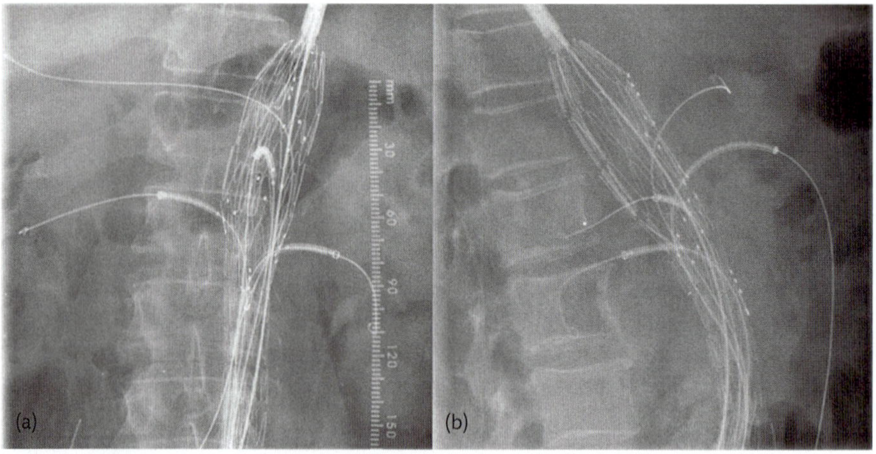


**Figure 3.6** Each visceral artery was cannulated in turn through the fenestration in the aortic stent graft and stents were placed within them: (a) AP and (b) lateral views.

Balloon moulding was performed to flare each visceral artery stent into the body of the stent graft. A bifurcated aortic stent graft was then deployed with each limb landing in the common iliac arteries. Post-procedure angiography (Figure 3.7) demonstrated good flow in all the visceral artery stent grafts and no endoleak within the aneurysm sac. The patient made a good recovery and was discharged on the third post-operative day. Repeat blood results showed a post-procedure creatinine of 98μmol/l and haemoglobin of 12.5g/dl with no blood transfusion being used. Follow-up CT at three months (Figure 3.8) demonstrated good stent graft position with all four visceral arteries patent and no endoleaks.

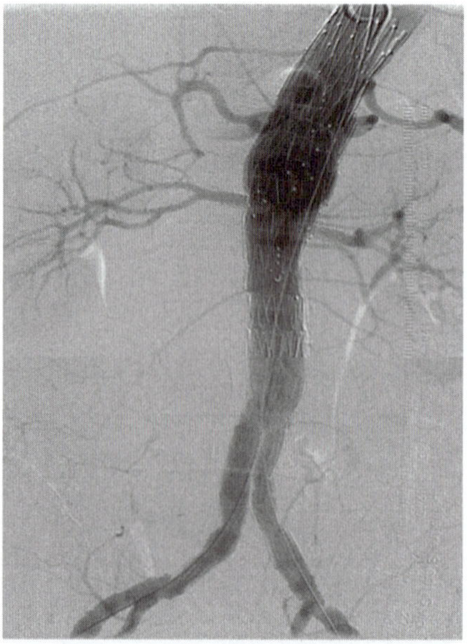

**Figure 3.7** Completion angiogram demonstrating good flow through all four visceral artery stent grafts and good flow through the bifurcated infrarenal stent graft.

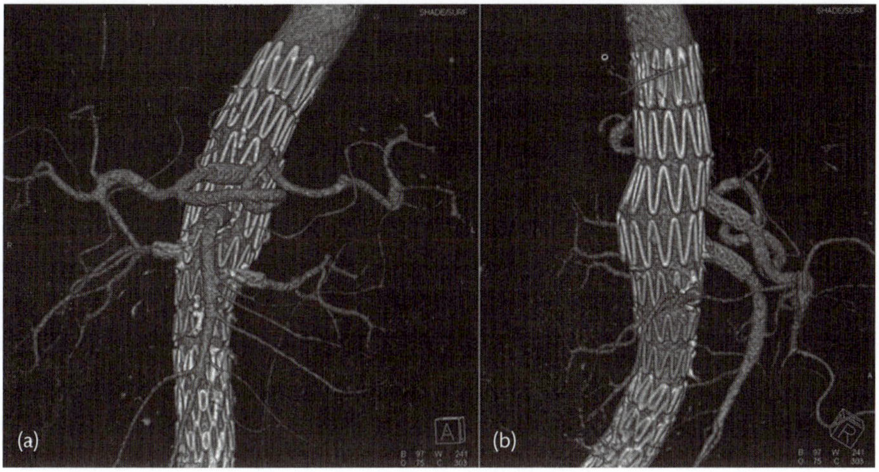


**Figure 3.8** (a) AP and (b) lateral CT VRT images three months after stent graft insertion demonstrating visceral artery patency.

# Discussion

## Limitations of conventional EVAR

Since the advent of endovascular aneurysm repair (EVAR) in the early 1990s [2] endovascular stenting has become the treatment of choice for many infrarenal AAAs. However, only 50–70% of patients with AAAs have anatomy that is suitable for conventional EVAR [3], with limitations imposed by inadequate landing zones and difficulty in obtaining access, typically because of unfavourable iliac artery anatomy. The advent of smaller and lower profile devices has improved the problem posed by tortuous iliac artery anatomy. Therefore, in recent years attention has shifted to finding techniques and devices to counter the problems associated with inadequate landing zones, particularly proximally.

The traditional teaching is that an infrarenal neck should be at least 15mm long and not angulated by more than 60° if it is to be considered 'acceptable' for EVAR More recently, the indications have been extended such that a neck length of greater than 10mm if straight or angulation up to 90° for neck lengths up to 20mm have been considered acceptable [4]. Furthermore, some centres have pushed the boundaries yet further by performing standard EVAR beyond these indications; however, it appears that, although technically feasible, such cases come at the expense of higher re-intervention rates [5].

Therefore it is apparent that, despite advances in equipment and technique, a proportion of patients have proximal anatomy that is unsuitable for conventional EVAR. In such patients, treatment options include conservative management, open or hybrid repair, or complex endograft repair. A number of potential solutions employing either custom-built fenestrated and branched endovascular stent grafts or standard infrarenal aortic stent grafts with adjunctive visceral artery stent grafting have been described.

## Customized devices

The two commonly described options are FEVAR or branch grafts. FEVAR was first developed in the mid-1990s [6] and classically described for use in juxtarenal aneurysms. FEVAR involves the use of fenestrations (holes in the stent graft) and scallops (gaps in the upper margin) in the graft material to preserve visceral artery supply. Each device is custom built using a prior CT to plan the position of the fenestrations or scallops in relation to the visceral artery origins. FEVAR may involve up to four fenestrations as seen in the case described, or more simply may involve one or both renal arteries. After the initial body is deployed by aligning radio-opaque markers with the vessel origins, each involved visceral artery is cannulated and a covered stent graft deployed. Scallops can be used to preserve supply to the SMA or coeliac, if needed, without the need to place a stent graft within the target artery.

Much of the evidence for FEVAR is based around individual or multicentre case series with a paucity of level 1 evidence. In addition, given that FEVAR is a relatively recent procedure, there is a lack of evidence in terms of long-term outcome. In view of the added complexity and procedure length of FEVAR compared with EVAR, one would expect that problems such as blood loss, limb ischaemia, and renal dysfunction would be greater in FEVAR, and therefore some of the advantages of endovascular repair over open repair would be lost (Table 3.1). In addition, given the increased number of components required, the risk of type III endoleaks is higher (although one would expect fewer type I endoleaks as the proximal part of the stent graft should be landing in a relatively long segment of normal aorta). However, overall, the data from multicentre studies from both the UK [7] and the USA [8] suggest that, at least in the short and medium term, FEVAR is a safe and effective procedure particularly when performed at centres with experience of the procedure.

**Table 3.1** Complications of FEVAR

| General | Specific |
|---|---|
| Myocardial infarction/cardiac failure | Renal failure |
| Pneumonia | Pseudoaneurysm formation |
| Sepsis | Stent occlusion/dislocation/fracture |
| Uterine tract infection | Arterial dissection |
| Wound infection | Spinal ischaemia |
| | Leg ischaemia |
| | Organ ischaemia/infarction |

A second type of customized device is a 'branched' aortic stent graft, which consists of an aortic stent graft with custom-made branches that are extended into the target visceral arteries. These devices were initially designed for use at the iliac bifurcation but have now been applied elsewhere, including the visceral segment of the abdominal aorta [9]. Branched EVAR is most commonly used in TAAs where the aneurysmal segment of the aorta extends to involve the visceral artery origins. These generally pass caudally so it is helpful to cannulate them via a brachial approach. The branches are then extended into the visceral arteries and continuation stents are deployed. These should be deployed in an anatomically favourable manner with no sharp angulations and with a considerable degree of overlap such that the risk of component separation, type III endoleaks, and protrusion of the branch stents into the main stent graft is minimized.

**Clinical tip** Chimneys, periscopes, and sandwiches

The 'chimney graft' technique was originally developed as a bail-out when standard EVAR stent grafts were placed a little too high, partially covering the renal artery origins [9]. Over time it has gained popularity as a treatment for juxtarenal aneurysms as well as being employed in the aortic arch during endovascular repair of the thoracic aorta. Essentially the technique involves cannulating the visceral arteries from above and deploying stent grafts such that the proximal ends of the visceral artery stent lie parallel to and above the proximal aspect of the aortic stent graft, thus maintaining flow within the target visceral artery. Although the evidence in the literature for such a technique is mainly limited to case series, a number of centres have reported satisfactory short- and medium-term results [10].

The main advantage of using such devices is that there is no need for a costly (in terms of both finance and time) customized device to be manufactured and shipped. This potentially means that it is possible to treat cases in an emergency situation that were previously deemed unsuitable for endovascular repair due to unfavourable anatomy. Critics of the technique point to the fact that, depending on anatomy; the technique may require formation of a seal between one or more visceral 'chimneys' and the main aortic stent graft. This may lead to the formation of 'gutters' between the various stents, which could cause type I endoleaks.

Various modifications of the chimney graft have been described. The 'periscope graft' technique describes insertion of a stent graft which, instead of extending beyond the proximal landing zone, is deployed parallel to the distal sealing zone and then provides retrograde filling to a visceral artery [11]. More recently, the 'sandwich technique' has been described whereby the visceral artery stent graft is 'sandwiched' between two pieces of aortic stent graft [12].

**Learning point** Surgical repair

Open surgery has been the mainstay of treatment for many years; however, it is complex and challenging, and often requires exposure through both thoracic and abdominal cavities and supracoeliac aortic cross-clamping. Despite improvements in post-operative care, surgery still carries a significant risk of morbidity and mortality. A more recent alternative treatment is 'hybrid' repair, where EVAR is combined with surgery. The technique involves surgical 'debranching' of the reno-visceral arteries and construction of an extra-anatomical bypass [13]. This provides the ability to place an aortic stent graft across the native visceral artery origins with impunity.

## A final word from the expert

There are a significant number of patients who have anatomy that is unsuitable for conventional EVAR. As described, several newer endovascular options are available which extend the indication for endovascular repair. FEVAR is now an established procedure in larger centres for treating juxtarenal and type IV TAAs. In an emergency setting where a custom device is not available, a chimney technique can be employed. Branched aortic stent grafts offer an endovascular solution for TAAs involving the visceral abdominal aorta. The sandwich technique has been described as an alternative to custom-made branched grafts.

Novel devices are coming on the market which will provide an off-the-shelf fenestrated option for the renal arteries with only a few stent graft configurations needed in order to treat the majority of anatomies. Other advances in technology, such as pre-cannulated fenestrations, also aim to significantly reduce procedure time.

Given the paucity of long-term follow-up of non-standard EVAR, one should still consider conventional open surgical repair in young patients who do not have significant comorbidity,. When considering the various endovascular options available, one must take into account the urgency of treatment (custom building often takes six weeks), the expense involved, and shelf stock availability.

## References


1. Huynh TT, Miller CC 3rd, Estrera AL, et al. Determinants of hospital length of stay after thoracoabdominal aortic aneurysm repair. *J Vasc Surg* 2002; 35(4): 648–53.
2. Parodi JC, Plamaz JC, Barone HD. Transfemoral intraluminal graft implantation for abdominal aortic aneurysms. *Ann Vasc Surg* 1991; 5: 491–9.
3. Green RM. Patient selection for endovascular abdominal aortic aneurysm repair. *J Am Coll Surg* 2002; 194: s67–73.
4. Cross J, Gurusamy K, Gadhvi V, et al. Fenestrated endovascular aneurysm repair. *Br J Surg* 2012; 99: 152–9.
5. Abu Rahma AF, Campbell J, Stone P, et al. The correlation of aortic neck length to early and late outcomes in endovascular aneurysm repair patients. *J Vasc Surg* 2009; 50(4): 738–48.
6. Park JH, Chung JW, Choo IW, et al. Fenestrated stent-grafts for preserving visceral arterial branches in the treatment of abdominal aortic aneurysms: preliminary experience. *J Vasc Interv Radiol* 1996; 7:8199–23.
7. British Society of Endovascular Therapy and the GLOBALSTAR Registry. Early results of fenestrated endovascular repair of juxtarenal aortic aneurysms. *Circulation* 2012; 125(22): 2707–15.
8. Greenberg RK, Sternbergh WC, Makaroun M, et al. Intermediate results of a US multicentre trial of fenestrated endograft repair for juxtarenal aortic aneurysms. *J Vasc Surg* 2009; 50(4): 730–7.
9. Greenberg RK, Clair D, Srivasta S, et al. Should patients with challenging anatomy be offered endovascular aneurysm repair? *J Vasc Surg* 2003; 38:990–6.
10. Chuter TA, Gordon RL, Reilly LM, et al. An endovascular system for thoraco-abdominal aortic aneurysm repair. *J Endovasc Ther* 2001; 8:25–33.
11. Hiramoto JS, Chang CK, Reilly LM, et al. Outcome of renal stenting for renal artery coverage during endovascular aortic aneurysm repair. *J Vasc Surg* 2009; 49:1100–6.
12. Lobato, AC. Sandwich technique for aortoiliac aneurysms extending to the internal iliac artery: a new endovascular approach to preserve pelvic circulation. *J Endovasc Ther* 2011; 18(1): 106–11.
13. Quinines-Baldrich WJ, Panetta TF, Vescera CL, et al. Repair of type IV TAA with a combined endovascular and surgical approach. *J Vasc Surg* 1999; 30: 555–60.

CASE

# 4 Management of endoleaks after abdominal aneurysm endovascular repair


**Raymond Chung**

**Expert commentary** Robert Morgan


## Case history

A 73-year-old female with a 5.5cm infrarenal abdominal aortic aneurysm underwent endovascular aneurysm repair (EVAR) with a bifurcated aortic stent graft. The post-operative abdominal radiograph showed the endograft to be in a satisfactory position. A duplex ultrasound showed a patent endograft and no visible endoleak (EL).

Routine follow-up ultrasound showed an increasing sac size at 17 months (5.7cm in the maximum AP dimension compared with 4.9cm immediately post EVAR). CT angiography (CTA) demonstrated an EL in the posterior aspect of the aneurysm sac (Figure 4.1) secondary to a left lumbar artery consistent with a type II EL.

In view of the increase in sac size, the patient was referred for EL embolization. A catheter was advanced into the left internal iliac artery via a left femoral access. Arteriograms confirmed a type II EL arising from a lumbar artery communicating with the left iliolumbar artery (Figure 4.2). The catheter was advanced into the aneurysm sac via the lumbar artery (Figure 4.3). The EL was successfully embolized (Figure 4.4) with 10ml ethylene–vinyl alcohol (Onyx; MicroTherapeutics, Irvine, CA). The patient was observed overnight and discharged the following day with no procedural complications.

Currently, the aneurysm sac size remains stable with no evidence of an EL at 14 months follow-up.

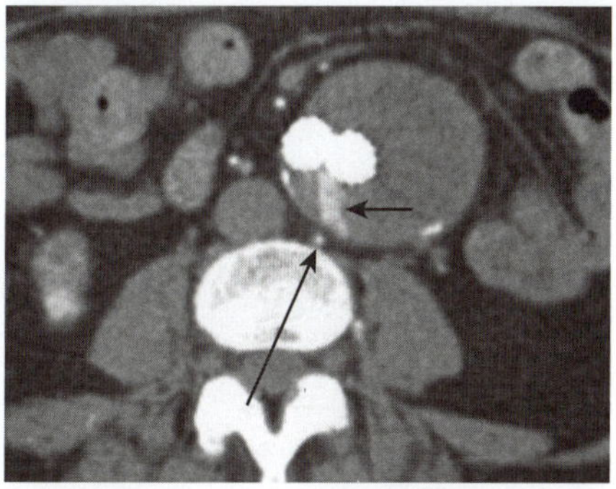

**Figure 4.1** CTA showing an endoleak in the posterior aspect of the aneurysmal sac (short arrow). The endoleak originates from a left lumbar artery (long arrow) and is a type II.

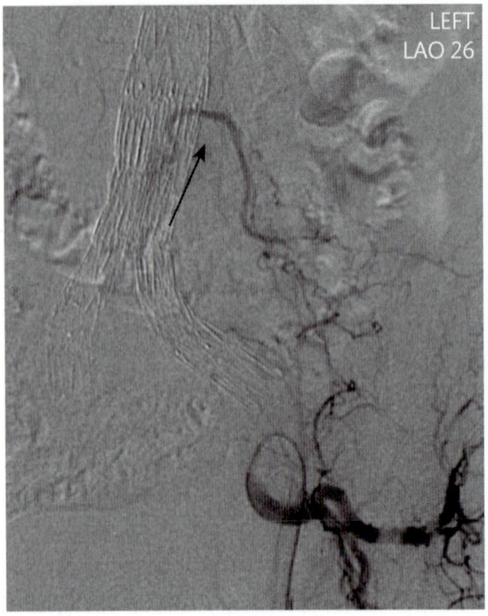


**Figure 4.2** Angiogram obtained with 26° left angulation. A catheter is advanced into the left internal iliac artery and the angiogram confirms the presence of a left lumbar artery that ends in the aneurysmal sac (arrow).

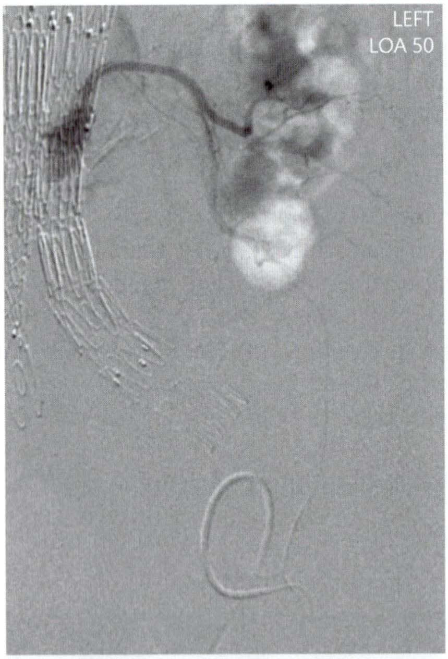


**Figure 4.3** Superselective catheterization of the lumbar artery with a microcatheter and confirmation of the contrast pooling within the aneurysmal sac.

**Expert comment**

This case highlights the fact that not all type II ELs are benign entities and can alone result in aneurysm sac growth. Our favoured treatment algorithm is via a transarterial approach, with direct sac puncture reserved for those with unfavourable arterial anatomy who undergo a failed attempt at transarterial embolization. Although coils have been used in the past, our embolic material of choice is now Onyx. With sufficient experience and modern microcatheters and guidewires, it is possible to achieve a high technical success rate using the transarterial route. However, because of the ongoing risk of late endoleak formation, continued surveillance is mandatory.

6. Pitton MB, Schweitzer H, Herber S, et al. MRI versus helical CT for endoleak detection after endovascular aneurysm repair. *AJR Am J Roentgenol* 2005; 185: 1275–81.
7. Lockstein RA, Goldman J, Pukin L, et al. Time-resolved magnetic resonance angiography as a noninvasive method to characterize endoleaks: initial results compared with conventional angiography. *J Vasc Surg* 2004; 39: 27–33.
8. Shah A, Stavropoulos SW. Imaging Surveillance following endovascular aneurysm repair. *Semin Intervent Radiol* 2009; 26(1): 10–16.
9. Faries PL, Cadot H, Agarwal G, et al. Management of endoleak after endovascular aneurysm repair: cuffs, coils, and conversion. *J Vasc Surg* 2003; 37: 1155–61.
10. Veith FJ, Baum RA, Ohki T, et al. Nature and significance of endoleaks and endotension: summary of opinions expressed at an international conference. *J Vasc Surg* 2002; 35: 1029–35.
11. van Marrewijk C, Buth J, Harris PL, et al. Significance of endoleaks after endovascular repair of abdominal aortic aneurysms: the EUROSTAR experience. *JVasc Surg* 2002; 35: 461–73.
12. Gelfand DV, White GH, Wilson SE. Clinical significance of type II endoleak after endovascular repair of abdominal aortic aneurysm. *Ann Vasc Surg* 2006; 20: 69–74.
13. Jones JE, Atkins MD, Brewster DC, et al. Persistent type 2 endoleak after endovascular repair of abdominal aortic aneurysm is associated with adverse late outcomes. *J Vasc Surg* 2007; 46: 1–8.
14. Greenhalgh RM, The United Kingdom EVAR Trial Investigators. Endovascular versus open repair of abdominal aortic aneurysm. *N Engl J Med* 2010; 362: 1863–71.
15. Hobo R, Buth J, EUROSTAR collaborators. Secondary interventions following endovascular abdominal aortic aneurysm repair using current endografts: a EUROSTAR report. *J Vasc Surg* 2006; 43(5): 896–902.
16. Gilling Smith G, Brennan J, Harris PL, et al. Endotension after endovascular aneurysm repair: definition, classification, and strategies for surveillance and intervention. *J Endovasc Surg* 1999; 6: 305–7.
17. Naughton PA, Garcia-Toca M, Rodriguez HE, et al. Endovascular treatment of delayed type 1 and 3 endoleaks. *Cardiovasc Intervent Radiol* 2011; 34: 751–7.
18. Sheehan MK, Barbato J, Compton CN, et al. Effectiveness of coiling in the treatment of endoleaks after endovascular repair. *J Vasc Surg* 2004; 40: 430–4.
19. Henrikson O, Roos H, Falkenberg M. Ethylene vinyl alcohol copolymer (Onyx) to seal type I endoleak: a new technique. *Vascular* 2011; 19(2): 77–81.
20. May J, White GH, Yu W, et al. Conversion from endoluminal to open repair of abdominal aortic aneurysms: a hazardous procedure. *Eur J Vasc Endovasc Surg* 1997; 14:4–11.
21. Patatas K, Ling L, Dunning J, et al. Static sac size with a type II endoleak post-endovascular abdominal aortic aneurysm repair: surveillance or embolization? *Interact Cardiovasc Thorac Surg* 2012; 15(3): 462–6.
22. Rial R, Serrano FJ, Vega M, et al. Treatment of type ii endoleaks after endovascular repair of abdominal aortic aneurysms: translumbar puncture and injection of thrombin into the aneurysm sac. *Eur J Vasc Endovasc Surg* 2004; 27: 333–5.
23. Richardson WS, Sternbergh WC 3rd, Money SR. Laparoscopic inferior mesenteric artery ligation: an alternative for the treatment of type II endoleaks. *J Laparoendosc Adv Surg Tech* 2003; 13(6): 355–8.
24. Ryu RK, Palestrant S, Ryu J, et al. Sac hygroma after endovascular abdominal aortic aneurysm repair: successful treatment with endograft relining. *Cardiovasc Intervent Radiol* 2007; 30: 488–90.
25. van Marrewijk CJ, Fransen G, Laheij RJ, et al. Is a type II endoleak after EVAR a harbinger of risk? Causes and outcome of open conversion and aneurysm rupture during follow-up. *Eur J Vasc Endovasc Surg* 2004; 27: 128–37.

CASE

# 5 Carotid artery stenting: how to treat restenosis

**Alessandro Cannavale**

**Expert commentary** Fabrizio Fanelli

## Case history

A 63-year-old female with history of arterial hypertension, type II diabetes mellitus, and smoking underwent carotid endarterectomy (CEA) of the left internal carotid artery (ICA) because of a symptomatic (transitory dysphasia and right facial weakness resolved within an hour) 75% stenosis. A few years previously the patient had had a right ischaemic stroke due to complete occlusion of the right ICA, which resulted in left-side hemiparesis that was partially improved with rehabilitation. The patient was under antiplatelet therapy with aspirin (100mg/day).

Ultrasound colour Doppler (USCD) confirmed occlusion of the right ICA and the presence of an irregular hypo-echoic plaque at the level of the left carotid bifurcation with 75% severe stenosis and a peak systolic velocity (PSV) of 250cm/s. The findings were also confirmed with computed tomography angiography (CTA) which revealed the presence of a soft ulcerated plaque. There was no sign of ischaemia at the level of the ipsilateral cerebral parenchyma There was a lacunar area at the level of the right parietal lobe. CEA was performed and the aspirin dose was increased to 325mg/day post-operatively.

A year later, the patient reported right hand shaking and transitory right arm weakness which resolved within 30 minutes. The episode was highly suspicious of a transient ischaemic attack (TIA), and a USCD was performed which revealed restenosis at the level of the previous CEA (80%). This time the patient underwent endovascular treatment with a balloon expandable stent which was deployed at the level of the recurrent stenosis. A few days later the patient was discharged in good clinical condition with the following antiplatelet therapy: clopidogrel 75mg/day for the first month, followed by aspirin 325mg/day indefinitely.

Seven months later, during clinical and imaging follow-up (Table 5.1), USCD revealed an increase in PSV at the proximal end of the stent (PSV of 325cm/s); the

**Table 5.1 Suggested imaging protocol before and after CEA and/or CAS**

| | Pre-procedure | Post-procedure | | | | | |
|---|---|---|---|---|---|---|---|
| | | 24 h | 1 month | 3 months | 6 months | 9 months | 12 months |
| Clinical evaluation | ✓ | ✓ | ✓ | ✓ | ✓ | ✓ | ✓ |
| Neurological examination | ✓ | ✓ | | | | | |
| USCD | ✓ | ✓ | ✓ | | ✓ | | ✓ |
| CTA | ✓ | In cases of doubt | | | | | |
| DSA | To be performed in case of abnormal findings or for stent and/or CEA revision | | | | | | |

Diagnostic DSA should be avoided in the pre-treatment evaluation because diagnostic angiography of the carotid arteries is correlated with 0.5% stroke and 2.5% procedure-related complications.

**Clinical tip** Imaging assessment in patients with carotid restenosis.

Imaging assessment is generally based on USCD and CTA; however, if there is still doubt on the exact grade of restenosis due to beam hardening artefacts (extensive calcified plaque, presence of stent) after USCD and CTA, DSA may be performed as reference standard diagnostic to determine whether any kind of operative treatment is necessary. Moreover, diagnostic DSA may be the test of choice in patients with renal dysfunction to limit the amount of contrast material required [2].

end diastolic velocity (EDV) was 110cm/s. These values suggested type I restenosis according to the classification by Lal et al. [1]. Moreover, the stent appeared collapsed in the same area. A complete neurological examination showed a National Institutes of Health Stroke Scale (NIHSS) score of 8, a Barthel index of 8, and a Rankin scale of 3 (moderate disability).

**Expert comment** Carotid DSA technique

From a conventional common femoral artery approach a 4Fr pigtail catheter is advanced into the ascending aorta. Images are acquired in the lateral anterior oblique (LAO) projection of 40° in order to have a better view of the aortic arch and the origin of the supra-aortic vessels. Non-ionic contrast media ($30cm^3$) is injected via an injector at a flow rate of $20cm^3/s$ and images are acquired at a frame rate of 3 frames/s. Then a selective injection of the common carotid artery (CCA) is suggested, preferably with a vertebral catheter.

**Evidence base**

Leading international guidelines [2–5] advise a close clinical imaging follow-up of patients who have undergone carotid revascularization. In particular, USCD is considered the first-line imaging tool after the intervention, and should be performed within at least one month, at six months, and annually thereafter.

USCD is considered to be the leading imaging tool to detect restenosis after CAS/CEA. However, USCD in-stent restenosis (ISR) criteria are not definitely established because of the reduced compliance of the stented vessel wall which may increase peak systolic velocity. Recent studies [1,6–10] suggest several morphological and velocity criteria (PSV, EDV, ICA/CCA ratio) to define ISR, and we may consider the following thresholds:

- stenosis <30%: PSV<100cm/s; EDV <40 cm/s
- stenosis 30–50%: PSV = 100–170cm/s; EDV = 80cm/s
- stenosis 50%–70%: PSV = 171–299cm/s; EDV = 90cm/s
- stenosis > 70%: PSV >300cm/s; EDV >120cm/s.

In general a value of PSV above a threshold of 300cm/s is now considered diagnostic for significant ISR (>70%) [8,9].

Lal et al. [1] described morphological classification of ISR as follows.

- Type I: focal end stent
- Type II: focal intra-stent
- Type III: diffuse intra-stent
- Type IV: diffuse proliferative
- Type V: total occlusion.

**Clinical tip** Clinical and neurological assessment

Clinical assessment includes complete neurological evaluation with the National Institute of Health Stroke Scale (NIHSS), the Barthel index, and the modified Rankin scale.

The NIHSS is a 15-item neurological examination scale used to evaluate the effect of acute cerebral attack on the levels of consciousness, language, neglect, visual field loss, extra-ocular movement, motor strength, ataxia, dysarthria, and sensory loss. A trained observer rates the patient's ability to answer questions and perform activities. Ratings for each item are scored with 3-5 grades with 0 as normal, and there is an allowance for untestable items. Assessment of a single patient requires less than 10 minutes to complete.

The Barthel index and the modified Rankin scale should also be used to evaluate the degree of disability or dependence in the daily activities, especially in patients with history of previous neurological symptoms.

The components of the Barthel index include feeding, moving from wheelchair to bed and returning, grooming, transferring to and from a toilet, bathing, walking on a level surface, going up and down

(continued)

stairs, dressing, and bowel and bladder continence. Each item is assessed by a score (1-2-3 or 5-10-15), reaching a potential maximum total of 20 or 100 scores depending on the institution. The Rankin scale runs from perfect health without symptoms (0) to death (6).

0 No symptoms.
1 No significant disability: able to carry out all usual activities, despite some symptoms.
2 Slight disability: able to look aftertheir own affairs without assistance, but unable to carry out all previous activities
3 Moderate disability: requires some help, but able to walk unassisted.
4 Moderately severe disability: unable to attend to own bodily needs without assistance, and unable to walk unassisted.
5 Severe disability: requires constant nursing care and attention, bedridden, incontinent.
6 Dead.

CTA revealed deformation of the stent at the level of its proximal part (Figure 5.1). Cerebral CT was also included in the pre-treatment protocol to assess recent/previous cerebral damages; no recent signs of cerebral ischaemia/haemorrhage were detected. The lacunar area in the right cerebral parenchyma was confirmed. To assess any eventual cerebral injury MRI was also performed using diffusion-weighted imaging (DWI) sequences, which did not show any acute ischaemic cerebral lesion (Figure 5.2).

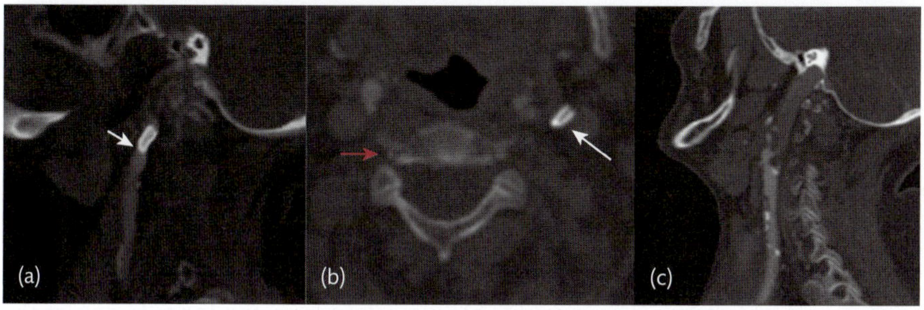


**Figure 5.1** CT angiography: (a, b) Multiple intensity projections (MIPs) and axial reconstructions of the left carotid artery show deformation of the proximal end of the stent (white arrow) with a severe restenosis (70%) of the internal carotid artery. Note also hypoplasia of the right vertebral artery (red arrow). (c) MIP reconstruction shows complete occlusion of the right internal carotid artery; the external carotid artery appears patent.

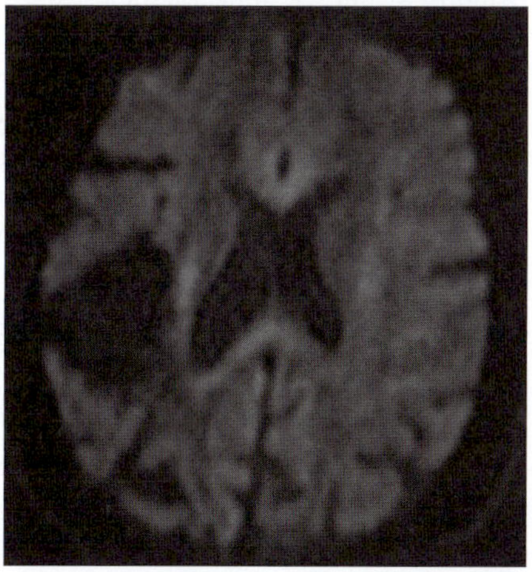

**Figure 5.2** Pre-operative brain MRI: DWI sequences confirmed the lacunar area within the right parietal lobe. There is no evidence of recent ischaemic lesions.

**Expert comment**

Evaluating the indications for re-intervention: this patient was asymptomatic but with significant restenosis (ISR >50%) and with deformation of the stent. Even though the guidelines are not completely clear for such cases [2–5], this is a high-risk patient, and new endovascular treatment is considered as the most appropriate approach in the case of restenosis after stenting/CEA.

Treatment with placement of a new carotid stent was decided after a multidisciplinary meeting. The patient was prepared in standard sterile condition. Aspirin (325mg/day) was maintained prior to the procedure, and 75mg clopidogrel was administered 24 hours before the procedure.

The procedure was performed without sedation to allow continuous monitoring of the patient's neurological conditions. The right common femoral artery was punctured in a retrograde fashion under local anaesthesia (mepivacaine 2%; Industria Farmaceutica Galenica Senese, Siena, Italy). A 7Fr introducer sheath (25cm) was placed through the common femoral artery and a bolus of 75IU/kg of heparin was administered. Left CCA catheterization was performed using a 'direct approach' technique with a 7Fr guiding catheter (Mach 1–40°; Boston Scientific, Natick, MA, USA). The guiding catheter was managed in combination with a standard 0.035 inch (180cm) angled-tip hydrophilic guidewire (Terumo Co, Tokyo, Japan) to enter the CCA. The activated clotting time (ACT) was kept between 275 and 300 seconds. To avoid thrombus formation, the guiding catheter was connected to a pressurized heparinized saline bag in order to flush its inner lumen continuously.

Angiography confirmed significant restenosis at the third proximal of the stent with deformation of the stent mesh (Figure 5.3a). AP and lateral angiography of the cerebral vascularity was then performed. Subsequently a filter device (Angioguard 6mm; Cordis Europe, Waterloo, Belgium) was advanced, crossing the stenosis into the third distal of the extra-cranial part of the ICA (Figure 5.3b). A 7mm × 3cm stent (Precise Rx; Cordis Europe, Waterloo, Belgium) was placed at the level of the lesion with its proximal end at the CCA level (Figure 5.3c). Post-dilation of the stent was performed using a low-profile rapid-exchange balloon (5.5mm in diameter) in accordance with the stent diameter (Figure 5.3d). Immediately before stent dilation, 1mg of atropine was injected intravenously to prevent sinus reflex. Temporary dysphasia, which resolved within 2 minutes, occurred immediately after stent dilation. After stent deployment and before filter removal, angiography was performed to 'clean' any possible plaque debris from the inner lumen of the stent (Figure 5.3e). After filter removal, final angiography showed no evidence of arterial spasms and good flow within the stent, with restoration of the normal vessel calibre. Finally an angiogram of the intracranial circle in two projections showed good flow within the arteries (Figure 5.3f). A vascular closure device (Angioseal 8Fr; St Jude Medical, St Paul, MN, USA) was used to seal the right common femoral access.

To assess any eventual cerebral injury DWI MRI was performed, which did not show any acute ischaemic cerebral lesion. Post-procedural care involved monitoring vital parameters for 24 hours (controlling blood pressure and heart rate) and performing a complete clinical–neurological examination. Neurological examination and NIHSS score (8 as before the procedure) did not reveal any changes compared with the neurological status of the patient before the procedure. The patient was discharged after 2 days in a stable clinical condition with antiplatelet therapy: aspirin 325mg/day indefinitely and clopidogrel 75mg/day for 4 weeks. She was followed up by regular clinical and imaging examinations. She remained asymptomatic and follow-up USCD over two years did not show any further ISR (Figure 5.4).

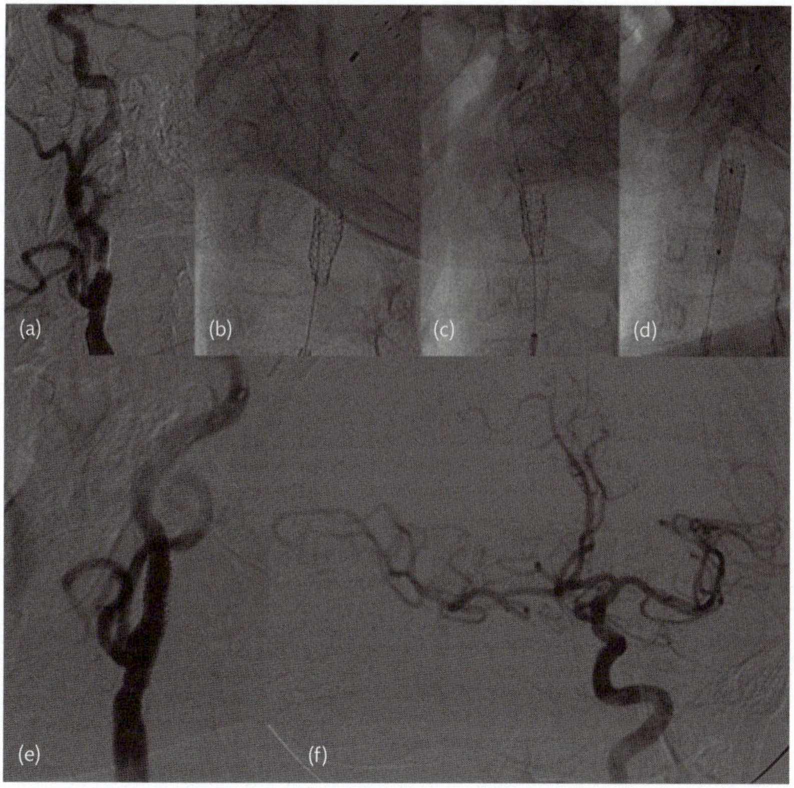


**Figure 5.3** (a) Selective angiography of the left common carotid artery confirms the deformation of the proximal end of the stent with the presence of severe in-stent stenosis. (b) A filter device is advanced through the stent until the third distal of the extracranial part of the internal carotid artery. (c, d) A self-expandable stent (7mm × 3cm; Precise Rx, Cordis) was released at the level of stenosis and then dilation with low-profile undersized balloon was performed. (e) A final angiogram before removal of the filter shows expansion of both stents with good flow along the entire internal carotid artery. (f) Arteriography of the intracranial circle shows good flow in the contralateral cerebral vessels.

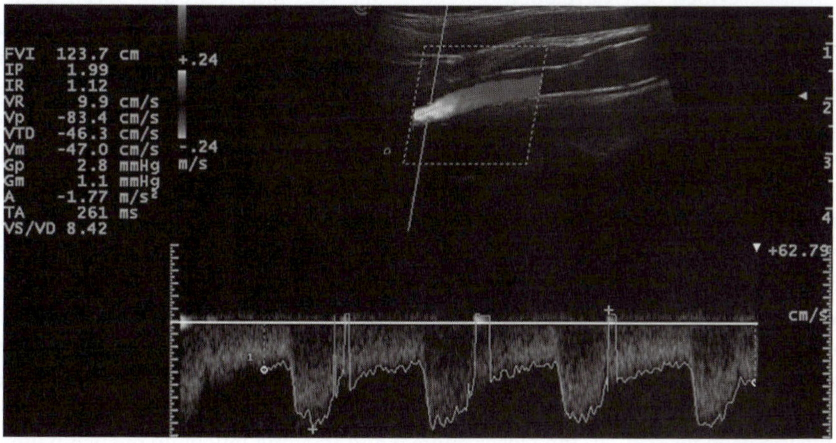


**Figure 5.4** After two years, USCD shows good flow within the stents with normal values of PSV (83.4cm/s) and EDV (46.3cm/s). Note minimal parietal intimal hyperplasia alongside the stent wall.

## Discussion

Recurrent stenosis after carotid artery stenting (CAS) is a relatively rare condition with 3–15% incidence in five years follow-up [1,2]. The majority of ISRs occur within the first year after intervention and they are mainly related to neo-intimal hyperplasia (early ISR) or recurrent atherosclerosis (late ISR). Restenosis rates appear to be significantly higher after CAS than after CEA; however, this is not always linked to symptoms [9,11,12].

**Landmark trial** CREST trial: restenosis after carotid artery stenting and endarterectomy [9].

A prospective randomized multicentre trial was performed at 117 clinical centres in the USA and Canada between 21 December 2000 and 18 July 2008 which included 2,191 patients (1,086 treated with CAS; 1,105 underwent CEA). Prospective USCD was performed at baseline and at 1, 6, 12, 24, and 48 months after revascularization. Sixteen Doppler waveform samples were obtained at every examination: eight samples were taken from each side of the neck, six at 1–2cm intervals along the common and internal carotid arteries, one from the external carotid artery, and one from the vertebral artery. Waveform: 60° angulation—highest PSV to identify restenosis with a threshold of 300cm/s.

- Secondary analysis of CREST trial, main endpoint: composite of restenosis (≥70% diameter reducing stenosis) or complete occlusion at two years.
- Two-year composite outcome (restenosis and occlusion): 120 patients (58 CAS; 62 CEA). Frequency of restenosis (Kaplan–Meier estimation) was 6.0% for CAS and 6.3% for CEA (hazard ratio (HR) 0.90, 0.95% CI 0.63–1.29; $p = 0.58$).
- Restenosis alone (113 patients): 56 CAS and 57 CEA Kaplan–Meier estimate of the two-year frequency of restenosis was 5.8%.
- Risk of neurological events: patients who had restenosis or occlusion within two years were at greater risk for ipsilateral stroke after the peri-procedural period up to the end of follow-up than those who did not have restenosis (HR 4.37, 95% CI 1.91–10.03; $p$=0.0005).

Recurrent stenosis after stenting may also be related to stent fracture or deformation, which may occur in 2–29% of patients treated with CAS [13]. Neo-intimal proliferation has been related to peri-interventional inflammation markers and may be influenced by stent size and geometry [12,14]. Open-cell stents and highly calcified plaques are considered independent predictors of stent deformation [13]. The patient described here developed restenosis one year after CEA and seven months after CAS. Both surgical and endovascular intervention represent a vessel injury which may lead to an inflammation process (increased values of plasma C-reactive protein have been found by Wasser et al. [15]) and neo-intimal proliferation through the stent mesh. Recent studies have highlighted potential clinical and technical risk factors for ISR after CAS: advanced age [12,14]; previous treatment for a radiogenic stenosis or a recurrent stenosis after CEA [12]; contralateral ICA occlusion [12]; significant residual stenosis after CAS (PSV >120cm/s)[16]; presence of cardiovascular risk factors such as tobacco use; diabetes mellitus; dyslipoproteinemia; and certain procedure-related factors (a narrow or long stent, insufficient stent adaptability after CAS or the use of multiple stents) [12]. In the case described here we found a history of contralateral ICA occlusion and previous stenting for restenosis after CEA, so that the increased PSV of 325cm/s at level of the proximal end of the stent, which appeared deformed, was highly suggestive for in-stent restenosis. This would reinforce the need for regular and closer clinical and imaging follow-up of such patients who are sometimes referred to the emergency department because of the sudden appearance of neurological symptoms.

CT angiography after USCD is considered the reference imaging examination for the assessment of post-CAS/CEA restenosis and the depiction of the anatomy of supra-aortic vessels in order to plan endovascular or surgical intervention. The role of MR angiography in patients with carotid stents is still controversial: poor lumen visibility is linked to carotid stainless steel stents, but the majority of (nitinol) stents can be assessed with MRI [17]. Cerebral-MRI is now in widespread use for pre- and post-procedure assessment of ischaemic neurological events.

Neurological assessment (general neurological examination, NIHSS scale, Barthel index, and Rankin scale) should be performed before and after every procedure so that improvement or lack of improvement can be noted. It is highly recommended that, as well as neurological evaluation, medical therapy should be adjusted before treating restenosis. In fact correct medical therapy is a leading method of preventing restenosis and thus the development of adverse neurological events such as TIA or ischaemic stroke.

**Clinical tip**

During clinical follow-up in these patients the physician should also consider specific issues.

- After first successful recanalization the mean arterial pressure should be reduced to 10–20% less than the baseline value.
- Presence of carotid sinus dysfunction: prolonged bradycardia and/or hypotension requiring intravenous vasopressors or ionotropic agents.
- Fluctuation of blood pressure: use 24 hour monitoring of pressure because of increased baroflex sensitivity in patients who have undergone CAS or CEA.
- Recent/previous TIA or stroke: our patient had a prior stroke event and subsequently two episodes of TIA related to the 'native' left ICA stenosis and then to restenosis of the CEA. However, the NIHSS score remained stable because TIA episodes usually do not have a permanent influence on neurological function. Some authors [18] have recently reported that in the case of unilateral ICA occlusion, contralateral endovascular treatment resulted in delayed cerebral blood flow haemodynamic improvement in both cerebral hemispheres.

**Learning point** Antiplatelet and anticoagulant therapy to prevent ISR and secondary neurological events.

Antiplatelet and anticoagulant therapy for secondary prevention of stroke has recently been addressed in current guidelines [19].

- Aspirin (50–325mg/day) monotherapy (Class I; Level of Evidence A); a combination of aspirin 25mg and extended-release dipyridamole 200mg twice daily (Class I; Level of Evidence B); clopidogrel 75mg monotherapy (Class IIa; Level of Evidence B) are all acceptable options for initial therapy.
- The addition of aspirin to clopidogrel increases risk of haemorrhage and is not recommended for routine secondary prevention after ischaemic stroke or TIA (Class III; Level of Evidence A).
- For patients who have an ischaemic stroke while taking aspirin, there is no evidence that increasing the dose of aspirin provides additional benefit (Class IIb; Level of Evidence C).

Considering our case, initial antiplatelet therapy alone (aspirin 100mg) after a previous right-sided stroke (occlusion of right ICA) was generally correct, obviously accompanied by control of hypertension and diabetes, and encouraging cessation of tobacco use. Moreover, she had a contralateral TIA treated with CEA; after that aspirin dosage was increased to 325mg/day. However, a non-definitive control of restenosis and neurological events was achieved, as stated in the guidelines.

After CEA restenosis was treated with stenting placement, antiplatelet therapy was switched to clopidogrel 75mg/day for the first month and then aspirin 325mg/day indefinitely. In this case the antiplatelet therapy followed the current guidelines [2], but after six months the patient experienced in-stent restenosis. Despite good antiplatelet therapy, other restenotic factors should be considered in our case: tobacco use has been related more to CEA restenosis than endovascular stenting [8], and diabetes mellitus and hypertension may also be related to the occurrence of restenotic events. Nevertheless, such factors seem to be weaker than those related to the technical procedure, which should be considered as leading restenotic risk factors in our case.

**Evidence base** Management of patients who experience recurrent stenosis after CAS/CEA: current guidelines

Current recommendations regarding patients who experienced restenosis are mainly outlined by ASA/ACCF/AHA guidelines, updated SVS guidelines, ESC guidelines, and Australasian guidelines. For the former guideline clinical behaviour in patients undergoing CAS or CEA similarly consists of three main steps (Class I: Level of Evidence C).

1. Before (usually 3 days before) and for a minimum of 30 days after CAS, dual antiplatelet therapy with aspirin (80–325mg daily) plus clopidogrel (75mg daily) is recommended. (Use ticlopidine 250mg twice daily if there is intolerance to clopidopgrel.)
2. Blood pressure control with antihypertensive medication.
3. Neurological examination 24 hours before and after the procedure.

Regarding indications in patients who have experienced restenosis, it is reasonable (Class IIa, Level of Evidence C) to repeat CEA or perform CAS in patients with symptomatic cerebral ischaemia and recurrent carotid stenosis due to intimal hyperplasia or atherosclerosis, or when duplex ultrasound and another imaging method identifies rapidly progressive restenosis that indicates a threat of complete occlusion.

Less evidence is required in the case of asymptomatic patients with recurrent stenosis. Intervention (CAS/CEA) may be considered using the same criteria as recommended for initial revascularization (Class IIb; Level of Evidence C).

Finally, it is considered high risk and unjustified (Class III Harm; Level of Evidence III) to re-intervene (either with CEA or CAS) in asymptomatic patients with less than 70% carotid stenosis which has remained stable over time.

Updated guidelines from the Society of Vascular Surgery [3] give some recommendations on imaging follow-up to diagnose recurrent stenosis after CEA/CAS.

- USCD is the diagnostic imaging test of choice for long-term follow-up of these patients.
- It is recommended 30 days after intervention to assess the status of the operated vessel.
- It is useful to monitor the contralateral disease progression.
- DSA, CT, and MRA are needed in addition to USCD when there is any suspicion of restenosis and are useful for planning operative therapy. DSA is particularly useful when non-invasive tests give conflicting findings.

The ESC Guidelines [4] do not make any recommendations regarding the management of the patient at risk of restenosis after CAS/CEA. They make recommendations on primary carotid stenosis and medical therapy, which should be followed in a patient with carotid artery stenosis. The Australasian guidelines [5] do not address the issue of restenosis after CAS/CEA extensively; however, they recommend that CAS is considered as a treatment option in patients who are unsuitable for surgery: following radiation therapy, block dissection of the neck, in situ tracheostomy, recurrent stenosis following previous CEA, severe cervical spine arthritis, surgically inaccessible carotid stenosis (i.e. obesity, high carotid bifurcation), contralateral recurrent laryngeal nerve injury, and contralateral internal carotid occlusion.

Procedure-related risk factors for early neurological events and late restenosis after CEA are female gender, small diameter ICA, and performing the standard technique with primary closure. Patch closure or an eversion technique has been found to have benefits over primary closure in patients undergoing standard CEA, regardless of the patch material used [3,20]. Other technical elements of CAS which have been related to restenosis are previous CEA, type of stent (a narrow or long stent, insufficient stent adaptation after CAS), the use of multiple stents, and residual stenosis after stent deployment [21,22]. The type of restenotic lesion (type IV) has also been defined as an independent predictor of high-grade recurrent ISR and re-intervention [1].

Some authors have suggested that, when multiple stents are used, in-stent restenosis may be due to a larger surface area covered with stent mesh or to the overlapping edges of the stent inducing well-defined intimal hyperplasia [22]. However, Wasser et al. [12] concluded that the use of multiple stents, stent type (open/closed cell mesh) and dimensions, pre-dilation, and post-dilation are not related to a higher risk of in-stent restenosis on multivariate analysis.

Regardless of the factors which determined restenosis, two different interventions are available to treat in-stent restenosis: endovascular or surgical. Generally speaking (>70% of cases), endovascular intervention is the initial approach for patients who develop significant ISR due to intimal hyperplasia (most commonly early) or atherosclerosis, [1,23,24]. Surgical revision of the stent, with stent removal and endarterectomy using eversion technique or other techniques, has recently been proposed, albeit with potential cerebral and bleeding complications [25,26]. Surgical treatment of ISR is mainly indicated in the following conditions: heavily calcified lesions with suboptimal primary stenting results, pre-occlusive lesions that no longer respond to or are approachable by angioplasty, technical failure of stent material, or primary stent thrombosis [1].

In the case described, we faced a contralateral ICA occlusion, restenosis of CEA treated with a balloon expandable stent, and multiple cardiovascular risk factors. In this situation the endovascular approach is the preferred choice because of the patient features. Furthermore CEA is not appropriate because of the presence of post-operative fibrosis of soft tissue, which may be associated with a higher risk of cranial nerve injury, as well as wound haematoma with a higher morbidity than primary surgery.

Different endovascular techniques have been described in the literature: angioplasty alone, cutting balloon angioplasty, stenting and angioplasty, brachytherapy, drug-eluting stents, and drug-eluting balloons (Table 5.2).

Some authors generally advise using angioplasty as the primary approach and releasing a stent in case of suboptimal result with residual stenosis [1,30]. The mechanism of lumen expansion in standard angioplasty consists of compressing the intimal hyperplasia against the stent mesh which leads to an enlargement of the stent diameter. If this is not sufficient, a stent should be released in order to resolve residual stenosis. Re-stenting may also be useful to resolve stent fracture and deformation, in order to restore the correct stent morphology and thus reduce the related risk of restenosis or stent occlusion.

The cutting-balloon mechanism for increasing the stent lumen is different from standard angioplasty. The microsurgical incisions of the cutting balloon result in a division of the neointimal hyperplastic tissue into small fragments which are more easily extruded out of the stent into the surrounding artery during inflation of the non-compliant balloon [30]. Case series have shown acceptable results in terms of immediate and mid-term stent patency after cutting balloon angioplasty [31–33].

**Table 5.2 Treatment options to approach restenosis**

| Endovascular technique | Advantage | Limitation |
|---|---|---|
| Standard angioplasty | Avoids re-stenting | Recurrence of stenosis/residual stenosis |
| Stenting ± angioplasty | Guarantees optimal result: remodelling stent geometry (i.e. stent deformation/fracture) | Risk of increasing the number of stents |
| Cutting balloon angioplasty | Good results<br>Also avoids re-stenting | Avoid in tortuous anatomy out of the limits of the stent |
| Brachytherapy | Avoid re-stenting | Small case series reported<br>Needs technical and skills improvement |
| Surgery | Stent occlusion<br>Tight stenosis<br>Tortuous anatomy | High risk patients<br>Previous CEA<br>Stent conformation<br>Carotid bifurcation anatomy |
| Drug-eluting stents [27,28] | Good mid-term patency rate (mean of 17 months)<br>Potential use in vasculitis | Ongoing studies<br>Some cases of stent thrombosis<br>Avoid use outside the carotid stent scaffold |
| Drug-eluting balloons [29] | Potential inhibition of neointimal hyperplasia<br>Avoids stenting | Only in vitro studies |

**Clinical tip** Using a cutting balloon for carotid in-stent restenosis

- Avoid using a cutting balloon in cases of tortuous anatomy.
- A cutting balloon is useful for avoidIng migration of the balloon during inflation at the level of the stent [31].
- Late hard in-stent intimal hyperplasia causing restenosis may be better remodelled using a cutting balloon.
- Always use cutting balloons inside the stented area. Therefore avoid their use when the intimal hyperplasia is at the end of the stent (Type I according to Lal et al. [1]) and partly in the non-stented area.

Only a few cases of ISR treated with brachytherapy have been described. Seeman et al. [34] and Chan et al. [35] reported good immediate and mid-term patency rates, but identified the need for larger studies and improvement of technique to confirm the efficacy of this revascularization technique.

The current literature does not identify a preferred technique. In our case it was reasonable to modify the geometry of the stent which was evidently altered. Placement of another stent with subsequent dilation until the stenosis was resolved was a reasonable approach.

In general when the stenosis is localized at the end of the stent, elongating the stented area may be useful for modifying the haemodynamic forces, which could favour the development of restenosis. If restenosis is multifocal or focal inside the stent, standard angioplasty or cutting balloon angioplasty may be suitable. Also, another stent may be added to solve a residual stenosis. However, because of the high risk of re-intervention in such patients [32] and the fact that repeated stenting does not guarantee longer-term patency rate, re-stenting should be reserved for cases where a sufficient immediate result cannot be obtained with angioplasty (standard or cutting balloon) alone (i.e. calcified lesions). The future of endovascular treatment of ISR is represented by the drug-eluting stent, which showed good results in terms of mid-term patency rate [27,28], nevertheless such stents are still only under investigation.

Finally, we recommend surgery with removal of the stent when an endovascular treatment cannot be performed due to tight stenosis which cannot be passed by the guidewire or in the case of complete acute or chronic stent thrombosis or occlusion (Type V of Lal et al. [1]) or plaque protrusion after a failed endovascular attempt [1,36,37].

## A final word from the expert

In patients who have undergone previous carotid intervention with multiple cardiovascular risk factors a multidisciplinary clinical–neurological and imaging assessment is essential not only to adjust medical therapy or imaging follow-up but also to better plan subsequent treatment. Endovascular therapy is the treatment of choice for in-stent restenosis because it is less invasive. Moreover, the presence of a stent increases the risk of surgical intervention and consequently the endovascular approach is paramount in those situations. The main issue in the case described here is the technical mistake of deploying a balloon-expandable stent within the internal carotid artery to treat CEA restenosis. The continuous movements of the neck may easily alter such a stent. Obviously the insertion of a longer and more flexible self-expandable stent can reduce the complications related to the deformation of the stent. This is confirmed by the clinical improvement of the patient and the long-term patency of the stent.

## References

1. Lal BK. Recurrent carotid stenosis after CEA and CAS: diagnosis and management. *Semin Vasc Surg* 2007; 20(4): 259–66.
2. Brott TG, Halperin JL, Abbara S, et al. ASA/ACCF/AHA/AANN/AANS/ACR/ASNR/CNS/SAIP/SCAI/SIR/SNIS/SVM/SVS guideline on the management of patients with extracranial carotid and vertebral artery disease. *Stroke* 2011; 42(8): e464–540.
3. Ricotta JJ, Aburahma A, Ascher E, et al. Updated Society for Vascular Surgery guidelines for management of extracranial carotid disease. *J Vasc Surg* 2011; 54: e1–e31.
4. Tendera M, Aboyans V, Bartelink ML, et al. ESC Guidelines on the diagnosis and treatment of peripheral artery diseases: document covering atherosclerotic disease of extracranial carotid and vertebral, mesenteric, renal, upper and lower extremity arteries. *Eur Heart J* 2011; 32: 2851–906.
5. Carotid Stenting Guidelines Committee. Guidelines for patient selection and performance of carotid artery stenting. *Int Med J* 2011; 41: 344–7.
6. Lal BK, Beach KW, Roubin GS, et al. Restenosis after carotid artery stenting and endarterectomy: a secondary analysis of CREST, a randomised controlled trial. *Lancet Neurol* 2012; 11(9): 755–63.
7. AbuRahma AF, Abu-Halimah S, Bensenhaver J, et al. Optimal carotid duplex velocity criteria for defining the severity of carotid in-stent restenosis. *J Vasc Surg* 2008; 48(3): 589–94.
8. Setacci C, Chisci E, Setacci F, et al. Grading carotid intrastent restenosis: a 6-year follow-up study. *Stroke* 2008; 39(4): 1189–96.
9. Bonati LH. Restenosis after carotid artery stenting: remaining issues. *Lancet Neurol* 2012; 11(9): 740–1.

10. Bonati LH, Ederle J, McCabe DJ, et al. Long-term risk of carotid restenosis in patients randomly assigned to endovascular treatment or endarterectomy in the Carotid and Vertebral Artery Transluminal Angioplasty Study (CAVATAS): long-term follow-up of a randomised trial. *Lancet Neurol* 2009; 8(10): 908–17.
11. MacDonald S. Carotid artery stenting trials: conduct, results, critique, and current recommendations. *Cardiovasc Intervent Radiol* 2012; 35: 15–29.
12. Wasser K, Gröschel S, Wohlfahrt J, Gröschel K. Predictors of carotid artery in-stent restenosis. *Perspect Med* 2012: 1; 122–8.
13. Chang CK, Huded CP, Nolan BW, Powell RJ. Prevalence and clinical significance of stent fracture and deformation following carotid artery stenting. *J Vasc Surg* 2011; 54: 685–90.
14. Zhou W, Lin PH, Bush RL, et al. Management of in-stent restenosis after carotid artery stenting in high-risk patients. *J Vasc Surg* 2006; 43: 305–12.
15. Wasser K, Schnaudigel S, Wohlfahrt J, et al. Inflammation and in-stent restenosis: the role of serum markers and stent characteristics in carotid artery stenting. *PLoS One* 2011; 6(7): e22683
16. Wasser K, Schnaudigel S, Wohlfahrt J, et al. Clinical impact and predictors of carotid artery in-stent restenosis. *J Neurol* 2012; 259(9): 1896–1902.
17. Burg MC, Bunck AC, Seifarth H, et al. MR Angiography of peripheral arterial stents: in vitro evaluation of 22 different stent types. *Radiol Res Pract* 2011; 2011:478175
18. Oka F, Ishihara H, Kato S, et al. Cerebral hemodynamic benefits after contralateral carotid artery stenting in patients with internal carotid artery occlusion. *AJNR Am J Neuroradiol* 2013; 34(3): 616–21.
19. Furie KL, Kasner SE, Adams RJ, et al. Guidelines for the prevention of stroke in patients with stroke or transient ischaemic attack: a guideline for healthcare professionals from the american heart association/american stroke association. *Stroke* 2011; 42(1): 227–76.
20. Bond R, Rerkasem K, Naylor AR, et al. Systematic Review of randomized controlled trials of patch angioplasty versus primary closure and different types of patch materials during carotid endarterectomy. *J Vasc Surg* 2004; 40: 1126–35.
21. Setacci C, Pula G, Baldi I, et al. Determinants of in-stent restenosis after carotid angioplasty: a case-control study. *J Endovasc Ther* 2003; 10(6): 1031–8.
22. Cosottini M, Michelassi MC, Bencivelli W, et al In stent restenosis predictors after carotid artery stenting. *Stroke Res Treat* 2010 14; doi 10.4061/2010/864724.
23. King BN, Scher LA, Lipsitz EC. Refractory in-stent restenosis following carotid artery stenting: a case report and review of operative management. *Vasc Endovasc Surg* 2009; 43(3): 306–11.
24. Zhou W, Lin PH, Bush RL, et al. Management of in-stent restenosis after carotid artery stenting in high-risk patients. *J Vasc Surg* 2006; 43(2): 305–12.
25. Jost D, Unmuth SJ, Meissner H, et al. Surgical treatment of carotid in-stent-restenosis: novel strategy and current management. *Thorac Cardiovasc Surg* 2012; 60(8): 517–24.
26. Reichmann BL, van Laanen JH, de Vries JP, et al. Carotid endarterectomy for treatment of in-stent restenosis after carotid angioplasty and stenting. *J Vasc Surg* 2011; 54(1): 87–92.
27. Iancu A, Lazar A. Carotid artery in-stent restenosis in a patient with contralateral total occlusion, resolved with drug-eluting stenting. *J Invasive Cardiol* 2007; 19(6): 275–9
28. Tekieli L, Pieniazek P, Musialek P, et al. Zotarolimus-eluting stent for the treatment of recurrent, severe carotid artery in-stent stenosis in the TARGET-CAS population. *J Endovasc Ther* 2012; 19(3): 316–24.
29. Gertz ZM, Wilensky RL. Local drug delivery for treatment of coronary and peripheral artery disease. *Cardiovasc Ther* 2011; 29(6): e54–66.
30. Reimers B, Tübler T, de Donato G, et al Endovascular treatment of in-stent restenosis after carotid artery stenting: immediate and midterm results. *J Endovasc Ther* 2006; 13: 429e35.
31. Shah QA, Georgiadis AL, Suri MF, et al. Cutting balloon angioplasty for carotid in-stent restenosis: case reports and review of the literature. *J Neuroimaging* 2008; 18(4): 428–32.
32. Heck D. Results of cutting balloon angioplasty for carotid artery in-stent restenosis in six patients: description of the technique, long-term outcomes, and review of the literature. *J Neurointerv Surg* 2009; 1(1): 48–50.

33. van Haaften AC, Bots ML, Moll FL, de Borst GJ. Therapeutic options for carotid in-stent restenosis: review of the literature. *J Vasc Interv Radiol* 2010; 21(10): 1471–7.
34. Seemann JH, Leppien A, Feyer P, Felix R. Peripheral vascular disease: carotid and vertebral brachytherapy for in-stent restenosis. *Catheter Cardiovasc Interv* 2005; 65(3): 412–15.
35. Chan AW, Roffi M, Mukherjee D, et al. Carotid brachytherapy for in-stent restenosis. *Catheter Cardiovasc Interv* 2002; 58: 86–92.
36. Takigawa T, Matsumaru Y, Kubo T, et al. Recurrent subacute in-stent restenosis after carotid artery stenting due to plaque protrusion. *Neurol Med Chir (Tokyo)* 2009; 49(9): 413–17.
37. Ferrero E, Ferri M, Viazzo A, Nessi F. Carotid stent removal of symptomatic plaque protrusion after carotid angioplasty stenting. *Interact Cardiovasc Thorac Surg* 2010; 11(3): 254–6.
38. Higashida RT, Meyers PM, Phatouros CC, et al. Reporting standards for carotid artery angioplasty and stent placement. *J Vasc Interv Radiol* 2009; 20(7 Suppl): S349–73.

CASE

# 6 Iliac artery occlusions: surgical bypass, covered and uncovered stents

**Andrew Christie**

**Expert commentary** Iain Robertson

## Case history

A 66-year-old woman presented to her general practitioner with rest pain in both feet of recent onset. Previous medical history revealed progressively worsening bilateral claudication stretching over many years and a history of bilateral common iliac artery (CIA) stenting for claudication performed in 1997 (with further angioplasty to the left-sided stent in 2005). Relevant medical history included stable angina and 10 cigarettes a day for approximately 50 years. She lives alone, and is fully independent.

Following vascular surgical referral, a magnetic resonance angiogram (MRA) was performed. This identified occlusion of the right external iliac artery (EIA).

**Learning point** Pre- treatment planning

Whilst the right EIA occlusion is contributory to the presentation, it is not clear from the MRA whether her symptoms of chronic claudication progressing to rest pain are partly explained by infra-inguinal run-off disease, particularly on the left side. Accurate assessment of potential in-stent stenosis/occlusion is not possible due to signal drop-out observed with a metallic artefact. Also, this case highlights a not uncommon problem of contrast-enhanced MRA, where simultaneous contrast depiction of the venous system obscures arterial interpretation—so-called venous 'contamination'. This problem is further exaggerated in the presence of critical ischaemia (foot pain at rest, as in this case) where rapid arteriovenous shunting occurs [1], which may partly explain the venous enhancement.

Several factors impaired MRA imaging; signal drop-out within the previous stents and heavy venous 'contamination' hampered interpretation in the femoro-popliteal and run-off segments (Figures 6.1 and 6.2). The patient was discussed at the regional multidisciplinary team meeting, and subsequently booked for endovascular treatment.

An interventional radiologist obtained informed consent, with emphasis made that further diagnostic imaging (catheter angiography) was required prior to any subsequent endovascular management in view of the limited information obtained from the MRA. All possible treatment scenarios were fully discussed, including potential complications (namely haematoma and pseudo-aneurysm in relation to the puncture site, arterial rupture, and distal embolization).

In view of the right EIA disease on MRA, aortic pigtail catheter angiography was performed from a retrograde left common femoral artery (CFA) puncture. This identified that both CIA stents were patent, entire right EIA occlusion and stenosis of the entire left EIA, left superficial femoral artery (SFA) occlusion reconstituting at the popliteal level, and good three-vessel run-off bilaterally.

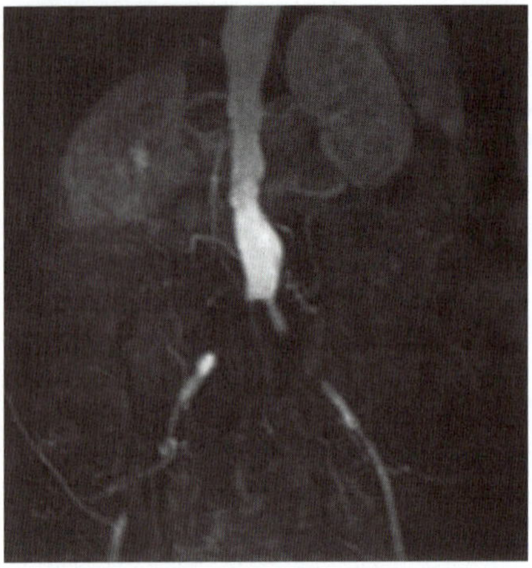

**Figure 6.1** Subtracted maximum intensity projection (MIP) of the aorto-iliac station using bolus chase contrast-enhanced MRA, showing signal loss relating to bilateral CIA stents and occlusion of the right EIA

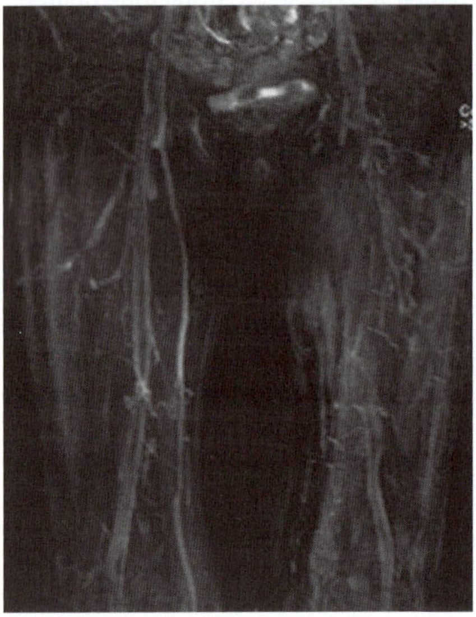

**Figure 6.2** MRA subtracted MIP projection at the femoro-popliteal station. Occlusion of the left SFA is suspected, but the images are largely non-diagnostic because of significant venous contamination. The below-knee station (not shown) also displayed venous contamination

**Evidence base** Transatlantic Inter-Society Consensus (TASC) [2,3]

- Derived from a multi-specialty working group, this consensus provides recommendations for management of peripheral vascular disease (PVD). It includes categorization of iliac lesions from A to D according to morphological complexity. Expansion in the capabilities of endovascular treatments is reflected in a revised document produced in 2007:

A. Should be treated only by endovascular means (e.g. short (<3cm) EIA stenosis).
B. Endovascular approach is preferred, unless open revascularization is required for a lesion in the same anatomical region (e.g. unilateral CIA occlusion).
C. Open revascularization is preferred, with endovascular treatment reserved for patients at high surgical risk (e.g. bilateral CIA occlusions).
D. Endovascular methods do not produce good enough results to justify them as primary treatment (e.g. unilateral CIA and EIA occlusion).

This case would be classified as TASC C

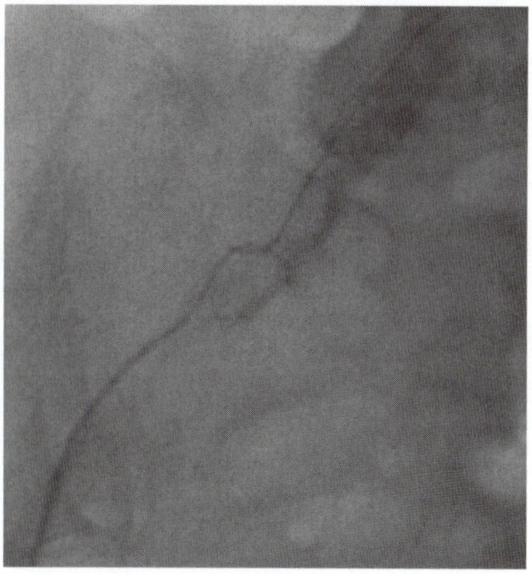

**Figure 6.3** Fluoroscopy. A 'through-and-through' wire technique crossing the right EIA occlusion subintimally from both sides. Note the previously stented right CIA.

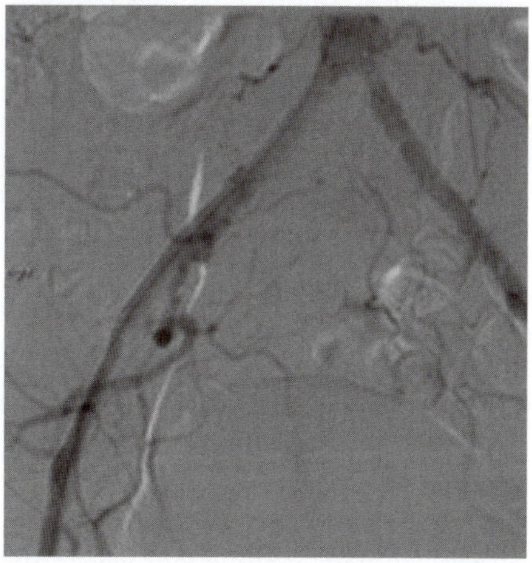

**Figure 6.4** Digital subtraction angiography (DSA): two stents covering the right EIA occlusion and a further stent treating the left EIA stenosis (in addition to bilateral CIA stents from a previous treatment).

The decision was taken to primary stent the bilateral EIA lesions, and 3000IU heparin was administered intra-arterially. The right EIA occlusion was addressed first via a retrograde CFA puncture. The intention was to cross the lesion intraluminally, but this was not achieved. A dissection plane was initiated, but again this could not be extended through the entire occlusion. Therefore a hydrophilic guidewire, aided by a hydrophilic catheter, was passed subintimally from the contralateral side so that both proximal and distal dissections were in continuity (Figure 6.3). This required the support of an 'over-the-top' long sheath (6Fr Flexor Introducer sheath; Balkan Up and Over Contralateral Design, Cook Medical UK Ltd). This facilitated the placement of two balloon expandable nitinol stents from the ipsilateral side following advancement of an Amplatz extra-stiff wire (Cook Medical) through the dissection path from that side. The left EIA stenosis was stented from the ipsilateral side, and finally all stents were remodelled with appropriate sized balloons (Figure 6.4).

**Evidence base** Recanalization of iliac artery occlusions by subintimal dissection using the ipsilateral and the contralateral approach [4]

- Iliac occlusions tend to be challenging because the retrograde guidewire makes a dissection readily, but re-entry is prohibited by the greater thickness of the intima as the aorta is approached.
- This causes a tendency for the dissection to extend into the aorta without making a successful re-entry.
- Initiating a dissection from a contralateral cross-over is not as problematic, as any force directed at the vessel wall causes the wire to take the path of least resistance, which is subintimal.
- The procedure should be abandoned if the antegrade dissection extends too near to the CFA bifurcation. Extending beyond this could compromise the profunda femoris or the SFA.

**Evidence base** Dutch Iliac Stent Trial [5,6]

- A randomized controlled trial (RCT) of primary stent placement versus percutaneous transluminal angioplasty (PTA) with selective stent placement in 279 patients.
- Only published RCT addressing this issue.
- Data collected at intervals extending to 8 years following initial treatment.
- No significant difference with regard to:
  - haemodynamic success (increase in ankle-brachial pressure index (ABI) of 0.10)
  - symptomatic success (increase of at least one Fontaine grade)
  - re-intervention rate and iliac patency.
- Major improvement of symptoms in the selective stent group.
- Conclusion: PTA and selective stent placement is at least as good as treatment with primary stent placement in the long term for iliac disease. Therefore, selective stenting should be the preferred treatment.

Completion angiography of the run-off vessels was performed as per routine practice. This identified distal embolization into the proximal run-off on the right (Figure 6.5). Given the relatively small clot burden the decision was taken not to proceed with catheter aspiration or thrombolysis. The patient was reviewed the following morning and was suffering no sequalae. She was reviewed at a vascular surgery outpatient clinic four weeks after the procedure and confirmed that her rest pain had improved.

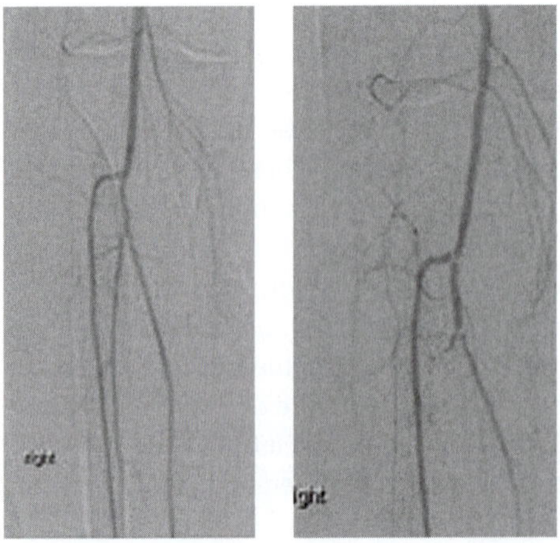

**Figure 6.5** DSA of the right leg run-off before (left-hand image) and after (right-hand image) the procedure. Emboli can be seen at the anterior tibial artery origin and the distal tibioperoneal trunk. The peroneal artery has become occluded shortly after its origin.

## Discussion

Most cases referred for endovascular treatment have diagnostic imaging confirming disease that is clearly attributable to their presentation. However, as in this case, the operator can be faced with partly non-diagnostic images, requiring an initial comprehensive catheter angiogram before forming a treatment strategy. Following the initial aorto-iliac angiogram showing a modest left-sided iliac stenosis, infra-inguinal disease was suspected to account for the rest pain. The integrity of the infra-inguinal run-off is probably the most important independent predictor of stent durability in the iliac arteries [7,8]. Continuing advancements in endovascular technology over recent years have initiated many studies measuring the short- and long-term patency rates of iliac stents as a means of justifying this treatment over established open techniques for more complex TASC C and D lesions. The initial TASC statement in 2000 provided a framework for deciding treatment options based on lesion length and morphology. Major changes in lesion classification came with the release of TASC II in 2007 as more lesions became treatable by endovascular means. TASC II states that for type C lesions 'open revascularization produces superior long-term results' and 'endovascular methods should only be used when there is high risk associated with open repair'.

However, data from studies addressing endovascular patency in type C and D lesions have shown that the TASC II statements no longer reflect modern practice [9,10]. Indeed, our case was not a high-risk surgical candidate and could equally have been offered open repair. The traditional surgical methods of managing iliac occlusive disease are thrombo-endarterectomy and, in particular, aorto-bifemoral (ABF) bypass graft (or iliofemoral graft depending on the extent of disease).

**Evidence base** Surgery versus endovascular treatment

Various review articles and meta-analyses have addressed the longevity of surgical bypass grafts versus endovascular treatment. The five-year primary patency rate for endovascular treatment of TASC C and D lesions, i.e. occlusive disease, has been consistently reported at around 65% [9,11,12]. This is significantly inferior to the 80–85% five-year patency reported for ABF grafts [13,14]. However, endovascular treatment is considered an easily repeatable procedure for restenosis, with long-term secondary patency rates reported to equal those of ABF grafts [9,11,13]. A meta-analysis found that re- intervention for TASC C and D lesions is not uncommon, at around 20% [9].

These figures reflect advances in stent technology as well as operator technique, resulting in a general trend away from open repair of iliac occlusive disease. With growing experience, technical success greater than 90% is achievable. Interesting, and rather surprisingly, the length of occlusion, TASC morphological classification, and whether there is combined occlusion of the CIA and EIA have all been shown to be unrelated to technical success [9,11,12]. The meta-analysis by Ye et al. [9] found similar technical success for TASC C compared with more complex TASC D lesions (93.7% versus 90.1%).

Morbidity and mortality also have to be considered when comparing surgical and endovascular treatments. Surgery is more invasive and has significantly higher complication rates [3]. The post- operative mortality for ABF grafts is around 4%, with major morbidity seen in 15–20% [11,14]. Procedure-related mortality for endovascular intervention is less than 1% [15], and major complications are around 5% [16]. We acknowledge that potential differences in patient selection, and differences in potential morbidity outcomes, make a direct comparison of these outcomes difficult. In high-risk patients, extra-anatomical bypass (axillofemoral and femorofemoral) avoids the need for an open abdominal procedure. However, these procedures have inferior long-term patency compared with endovascular treatment [13].

Primary and secondary patency rates are the most commonly adopted marker of outcome in peripheral endovascular intervention. This method has come under some criticism because it is not patient centred, with no reflection on the symptomatic success of procedures [17]. The Dutch Iliac Stent trial—the largest RCT of its kind—did measure quality of life (along with standard patency outcomes) in patients randomized to either primary or selective stent placement [5,6]. Whilst the results did not show a significant difference in long-term patency or re-intervention rates, the patients treated with angioplasty and selective stenting had a clinically better outcome. It also found considerable cost savings, as only 40% of the patients actually needed stenting, and thus concluded that selective stent placement should be the treatment of choice for iliac lesions. However, this study of 279 patients had strict criteria as it included only stenoses that were less than 10cm and occlusions that were less than 5cm, essentially excluding most TASC C and D lesions. A large meta-analysis involving almost 1000 patients with either TASC C or D lesions concluded that primary stenting gave superior long-term patency rates [9]. Interestingly, in the small group of iliac occlusions in the Dutch trial, 10 of 12 patients initially treated with angioplasty alone eventually required stent placement. In our practice, we preferentially adopt primary stenting after recanalization of occluded iliac segments. Benefits of primary stenting have been demonstrated. Contrary to the other findings in the Dutch trial, the complication rate in the angioplasty with provisional stenting was higher than in the primary stenting group (7% versus 4%) because of the complications of the initial angioplasty. In addition, primary stenting has been found to have a higher technical success rate [9].

Furthermore, the technical success of recanalization of an iliac occlusion seems to be higher with an antegrade approach (i.e. over the aorta from a contralateral puncture) than with a retrograde approach [11]. This study also found the major complication rate to be higher with the retrograde approach. As described by Bolia and Fishwick [4], a guidewire easily makes a dissection from the ipsilateral side, but re-entry is difficult closer to the aorta because the intima becomes thicker. Therefore this can lead to subintimal stent placement, which has a high stent thrombosis rate. This obviously applies more in CIA occlusions, but there should also be a low threshold to making a contralateral puncture for the EIA, as in our case presentation.

Our decision to primary stent the left EIA stenosis is certainly more contentious, with no clear supporting evidence. A strategy of provisional angioplasty followed by pressure gradient measurement across the lesion (with a gradient of >10mmHg requiring a stent) is often awkward and time consuming, but is probably underutilized in our, and many other, practices and would potentially avoid unnecessary stenting in stenotic disease. Endovascular treatment of EIA lesions has long been questioned [18]; in particular, long-segment EIA disease predicts a higher likelihood of restenosis [19]. Whereas the CIA is a straight and immobile vessel, the EIA is much more tortuous and stretches during hip extension, and is therefore better served with self-expandable stents [20]. In the case presented here, the combined stented segment on the right extended uninterrupted from the CIA origin to the CFA origin. In support of our decision, a large study found similar patient outcomes (in terms of morbidity and need for re-intervention) for isolated CIA and EIA stents compared with those with combined ipsilateral CIA and EIA stents [21].

As the preceding discussion suggests, bypass surgery has essentially become limited to certain TASC D sub-categories, including flush aortic occlusion, associated aorto-iliac aneurysmal disease, and severe contiguous involvement of the CFA. Synchronous disease involving the CFA is not uncommon in iliac occlusive disease, with about 65% presenting with disease above and below the inguinal ligament [22].

**Learning point** Alternative techniques

Hybrid repair combining endovascular iliac stenting with common femoral endarterectomy/profundoplasty is gaining popularity as an alternative to open reconstruction, with comparable outcomes over all TASC classifications [8], but this approach is largely restricted to instances where there is sparing of the distal EIA to allow a disease-free landing zone of the iliac stent. However, an approach that combines inline stenting across the inguinal ligament into a contiguous diseased CFA with no increased incidence of stent fracture or in-stent thrombosis has been described [22]. Animal studies have shown a lower risk of fracture with covered Wallstents compared with bare metal stents (BMSs) deployed across the hip joint. Whilst this has failed to gain acceptance in humans, the use of covered stents rather than BMSs in complex iliac occlusions is advocated by some in view of the potentially disastrous outcome of vessel rupture at this site. There has only been one published RCT comparing covered stents with BMSs in aorto-iliac occlusive disease, involving 125 patients followed for 18 months. This found similar results for TASC B lesions, but better outcomes with covered stents for TASC C and D lesions [23].

**Expert comment**

Imaging of lower limb vascular disease has been revolutionized by non-invasive imaging. The vast majority of patients will get an accurate assessment of their disease and treatment options with good quality MRA. In particular, patients with likely distal vessel disease and calcification are better assessed with MRA than with CT. However, there are potential limitations including signal drop-out from stents and other metallic structures such as clips, hip prostheses, etc. It is essential that the operator has a thorough knowledge of potential artefacts and reviews the source axial images as well as MIP angiographic images. In reality, there is little that can be done from a technical perspective to reduce metallic artefacts from the metal alloys currently used in stents, and an alternative form of imaging may be required. It is certainly possible to significantly improve the quality of run-off imaging and reduce venous contamination with the use of blood pool agents and a technique of steady state-extended phase imaging [24].

Critical limb ischaemia is most frequently secondary to multilevel disease. Treatment of inflow disease may be enough to alleviate symptoms or heal ulceration, or may permit further infrainguinal intervention. Endovascular intervention offers patients durable results in the iliac segment with a primary technical success rate of 81–97% and primary patency rates up to 60–80% even in patients with critical limb ischaemia. Although this patient had a TASC II C lesion, an attempt at endovascular therapy was considered appropriate by the clinical team and was acceptable to the patient because of the reduced morbidity associated with an endovascular procedure.

The treatment of iliac occlusions can be challenging and there is a well-founded perception that external iliac lesions are more prone to complications, including rupture. The use of a cross-over sheath can be invaluable in stabilizing position and permitting intermittent angiographic runs to guide further intervention. Antegrade recanalization from the common iliac avoids the potential difficulties of entering above the common iliac and if subintimal is often easier to re-enter the lumen distally. While the recorded complication rate from subintimal iliac angioplasty is acceptable, availability of appropriately sized stent-grafts is essential prior to any iliac intervention. Stable access and immediately available stent grafts should readily treat complications such as rupture. Modern balloon-deployable stent designs permit conformity to vessel wall and tracking over the bifurcation. However, self-expanding stents are often used in this location.

## A final word from the expert

This case was also complicated by an embolus to the run-off vessels of the right calf. Run-off views of the distal circulation are essential after intervention. Distal embolization is a well-recognized complication with an incidence of 1.6% recorded within the CIRSE Quality Improvement Guidance for Iliac Occlusive Disease [25]. The recommended treatment for small thrombi is clot aspiration, and every department undertaking endovascular treatment should have detachable hub sheaths and aspiration catheters available as this simple technique can rapidly rescue run-off. This particular case illustrates the need to balance the angiographic and clinical findings. The patient had preserved single-vessel run-off and a clearly viable foot, and therefore immediate clot aspiration was not undertaken. These decisions can be difficult and should be taken by the multidisciplinary team with arrangements made for close observation in an environment with experience of vascular disease and monitoring and with direct vascular surgical and interventional radiology review. Anticoagulation with heparin is valuable as it prevents further clot propagation and may allow natural lysis of small thrombi.

## References


1. Prince MR, Chabra SG, Watts R, et al. Contrast material travel times in patients undergoing peripheral MR angiography. *Radiology* 2002; 224: 55–61.
2. Dormandy JA, Rutherford RB. Management of peripheral arterial disease (PAD). TransAtlantic Inter-Society Consensus (TASC). *J Vasc Surg* 2000; 31: S1–S296.
3. Norgren L, Hiatt WR, Dormandy JA et al. Inter-Society Consensus for the Management of Peripheral Arterial Disease (TASC II). *J Vasc Surg* 2007; 45: S5–67.
4. Bolia A, Fishwick G. Recanalization of iliac artery occlusion by subintimal dissection using the ipsilateral and the contralateral approach. *Clin Radiol* 1997; 52: 684–7.
5. Tetteroo W, van der Graaf Y, Bosch JL, et al. Randomised comparison of primary stent placement versus primary angioplasty followed by selective stent placement in patients with iliac artery occlusive disease. *Lancet* 1998; 351: 1153–9.
6. Klein WM, van der Graaf Y, Seegers J, et al. Dutch Iliac Stent Trial: long term results in patients randomized for primary or selective stent placement. *Radiology* 2006; 238(2): 734–44.
7. Timaran CH, Prault TL, Stevens SL, et al. Iliac artery stenting versus surgical reconstruction for TASC (TransAtlantic Inter-Society Consensus) type B and C iliac lesions. *J Vasc Surg* 2003; 38(2): 272–8.
8. Piazza M, Ricotta JJ, Bower TC, et al. Iliac artery stenting combined with open femoral endarterectomy is as effective as open surgical reconstruction for severe iliac and common femoral occlusive disease. *J Vasc Surg* 2011; 54(2): 402–11.
9. Ye W, Liu CW, Ricco JB, et al. Early and late outcomes of percutaneous treatment of TransAtlantic Inter-Society Consensus class C and D aorto-iliac lesions. *J Vasc Surg* 2011; 53(6): 1728–37.
10. Leville CD, Kashyap VS, Clair DG, et al. Endovascular management of iliac artery occlusions: extending treatment to TransAtlantic Inter-Society Consensus class C and D patients. *J Vasc Surg* 2006; 43(1): 32–9.
11. Ozkan U, Oguzkurt L, Tercan F. Technique, complications, and long-term outcome for endovascular treatment of iliac artery occlusion. *Cardiovasc Intervent Radiol* 2010; 33: 18–24.

12. Gandini R, Fabiano S, Chiocchi M, et al. Percutaneous treatment in iliac artery occlusion: long-term results. *Cardiovasc Intervent Radiol* 2008; 31: 1069–76.
13. Ruggiero NJ, Michael RJ. The current management of aortic, common iliac, and external iliac artery disease: basic data underlying clinical decision-making. *Ann Vasc Surg* 2011; 25: 990–1003.
14. De Vries S and Hunink M. Results of aortic bifurcation grafts for aortoiliac occlusive disease: a meta-analysis. *J Vasc Surg* 1997; 26: 558–69.
15. Belli AM, Cumberland DC, Knox AM, et al. The complication rate of percutaneous peripheral balloon angioplasty. *Clin Radiol* 1990; 41: 380–3.
16. Ratnam L, Raza SA, Horton A, et al. Outcome of aortoiliac, femoropopliteal and infrapopliteal endovascular interventions in lesions categorized by TASC classification. *Clin Radiol* 2012; 67: 949–54.
17. Conte MS, Bandyk DF, Clowes AW et al. Results of PREVENT III: a multicenter, randomized trial of edifoliglide for the prevention of vein graft failure in lower extremity by-pass surgery. *J Vasc Surg* 2006; 43: 742–51.
18. Timaran CH, Stevens SL, Freeman MB. External iliac and common iliac artery angioplasty and stenting in men and women. *J Vasc Surg* 2001; 34: 440–6.
19. Powell RJ, Fillinger M, Walsh DB, et al. Predicting outcome of angioplasty and selective stenting of multisegment iliac artery occlusive disease. *J Vasc Surg* 2000; 32(3): 564–9.
20. Dyet JF, Watts WG, Ettles DF, et al. Mechanical properties of metallic stents: how do these properties influence the choice of stent for specific lesions? *Cardiovasc Intervent Radiol* 2000; 23(1): 47–54.
21. Danczyk RC, Mitchell EL, Burk C, et al. Comparing patient outcomes between multiple ipsilateral ilica artery stents and isolated iliac artery stents. *J Vasc Surg* 2012; 55(6): 1637–46.
22. Sharafuddin MJ, Kresowik TF, Hoballah JJ, et al. Combined direct repair and inline inflow stenting in the management of aortoiliac disease extending into the common femoral artery. *Vasc Endovasc Surg* 2011; 45(3): 274–82.
23. Mwipatayi BP, Thomas S, Wong J, et al. A comparison of covered vs bare expandable stents for the treatment of aortoiliac occlusive disease. *J Vasc Surg* 2011; 54(6): 1561–70.
24. Christie A, Chandramohan S, Roditi G. Comprehensive MRA of the lower limbs including high-resolution extended-phase infra-inguinal imaging with gadobenate dimeglumine: initial experience with inter-individual comparison to the blood-pool contrast agent gadofosveset trisodium. *Clin Radiol* 2013; 68(2): 125–30.
25. CISRE Standards of Practice; Quality Improvement Guidelines for Endovascular Treatment of Iliac Artery Occlusive Disease <http://www.cirse.org/files/File/SOP/>

CASE

# 7 SFA endoluminal bypass: the new era of critical limb ischaemia treatment

Aidan Shaw

Expert commentary Irfan Ahmed

## Case history

A 62-year-old man presented to A&E with a two-week history of rest pain in his right leg. He described the pain as constant, but improved by hanging his leg out of the bed at night. Two years previously he had undergone a redo right femoral to tibioperoneal bypass with a PTFE graft following a failed vein graft.

There was a history of hypertension and hypercholesterolaemia; he was still smoking (20 per day) and drank under 10 units of alcohol a week. There was a family history of coronary artery disease, with his father passing away from a myocardial infarction.

On examination, the patient was comfortable at rest and haemodynamically stable. The right leg was paler and cooler than the left, and there was a palpable right femoral artery pulse but no palpable popliteal, posterior tibial, or dorsalis pedis pulses. The ankle–brachial pressure index was 0.6. Mixed aetiology ulcers, located over the heel and medial malleolus, were present. The patient was grade III according to the Rutherford classification and stage IV according to the Fontaine classification (Table 7.1).

**Clinical tip** Interpreting ankle-brachial pressure index (ABPI or ABI) results

The ABI is a non-invasive method of identifying arterial insufficiency within a limb. It is obtained by placing a blood pressure cuff around the calf and measuring the peak systolic pressure at the dorsalis pedis (DP) and posterior tibial (PT) arteries with a hand-held doppler machine. The peak systolic pressure of the brachial arteries is then measured in both arms:

$$\text{ABPI} = \frac{\text{highest ankle systolic pressure (DP or PT)}}{\text{highest brachial systolic pressure (either arm)}}$$

- >1.2: abnormal due to heavy vessel calcification
- 0.9–1.2: normal
- 0.75–0.9: moderate disease
- 0.5–0.75: severe disease

**Clinical tip** Arterial and venous ulcers

Arterial ulcers are usually located on the tips of or between the toes and in extremities where the skin is often cold, shiny, and without hair. They are normally round with smooth punched out edges and no discernible odour. Venous ulcers can occur anywhere between the knee and the ankle, with the medial malleolus being the most common site. They are usually superficial, have irregular sloping borders and are associated with oedema and hyperpigmentation.

**Learning point** Rutherford and Fontaine Classifications

The Rutherford and Fontaine [1,2] classifications (Table 7.1) are the two clinical classifications of peripheral arterial disease (PAD), with the former more commonly cited in newer publications.

**Table 7.1 Rutherford and Fontaine classifications**

| Fontaine | | Rutherford | | |
|---|---|---|---|---|
| Stage | Clinical | Grade | Category | Clinical |
| I | Asymptomatic | 0 | 0 | Asymptomatic |
| IIa | Mild claudication (>200m) | I | 1 | Mild claudication |
| IIb | Moderate to severe claudication (<200m) | I | 2 | Moderate claudication |
| III | Ischaemic rest pain | II | 3 | Severe claudication |
| IV | Ulceration or gangrene | II | 4 | Ischaemic rest pain |
| | | III | 5 | Minor tissue loss |
| | | III | 6 | Major tissue loss |

A computed tomography (CT) angiogram was performed and demonstrated complete occlusion of the native right superficial femoral artery extending into the distal popliteal artery, as well as occlusion of the PTFE bypass graft. This was classified as a TASC D lesion Figure 7.2.

**Learning point** The Inter-Society Consensus (TASC) II guidelines

The Inter-Society Consensus (TASC) II guidelines [3] were developed to provide an international consensus on the diagnosis and treatment of PAD (Table 7.2). To keep abreast of the changing clinical landscape, the TASC II documentation is constantly evolving to encompass the latest clinical and technical updates in PAD. Therefore the guidelines provide healthcare workers with the only international consensus that gives dynamic information on the diagnosis and treatment of PAD.

**Table 7.2 The Inter-Society Consensus (TASC) II guidelines**

| Lesion type | Description |
|---|---|
| A | • Single stenosis <10cm<br>• Single occlusion <5cm |
| B | • Multiple lesions (stenoses or occlusions), each <5cm<br>• Single stenosis or occlusion <15cm not involving the infrageniculate popliteal artery<br>• Single or multiple lesions in the absence of continuous tibial vessels to improve inflow for a distal bypass<br>• Heavily calcified occlusion >5cm<br>• Single stenosis of the popliteal artery |
| C | • Multiple stenoses or occlusions totalling >15cm, with or without heavy calcification<br>• Recurrent stenoses or occlusions that need treatment after two endovascular interventions |
| D | • Chronic total occlusions of the common femoral artery or superficial femoral artery (>20cm, including the popliteal artery)<br>• Chronic total occlusion of the popliteal artery and the proximal trifurcation vessels |

Source data from Norgren L, Hiatt W, Dormandy J, et al. Inter-Society Consensus for the Management of Peripheral Arterial Disease (TASC II). Eur J Vasc Endovasc Surgery 2007; 33 (Suppl 1): S1-S75.

**Expert comment**

According to TASC II guidelines, the first-line treatment for this patient would be bypass surgery. However, in view of the two failed surgical bypasses and absence of veins for harvesting, endovascular treatment would appear appropriate.

After multidisciplinary discussion, it was decided to proceed with an endovascular approach. After obtaining informed consent, an antegrade puncture of the right common femoral artery was obtained using local anaesthetic and ultrasound guidance and a 4Fr sheath was sited. An angiogram confirmed the CT findings of total occlusion of the right superficial femoral artery (SFA) extending into the distal popliteal artery (Figures 7.1 and 7.2). The lesion was crossed with a hydrophilic wire via a subintimal approach and the lumen re-entered at the distal popliteal artery (P 3) distal to the lesion with a re-entry catheter (Cordis Outback®) and confirmed

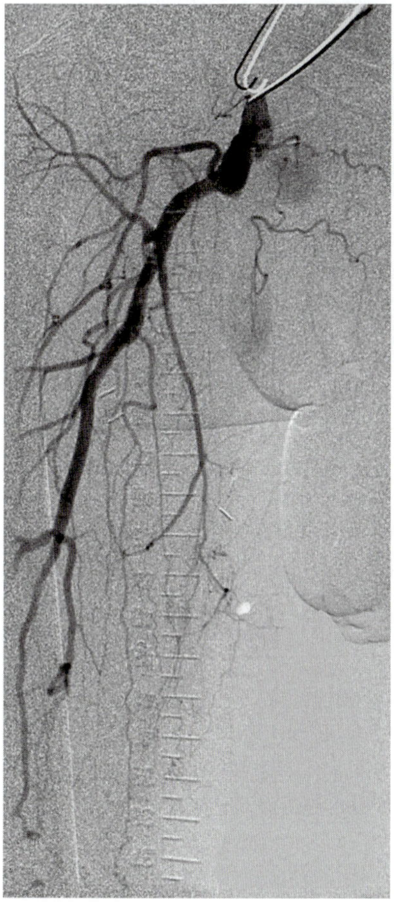

**Figure 7.1** Digital subtraction angiogram (DSA) demonstrating a flush occlusion of the right superficial femoral artery (SFA).

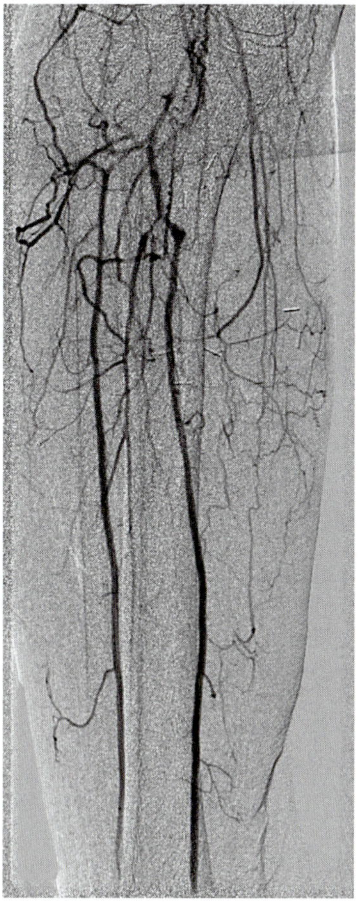

**Figure 7.2** DSA demonstrating the occlusion to extend into the popliteal artery with flow re-forming in the distal popliteal artery (P3 segment).

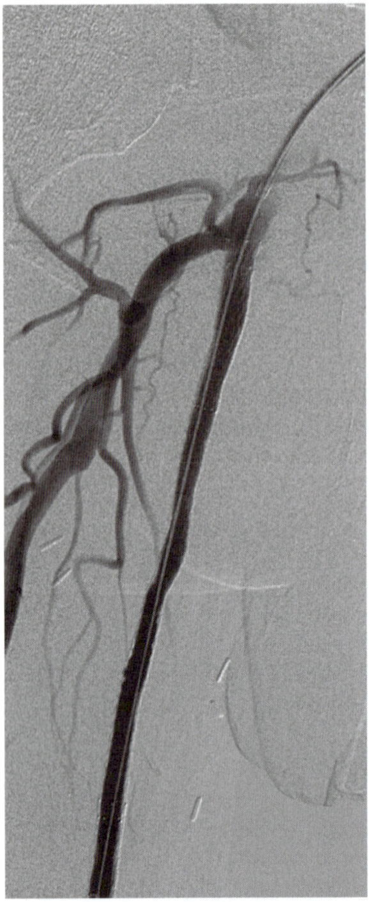

Figure 7.3 DSA demonstrating in-line flow down the SFA following stent placement.

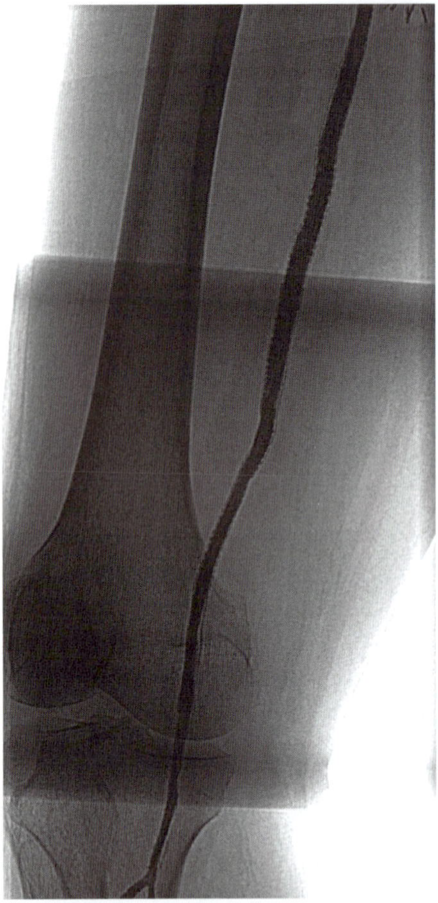

Figure 7.4 DSA demonstrating in-line flow down the SFA through to the popliteal artery and tibioperoneal trunk following stent placement.

**Clinical tip** Re-entry devices

Re-entering the lumen can be problematic in the presence of heavy calcification, and devices such as the Cordis Corporation Outback® or the Medtronic Pioneer® re-entry catheters, which utilize an angled needle to puncture back into the true lumen, have been developed. Both have been shown to be safe and effective in managing peripheral chronic occlusions with a symptom-free interval of 12 months and no procedural or post-procedural complications [4].

**Expert comment**

Stenting into the popliteal artery can be problematic because of the repeated external compression of the stent when placed at flexion points of the vessel, leading to stent fracture. The IDEV Supera® interwoven nitinol stent has recently shown promising results in the popliteal segment with no stent fractures at one year in the SUPERB trial or at two years in a recent study [5] with significant improvements in symptom classification.

**Clinical tip** Antiplatelet therapy

A recent study has shown that dual antiplatelet therapy was associated with reduced peri-interventional platelet activation and a reduced need for target lesion revascularization [6].

with contrast injection. The existing sheath was exchanged for a 6Fr sheath and multiple 7mm self-expanding nitinol stents (Covidien EverFlex®) were placed with a satisfactory angiographic result with no complications (Figures 7.3 and 7.4). Manual compression to the puncture site followed.

A 300mg loading dose of clopidogrel was administered in recovery and dual antiplatelet therapy with aspirin 75mg od and clopidogrel 75mg od prescribed after the procedure. Follow-up at three months demonstrated improved symptoms and ulcer healing, with a duplex examination showing stent patency with no in-stent restenosis.

## Discussion

The prognosis for patients presenting with critical limb ischaemia (CLI) is poor not only for the limb but also for life. A year after diagnosis 25% of patients will have died and 30% will have required a major amputation [7,8]. Vascular death had occurred in about 25% of patients five years after bypass surgery and in nearly 50% of patients after ten years, with the primary cause of death being vascular death [9].

The optimal treatment for patients presenting with CLI is revascularization, as it is associated with a much greater perioperative mortality and morbidity than amputation [10]. Extent of disease, morphology of the lesion(s), and distal run-off combined with patient comorbidities determine the method and success of revascularization. TASC guidelines [3] currently recommend that patients presenting with simple occlusive lesions (TASC A) are treated with endovascular therapy and those presenting with advanced occlusive lesions (TASC D) are treated with surgical bypass as a first-line treatment. Endovascular procedures are only recommended for patients who have a low healing potential following surgical revascularization with TASC C lesions, and treatment recommendations for type B and type C lesions are based on the patient's comorbidities, fully informed patient preference, and the local operator's long-term success rates [3].

Endovascular therapy has shorter recovery times and lower morbidity and mortality rates than surgery. Techniques and technology continue to improve and expand, making the treatment and outcomes for advanced disease more achievable by endovascular therapy. There are now many different percutaneous treatment options and methods available for recanalization of long-segment SFA occlusions including re-entry catheters, PTA with or without drug-eluting balloons, or self-expanding PTFE and drug-eluting stents. Re-entry catheters also allow accurate re-entry into the lumen following a subintimal approach with reduced risk of damaging healthy native vessel. Recent developments in stent technology for complex femoropopliteal lesions have been promising, with stenting shown to be superior to balloon angioplasty for long lesions. The latest generation of stents, including stent grafts, are of increased length (up to 20cm), have superior fracture resistance, allow complex long lesions to be treated endovascularly, and have comparable outcomes to artificial femoropopliteal bypass surgery. With the ever-increasing evolution of drug-eluting technology to further reduce in-stent restenosis rates and increase stent patency, it may be just a matter of time until TASC C and D lesions are primarily treated with endovascular techniques.

**Evidence base** Angioplasty for the SFA

- Technical and clinical success >95% [11].
- One-year patency 77% following angioplasty of the stenosis and 65% following recanalization [3].
- At three and five years, patency rates decrease to 40–50% [3]

Sub-intimal angioplasty (SIA):

- technical success reported to be between 74% and 92% [12,13]
- shown to be effective even with unfavourable anatomy with up to 83% of limb salvage [14]
- risk of vessel perforation is higher for SIA than for conventional PTA with an overall risk of 5–8%, particularly in heavily calcified vessels [15]

**Evidence base** DEB for the SFA

Drug-eluting balloons (DEBs) coated with paclitaxel are showing promising results, as demonstrated in the following trials.

- The Thunder trial (Paccocath-Cotavance technology) demonstrated that the use of paclitaxel-coated angioplasty balloons during the treatment of femoropopliteal arterial disease was associated with significant reductions in late lumen loss and target-lesion revascularization (TLR) (TLR at 24 months was 37% in standard balloon angioplasty versus 15% in the drug-coated balloon group) [16].
- The FemPac trial (Paccocath-Cotavance technology) demonstrated reduced restenosis in patients undergoing angioplasty of femoropopliteal arteries (TLR at 18–24 months was 50% in the standard balloon angioplasty versus 13% in the drug-coated balloon group) [17].
- Levant 1 trial (Lutonix Moxy™ paclitaxel-coated balloon): the six-month average late lumen loss, the trial's primary end point, was 0.46mm in patients in the paclitaxel-coated balloon group compared with 1.09mm for the conventional angioplasty control group ($p$=0.016). There was also a non-significant trend in favour of the druft5>g-coated balloon for target lesion revascularization (13% versus 22%).
- The Pacifier trial (Medtronic In.Pact Pacifier™ paclitaxel-coated balloon) demonstrated a lower rate of late lumen loss (0.01mm) associated with the use of the drug-eluting balloon compared with patients treated with an uncoated balloon (0.65mm). TLR at one year was 7.1% for the DEB versus 34.9% for the uncoated balloon.

**Evidence base** Surgery for the SFA

The large UK Bypass versus Angioplasty in Severe Ischaemia of the Leg trial compared bypass surgery with PTA/SIA for patients with femoropopliteal disease and severe limb ischaemia [25].

- The primary outcome, amputation-free survival after 6 months, did not differ between groups.
- There was no difference in all-cause mortality or quality of life at two years between the groups.
- Surgical therapy was more expensive than endovascular treatment.
- Re-intervention rates were significantly higher in the angioplasty group (28% versus 17%).

**Evidence base** Stents for the SFA

- Late restenosis secondary to intimal hyperplasia remains the Achilles heel of stenting.
- Four randomized trials (Absolute, Fast, Resilient, Scirocco II) for PTA versus stent have not shown a convincing advantage in favour of stents for short femoropopliteal stenoses (<10cm).
- New generation stents are designed to try and combat the problems of restenosis and stent fracture.
- 67% one-year restenosis with angioplasty compared with 37% for nitinol stent deployment [18.]
- New PTFE-lined stents have been designed to try and prevent in-stent restenosis through ingrowth
- Studies have demonstrated comparable patency rates over one, two, and 4 years between PTFE-lined stents (Gore Viabahn™) and surgical bypass with synthetic material (Dacron or PTFE) [19–21] with significantly reduced hospital stay for the covered stent group (0.9 versus 3.1 days) [19].

**Evidence base** DES for the SFA

- Sirolimus-coated stents
  - The SIROCCO trials [22,23] compared sirolimus-coated stents with bare metal stents. They failed to show a demonstrable efficacy of DESs compared with bare metal nitinol stents.
- Everolimus-coated stents
  - The STRIDES trial suggested improved patency of everolimus-coated stents versus bare metal stents at six months but this was not sustained at 12 months.
- Paclitaxel-coated stents
  - Recent trials evaluating paclitaxel-eluting stents for above knee lesions demonstrated promising anatomical and clinical results with 86% primary patency rate at 12 months [24]
  - Recently released but unpublished three-year data from the Zilver PTX (Cook Medical) randomized controlled trial of paclitaxel-eluting stents for femoropopliteal disease have shown 70.7% primary patency in the SFA at 36 months for patients treated with the Zilver PTX paclitaxel-eluting stent. This compares with 49.1% patency for patients with percutaneous transluminal angioplasty nd provisional bare metal stent placement in the study of 479 patients.

## A final word from the expert

This case study highlights the increasing practice of treating TASC C and D lesions with endovascular techniques. Unfortunately, traditionally many centres have poorly monitored theses patients post procedure. Medium to long term patency of an 'endoluminal bypass' can be improved if a more robust regime of follow up is pursued with regular duplex imaging and secondary interventions performed where required in the manner that most vascular surgeons follow up and maintain patency of bypass grafts. If such an approach is more widely adopted it is only a matter of time before endovascular therapy is considered the primary treatment of choice.

## References

1. Rutherford RB, Baker JD, Ernst C, et al. Recommended standards for reports dealing with lower extremity ischemia: revised version. *J Vasc Surg* 1997; 26(3): 517–38. Erratum. *J Vasc Surg* 2001; 33(4): 805.

2. Fontaine R, Kim M, Kieny R. [Surgical treatment of peripheral circulation disorders.] *Helv Chir Acta* 1954; 21(5-6): 499–533 (in German).
3. Norgren L, Hiatt W, Dormandy J, et al. Inter-Society Consensus for the Management of Peripheral Arterial Disease (TASC II). *Eur J Vasc Endovasc Surgery* 2007; 33(Suppl 1): S1–S75.
4. Smith M, Pappy R, Hennebry T. Re-entry devices in the treatment of peripheral chronic occlusions. *Tex Heart Inst J* 2011; 38(4): 392–7.
5. Scheinert D, Grummt L, Piorkowski M, et al. A novel self-expanding interwoven nitinol stent for complex femoropopliteal lesions: 24-month results of the SUPERA SFA registry. *J Endovasc Ther* 2011; 18(6): 745–52.
6. Tepe G, Bantleon R, Brechtel K, et al. Management of peripheral arterial interventions with mono or dual antiplatelet therapy—the MIRROR study: a randomized and double-blinded clinical trial. *Eur Radiol* 2012; 22(9):1998–2006.
7. Norgren L, Hiatt WR, Dormandy JA, et al., Inter-Society Consensus for the Management of Peripheral Arterial Disease (TASC II). Available at: <www.tasc-2-pad.org> (accessed October 2007).
8. Gottsater A. Managing risk factors for atherosclerosis in critical limb ischaemia. *Eur J Vasc Endovasc Surg* 2006; 32(5): 478–83.
9. Van Hattum ES, Tangelder MJ, Lawson JA, et al. Long-term risk of vascular events after peripheral bypass surgery. A cohort study. *Thromb Haemost* 2012; 108(3): 543–53.
10. Santilli JD, Santilli SM. Chronic critical limb ischemia: diagnosis, treatment and prognosis. *Am Fam Physician* 1999; 59(7): 1899–1908.
11. Muradin GS, Bosch JL, StijnenT, Hununk MG. Balloon dilation and stent implantation for treatment of femoropopliteal arterial disease: meta-analysis. *Radiology* 2001; 221:137–45.
12. Yilmaz S, Sindel T, Yegin A, et al. Subintimal angioplasty of long superficial femoral artery occlusions. *J Vasc Interv Radiol* 2003; 14: 997–1010.
13. Flørenes T, Bay D, Sandbaek G, et al. Subintimal angioplasty in the treatment of patients with intermittent claudication: long term results. *Eur J Vasc Endovasc Surg* 2004; 28: 645–50.
14. Kim JS, Kang TS, Ahn CM, et al. Efficacy of subintimal angioplasty/stent implantation for long, multisegmental lower limb occlusive lesions in patients unsuitable for surgery. *J Endovasc Ther* 2006; 13: 514–21.
15. Hayes PD, Chokkalingam A, Jones R, et al. Arterial perforation during infrainguinal lower limb angioplasty does not worsen outcome: results from 1409 patients. *J Endovasc Ther* 2002; 9: 422–7.
16. Tepe G, Zeller T, Albrecht T, et al. Local delivery of paclitaxel to inhibit restenosis during angioplasty of the leg. *N Engl J Med* 2008; 358(7): 689–99.
17. Werk M, Langner S, Reinkensmeier B, et al. Inhibition of restenosis in femoropopliteal arteries: paclitaxel-coated versus uncoated balloon: femoral paclitaxel randomized pilot trial. *Circulation* 2008 23; 118(13): 1358–65.
18. Schillinger M, Sabeti S, Loewe C, et al. Balloon angioplasty versus implantation of nitinol stents in the superficial femoral artery. *N Engl J Med* 2006; 354: 1879–88.
19. Kedora J, Hohmann S, Garrett W, et al. Randomized comparison of percutaneous Viabahn stent grafts vs prosthetic femoral-popliteal bypass in the treatment of superficial femoral arterial occlusive disease. *J Vasc Surg* 2007; 45: 10–16.
20. McQuade K, Gable D, Hohman S, et al. Randomized comparison of ePTFE/nitinol self-expanding stent graft vs prosthetic femoral-popliteal bypass in the treatment of superficial femoral artery occlusive disease. *J Vasc Surg* 2009; 49(1): 109–16.
21. McQuade K, Gable D, et al. Four-year randomized prospective comparison of percutaneous ePTFE/nitinol self-expanding stent graft versus prosthetic femoral-popliteal bypass in the treatment of superficial femoral artery occlusive disease. *J Vasc Surg* 2010; 52(3): 584–91.

22. Duda SH, Bosiers M, Lammer J, et al. Drug-eluting and bare nitinol stents for the treatment of atherosclerotic lesions in the superficial femoral artery: long-term results from the SIROCCO trial. *J Endovasc Ther* 2006; 13: 701–10.
23. Duda SH, Bosiers M, Lammer J, et al. Sirolimus-eluting versus bare nitinol stent for obstructive superficial femoral artery disease: the SIROCCO II trial. *J Vasc Interv Radiol* 2005; 16: 331–8.
24. Dake MD, Scheinert D, Tepe G, et al; Zilver PTX Single-Arm Study Investigators. Nitinol stents with polymer-free paclitaxel coating for lesions in the superficial femoral and popliteal arteries above the knee: twelve-month safety and effectiveness results from the Zilver PTX single-arm clinical study. *J Endovasc Ther* 2011; 18(5): 613–23.
25. Adam DJ, Beard JD, Cleveland T, et al. Bypass versus Angioplasty in Severe Ischaemia of the Leg (BASIL): multicentre randomised controlled trial. *Lancet* 2005; 366: 1925–34.

CASE

# 8 Below the knee angioplasty: bare versus drug-eluting stents

**Stavros Spiliopoulos**

**Expert commentary** Dimitrios Siablis

## Case history

A 74-year old patient suffering from critical limb ischaemia (CLI) of the left lower limb was scheduled to undergo angiographic evaluation of the peripheral arterial bed and subsequent percutaneous endovascular revascularization attempt in the interventional radiology department. The patient's baseline symptomatology was severe rest pain that was not responding to common analgesics, while physical examination revealed dry gangrene of the left toe and stage 5 CLI according to the Rutherford–Becket classification of peripheral arterial occlusive disease (PAOD). The ankle–brachial index (ABI) at presentation was 0.60.

**Learning point**

CLI is a manifestation of PAOD that describes patients with typical chronic ischaemic rest pain or with ischaemic skin lesions, either ulcers or gangrene (Fontaine III–IV and Rutherford–Becker 4–6 classifications). The diagnosis of CLI should be confirmed by the ABI and toe systolic pressure. Ischaemic rest pain most commonly occurs with an ABI ≤50mmHg or toe pressure ≤30mmHg. In the presence of ulcers or gangrene, CLI is suggested by an ABI <70mmHg or a toe systolic pressure <50mmHg. However, currently there is no consensus regarding the vascular haemodynamic parameters required to make the diagnosis of CLI. Moreover, ABI measurement can produce false-positive outcomes in diabetic patients because the reduced vessel wall elasticity results in increased ABI values. Finally, it should be noted that, by definition, the term CLI refers to patients with chronic ischaemia (presence of symptoms for more than two weeks) [1].

The patient suffered from multiple comorbidities including ischaemic coronary disease, chronic kidney failure under dialysis, and insulin-dependent diabetes mellitus and was judged unfit for surgery by the vascular surgery department. The decision to attempt a percutaneous endovascular approach was taken in a multidisciplinary meeting between interventional radiologists, vascular surgeons, and nephrologists. No history of allergies, coagulation disorder, or other contraindication to percutaneous endovascular treatment was present. Baseline demographics are reported in Table 8.1.

Pre-procedural Doppler examination revealed haemodynamically significant multilevel disease of the left superficial femoral artery (SFA) and below the knee (BTK) vessels, but no significant lesions were detected in the left iliac and common femoral arteries.

**Table 8.1** **Patient's baseline demographics and procedural details**

| | |
|---|---|
| Gender | Male |
| Age (years) | 74 |
| Baseline Rutherford–Becket classification of PAOD | 5 |
| Baseline ankle-brachial index (ABI) | 0.65 |
| Body mass index (BMI) | 22.5 (normal) |
| Comorbidities | Coronary disease<br>Insulin-dependent diabetes mellitus<br>Hypercholesterolaemia<br>Chronic renal failure (dialysis) |
| Medication | Insulin, β-blockers, statins, clopidogrel |
| Index lesion length | 90mm |
| Stented lesion | 94mm |
| Pre-procedural minimum vessel diameter | 1.0mm |
| Post-procedural minimum vessel diameter | 3.0mm |
| Remaining stenosis | 0% |

**Clinical tip**

Pre-procedural imaging prior to BTK interventions should provide accurate information about the inflow and the infrapopliteal arterial status and includes multidetector computed tomography angiography (MDCTA), contrast-enhanced magnetic resonance angiography (CEMRA), high-frequency duplex ultrasound (HFDU), and digital subtractive angiography (DSA) [1–3]. Choosing which imaging modality should be performed is case sensitive as each method presents specific advantages and disadvantages. Nonetheless, appropriate procedural planning necessitates detailed pre-procedural evaluation of the iliac arteries, the common femoral arteries, the SFA, the popliteal and infrapopliteal arteries, and the distal foot vasculature.

Pre-procedural laboratory examinations included baseline complete blood count, platelets, and clotting profile (INR, prothrombin time, partial thromboplastin time). The patient was already under antiplatelet therapy with clopidogrel 75mg 1 × 1 due to coronary disease.

Based on the pre-procedural imaging a decision was taken to perform a direct antegrade common femoral artery access as it allows easier catheter manoeuvres as well as better pushability and trackability of all the endovascular materials, especially when dealing with calcified distal occlusions. In our department local anaesthesia and arterial puncture is obtained under ultrasound guidance as it has been reported to produce a superior analgesic effect [5]. A 4Fr sheath was positioned in order to perform a selective diagnostic DSA, which revealed multiple significant stenosis (up to 80%) of the left SFA. The sheath was upgraded to 6Fr and the lesions were negotiated using a standard straight hydrophilic guidewire and a 4Fr vertebral catheter which was subsequently used to perform an angiographic evaluation of the BTK arteries. Selective DSA revealed occlusions from the origin of the anterior and posterior arteries, significant tortuous stenosis (50–60%) and one near-occlusion at the first segment of the peroneal artery, which was the only patent infrapopliteal vessel (Figure 8.1a). The arterial supply of the distal foot was maintained by the distal peroneal collateral network (Figure 8.1e). The peroneal artery demonstrated marked calcifications of the vessel wall, typical of

**Expert comment**

In patients who are not already under antiplatelet therapy, dual antiplatelet therapy with oral clopidogrel (75mg/day) and aspirin (100mg/day) is recommended at least three days prior to infrapopliteal intervention. In cases where this three-day antiplatelet regiment is not applied, a loading dose of clopidogrel 300mg (12 hours before the procedure) or clopidogrel 600mg (2 hours before the procedure) can be administered [4].

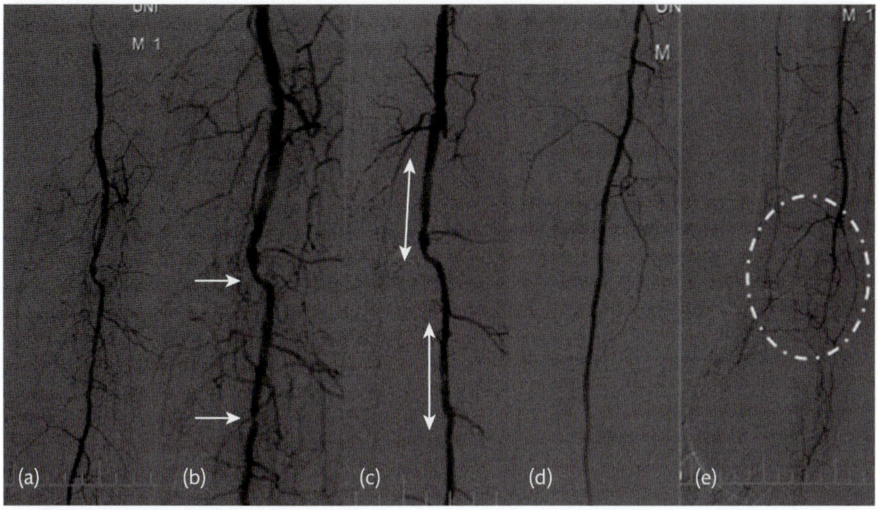


**Figure 8.1** (a) Baseline selective angiogram of the infrapopliteal arteries. Occlusion of the anterior and posterior tibial arteries is noted. The peroneal artery is the only patent vessel to the distal foot. (b) Magnified picture demonstrating a 50–60% stenosis (arrow) and a near-occlusion (distal arrow) at the proximal segment of the peroneal artery. (c) DSA at an angle of 45° with respect to the previous DSA, demonstrating areas of turbulent flow (double arrows) indicating marked atherosclerosis. (d) No other significant lesions were detected in the mid and distal segments of the peroneal artery; (e) the arterial supply of the distal foot was preserved by collaterals.

**Expert comment**

Decreased contrast media enhancement of a specific infrapopliteal arterial segment combined with decreased arterial flow should be considered as a radiological sign of flow-limiting atherosclerotic disease and treated appropriately.

patients who undergo dialysis, while the whole proximal peroneal segment gave the impression of diffuse atherosclerotic disease in various runs performed at different angles (Figures 8.1b, c).

A decision was taken to perform direct overlapping stenting of the entire proximal peroneal segment using balloon-expandable sirolimus-eluting stents (CYPHER Select©, Cordis, NJ, USA). A bolus dose of 5000IU of heparin was administered intra-arterially and balloon angioplasty of the SFA was successfully performed. The BTK lesions were crossed successively using a 0.014 inch guidewire (PT2® Guide Wire, Boston Scientific, MA, USA). The first stent (3 × 33mm) was deployed in the proximal segment (Figure 8.2a). A check angiogram after the deployment of the first stent demonstrated elastic recoil of the previously pre-dilated near-occlusion. The remaining segment was treated using two DESs (2.75 × 33mm and 2.75 × 28mm), again in an overlapping manner (Figure 8.2b). At the end of the procedure a straight arterial line of high antegrade flow down to the distal foot was achieved (Figure 8.2c).

Quantitative-vessel analysis using integrated semi-automated software (Allura Xper FD20, Philips, Amsterdam, The Netherlands) demonstrated 0% remaining stenosis at the end of the procedure, and the minimum diameter of the treated arterial vessel increased from 1.0mm to 3.0mm after stenting. Arterial haemostasis was obtained using an extra-luminal clip-based vascular closure device (StarClose®, Abbott Vascular Devices, CA, USA) and no immediate or short-term complications were noted. Dual antiplatelet therapy with aspirin 100mg 1 × 1 and clopidogrel 75mg 1 × 1 for six months followed by clopidogrel 75mg 1 × 1 for life was prescribed, and

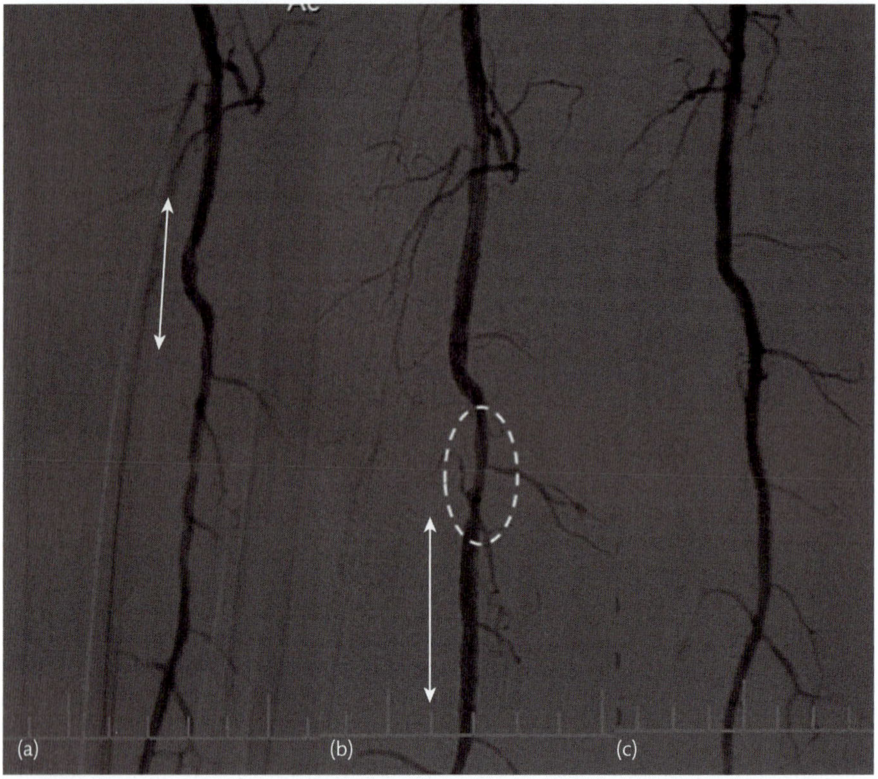


**Figure 8.2** Stenting procedure. (a) DSA image following the deployment of a 3 × 33mm DES in the proximal segment of the lesion (double arrow). (b) A second 2.75 × 33mm DES was deployed across the distal part of the lesion (double-headed arrow). The arterial segment between the two stents (circled area) was subsequently covered with a 2.75 × 28mm DES. The lesion was post-dilated with a 3.5 × 80mm balloon. (c) Final check angiogram demonstrating a straight arterial flow with no evidence of dissection or remaining stenosis along the treated area. Note the increased contrast enhancement compared with Figure 1c.

the patient was discharged after overnight hospitalization. Post-procedural surgical care was advised with clinical follow-up of regular visits at one and six weeks, six and twelve months, and annually thereafter. Imaging follow-up included Doppler ultrasound at three and six months, as well as annual DSA. After three months follow-up the ABI gradually reached 0.8 which permitted the vascular surgeon to safely perform surgical debridement to induce better wound healing. During the three- and six-month follow-up periods there were no signs of SFA or peroneal restenosis on Doppler ultrasound. The Rutherford–Becker classification at six and twelve months follow-up improved from 5 to 2 (moderate claudication). Complete wound healing was noted after twelve months follow-up (Figure 8.3). Follow-up angiography after two years revealed a patent peroneal artery with no evidence of in-stent restenosis (Figure 8.4). After three years clinical follow-up the patient is alive and has not suffered any major or minor amputation, and there are no signs of clinical relapse.

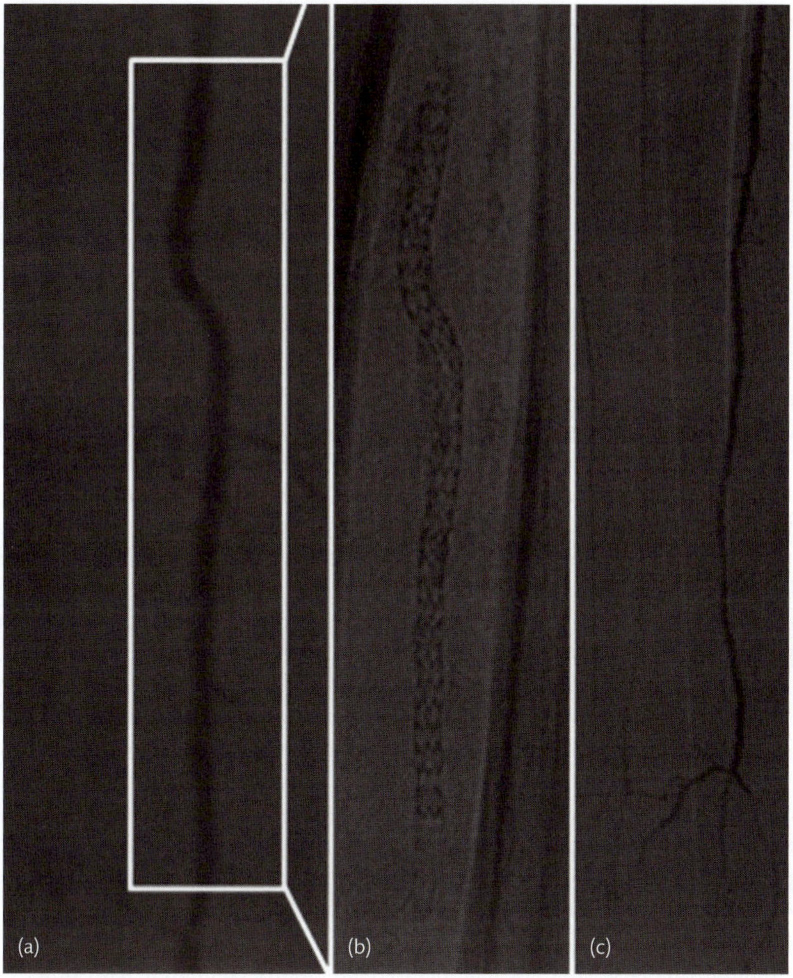


**Figure 8.3** Follow-up. (a) Magnified DSA image after two years follow-up shoeing a completely patent peroneal artery with no evidence of in-stent restenosis. (b) Magnified single-exposure picture demonstrating the stent's integrity. Note the heavily calcified arterial wall, typical of dialysis patients. (c) The peroneal artery is patent to the distal foot.

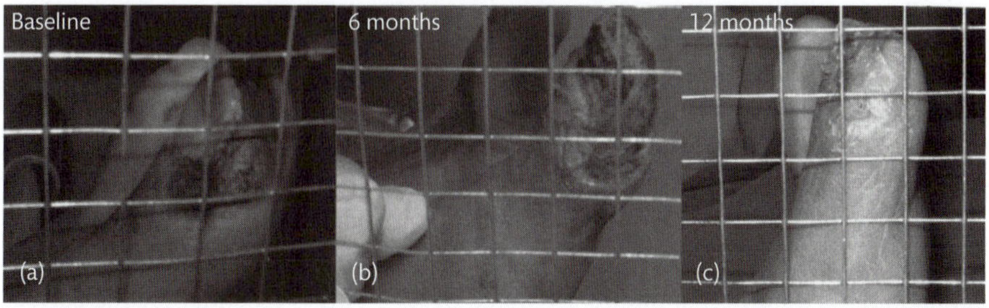


**Figure 8.4** Photographic documentation of wound status. (a) Pre-procedural gangrene. (b) Photo taken six months after the procedure, following surgical debridement. (c) Complete wound healing after follow-up for one year.

## Discussion

Infrapopliteal PAOD is a leading cause of CLI (Rutherford–Becker categories 4–6), a limb-threatening situation that may result in major amputation, especially if revascularization attempts fail [6]. Balloon angioplasty is considered as the main percutaneous method for the treatment of BTK disease, and has technical success rates between 80% and 100% and two-year limb salvage rates of up to 80% depending on the degree of infrapopliteal disease. Stenting is usually reserved as a bail-out option following suboptimal or complicated angioplasty [7,8]. However, the introduction of drug-eluting stents (DES) has transformed modern endovascular treatment protocols and provided excellent clinical and angiographic outcomes [4,9]. As initial reports from single-centre series provided sufficient data supporting the mid-term safety and effectiveness of infrapopliteal DES, larger multicentre randomized controlled trials (RCTs) were conducted in order to compare DES with balloon angioplasty and bare metal stents (BMSs) in the treatment of BTK arterial disease. Three recently published large-scale randomized trials have provided level A scientific evidence for the angiographic and clinical superiority of DES versus both angioplasty and BMS, supporting the primary use of olimus-eluting stents for infrapopliteal lesions up to 90mm [10]. In this case the decision to perform direct drug-eluting stenting was based on the superior primary patency rates and target lesion re-intervention free interval and composite clinical endpoints reported following the deployment of sirolimus-eluting stents compared with angioplasty and/or BMSs. Another valid decision would be to carry out balloon angioplasty first using a low-profile new generation dedicated infrapopliteal balloon catheter 3 × 100mm, and then perform bail-out stenting using DESs if necessary. Indeed, although balloon angioplasty can be still considered as an effective treatment of CLI, especially in long infrapopliteal lesions, as it is low cost, can be repeated with relative safety, does not preclude any future surgical treatment, and results in high long-term limb-salvage rates, the same does not apply for BMS. According to the data obtained from infrapopliteal trials, DES bail-out stenting provides superior outcomes, while primary bare metal stenting is no longer scientifically justified [10,11].

Although this case was not technically challenging compared with other cases presenting with long occlusions, bifurcation lesions, or distal pedal disease, it was described because it summarizes the essence of percutaneous treatment and also includes some technical key points crucial for the achievement of long-term clinical success. First, the patient was suffering from limb-threatening ischaemia (rest pain and possibly irreversible gangrene of the toe) caused by long multilevel stenotic femoropopliteal and infrapopliteal disease with poor distal run-off (Figure 8.1). Modern treatment protocols consider the endovascular approach as the treatment of choice in these cases [1]. Moreover, the patient was not fit for surgery and consequently percutaneous treatment was the only valid revascularization option. The first step to accomplishing technical and clinical success in infrapopliteal endovascular revascularization is excellent radiological assessment of the BTK vasculature and the choice of the target vessel(s). Following balloon angioplasty of the SFA, a selective angiogram with the catheter at the level of the tibial trifurcation was performed under magnification and at two different angles separated by 45°. This is essential for the correct evaluation of infrapopliteal disease, as non-selective angiograms performed through the sheath, especially prior to inflow correction, do not provide adequate visualization of the atherosclerotic BTK lesions and the distal run-off status, while a single projection might miss even an obvious lesion. Note that the obvious near-occlusion of the proximal peroneal segment (Figure 8.1b), is not visible in the DSA run performed in different angle (Figure 8.1c). This is why infrapopliteal endovascular procedures should be performed using dedicated DSA C-arm units adequately equipped with a large matrix in order to provide high-quality imaging and sufficient magnification. The total extent of these peroneal atherosclerotic lesions (Figures 8.1 and 8.2) would probably have been underestimated or even missed without selective magnified runs at two different angles or if a conventional C-arm had been used.

The second key point was the decision to perform direct stenting using sirolimus-eluting stents in a long lesion (9cm). This decision was based on the exceptional reported outcomes of bail-out drug-eluting stenting in short lesions and the initial positive results obtained by direct stenting of long lesions in our department [8,11–14]. DES placement was also decided because of the proximal location of the lesion, as distal infrapopliteal stenting has been reported to perform poorly because of the increased risk of fractures and/or deformation associated with reduced patency [15]. The long-term clinical and angiographic outcomes achieved in this case, as well as the results of recent multicentre RCTs, validated this treatment choice.

**Evidence base** ACHILLES trial [10]

- Seventeen European centres, randomized trial (1:1). Sponsors: Cordis, Johnson & Johnson.
- Percutaneous transluminal angioplasty (PTA) (101 patients, 113 lesions) versus sirolimus-eluting stents (SESs) (Cypher Select Plus©) (99 patients, 113 lesions).
- Mean total lesion length was 26.9 mm. Lesions of length up to 90mm were treated.
- At one year follow-up:
  - in-segment binary restenosis (by quantitative angiography), 22.4% for SES vs 41.9% for PTA ($p = 0.019$)
  - vessel patency, 75% for SES vs 57.1% for PTA ($p = 0.025$)
  - post hoc analysis of the composite endpoint including freedom from death, target lesion revascularization, bypass/amputation and Rutherford Class ≥4 significantly favoured the SES group over PTA treatment ($p = 0.0284$)
  - a trend towards improved wound healing was detected in the DES arm (61.7% vs 41.3%; $p = 0.0628$).

**Evidence base** Destiny Study [16]

- Seven European centres randomizing 140 CLI patients. Sponsor: Abbott.
- Compared 66 patients treated with bare metal stents (Multi link Vision) with 74 patients treated with everolimus-eluting stents (Xience V©).
- Maximum lesion length, 40mm.
- At one-year follow-up:
  - freedom from target lesion revascularization, 91% for Xience V vs 66% for BMS ($p = 0.001$)
  - primary patency, 85.2% for Xience V vs 54.4% for BMS ($p = 0.0001$
  - similar limb salvage rates in both arms.

**Evidence base** YUKON-BTX trial [17]

- Multicentre randomized trial. Sponsor: Translumina GmbH.
- Polymer-free sirolimus-eluting Yukon-BTX stent vs uncoated balloon expandable Yukon stent.
- 161 patients with CLI or intermittent claudication.
- Maximum lesion length, 45mm.
- At one-year follow-up:
  - superior clinical improvement of the patients enrolled in the DES Yukon BTX arm (Rutherford class ≤2, 78.8% in the DES arm vs 63.9% in the BMS arm; $p = 0.04$)
  - Primary patency 80.6% for DES vs 55.6% for BMS ($p = 0.004$).

One could argue that limb salvage rates following infrapopliteal plain balloon angioplasty remain similar to those achieved with DES. Nonetheless, inhibition of re-stenosis by DES results in not only superior vessel patency, but also sustained clinical improvement as demonstrated by the recent RCTs, which indicate that the patient's quality of life can be radically improved by preventing recurrent ischaemia, leading to numerous re-interventions, or improving healing of ischaemic ulcers [18]. In this case a specially designed questionnaire was used to evaluate our patient's pre- and post-procedural quality of life. On a 0–10 scale the patient rated his pre-procedural health status as 4/10, while aftera a one-year follow-up his health status improved by four points (8/10). He also stated that he no longer experienced pain or lifestyle-limiting claudication after three years follow-up.

## A final word from the expert

Over the last decade, several investigators have reported the infrapopliteal application of DES, usually for critical limb ischaemia treatment. Recent RCTs such as the ACHILLES trial (sirolimus-eluting stents versus standard balloon angioplasty of the infrapopliteal arteries) and the DESTINY trial (everolimus-eluting stents versus bare metal stents in the infrapopliteal arteries) have reported significantly improved patency of the target lesions at one-year follow-up. Additionally, in the ACHILLES trial a significantly improved composite endpoint of event-free survival and a trend towards improved wound healing were detected following DES application compared with balloon angioplasty. However, these results refer to relatively short lesions, with the exception of results obtained recently by Katsanos et al. [10] who reported encouraging long-term outcomes after full DES coverage of long infrapopliteal lesions of up to 28cm (average, 7.7cm). It should be noted that cost issues arise with the use of multiple DES in long lesions even though a relatively low number needed to treat (NTT) and incremental cost-effectiveness ratios (ICERs) following infrapopliteal DES use have been reported [19]. Other issues with infrapopliteal stenting include strict clinical and imaging follow-up protocols to avoid occlusions where re-canalization is more demanding, and care should be taken that DES placement does not impede any future bypass surgery option where healthy unstented arterial segments are needed.

Current data conclusively demonstrate that the infrapopliteal use of DES significantly reduces restenosis and clinically driven revascularization procedures compared with balloon angioplasty and bare metal stenting, justifying their primary BTK application. Moreover, DES utilized as a bail-out following suboptimal angioplasty result in superior long-term primary patency rates compared to bail-out BMS. Balloon-expandable DES should not be used for distal foot anatomical areas. In such cases, alternatives such as the emerging drug-coated balloon technology should be considered.

## References


1. Norgren L, Hiatt WR, Dormandy JA, et al. Inter-Society Consensus for the Management of Peripheral Arterial Disease (TASC II). *Eur J Vasc Endovasc Surg* 2007; 33 (Suppl 1): S1–75.
2. Rooke TW, Hirsch AT, Misra S, et al. 2011 ACCF/AHA focused update of the guideline for the management of patients with peripheral artery disease (updating the 2005 guideline). *Vasc Med* 2011; 16(6): 452–76.

3. Haider CR, Riederer SJ, Borisch, et al. High temporal and spatial resolution 3D time-resolved contrast-enhanced magnetic resonance angiography of the hands and feet. *J Magn Reson Imaging*; 2011; 34(1): 2–12.
4. Karnabatidis D, Spiliopoulos S, Katsanos K, Siablis D. Below the knee drug-eluting stents and drug-coated balloons. *Expert Rev Med Devices* 2012; 9(1): 85–94.
5. Spiliopoulos S, Katsanos K, Diamantopoulos A, et al. Does ultrasound-guided lidocaine injection improve local anaesthesia before femoral artery catheterization? *Clin Radiol* 2011; 66(5): 449–55.
6. Novo S, Coppola G, Milio G. Critical limb ischemia: definition and natural history. Curr Drug Targets Cardiovasc *Haematol Disord* 2004; 4(3): 219–25.
7. Romiti M, Albers M, Brochado-Neto FC, et al. Meta-analysis of infrapopliteal angioplasty for chronic critical limb ischemia. *J Vasc Surg* 2008; 47(5): 975–81.
8. Siablis D, Karnabatidis D, Katsanos K, et.al Infrapopliteal application of sirolimus-eluting versus bare metal stents for critical limb ischemia: analysis of long-term angiographic and clinical outcome. *J Vasc Interv Radiol* 2009; 20(9): 1141–50.
9. Ong AT, Serruys PW. Technology insight: an overview of research in drug-eluting stents. *Nat Clin Pract Cardiovasc Med* 2005; 2(12): 647–58.
10. Katsanos K, Spiliopoulos S, Krokidis M, et al. Does below-the-knee placement of drug-eluting stents improve clinical outcomes? *J Cardiovasc Surg (Torino)* 2012; 53(2): 195–203.
11. Karnabatidis D, Spiliopoulos S, Diamantopoulos A, et al. Primary everolimus-eluting stenting versus balloon angioplasty with bailout bare metal stenting of long infrapopliteal lesions for treatment of critical limb ischemia. *J Endovasc Ther* 2011; 18(1): 1–12.
12. Bosiers M, Deloose K, Verbist J, Peeters P. Percutaneous transluminal angioplasty for treatment of 'below-the-knee' critical limb ischemia: early outcomes following the use of sirolimus-eluting stents. *J Cardiovasc Surg (Torino)* 2006; 47: 171–6.
13. Commeau P, Barragan P, Roquebert PO. Sirolimus for below the knee lesions: mid-term results of SiroBTK study. *Cathet Cardiovasc Interv* 2006; 68:793–8.
14. Scheinert D, Ulrich M, Scheinert S, et al. Comparison of sirolimus-eluting vs bare-metal stents for the treatment of infrapopliteal obstructions. Eurointervention 2006; 2:169–174.
15. Karnabatidis D, Katsanos K, Spiliopoulos S, et al. Incidence, anatomical location, and clinical significance of compressions and fractures in infrapopliteal balloon-expandable metal stents. *J Endovasc Ther* 2009; 16(1): 15–22.
16. Bosiers M, Scheinert D, Peeters P, et al. Randomized comparison of everolimus-eluting versus bare-metal stents in patients with critical limb ischemia and infrapopliteal arterial occlusive disease. *J Vasc Surg* 2012; 55(2): 390–8.
17. Rastan A, Tepe G, Krankenberg H, et al. Sirolimus-eluting stents vs. bare-metal stents for treatment of focal lesions in infrapopliteal arteries: a double-blind, multi-centre, randomized clinical trial. *Eur Heart J* 2011; 32(18): 2274–81.
18. Karnabatidis D, Katsanos K, Siablis D. Infrapopliteal stents: overview and unresolved issues. *J Endovasc Ther* 2009; 16 (Suppl 1): I153–62.
19. Katsanos K, Karnabatidis D, Diamantopoulos A, et al. Cost-effectiveness analysis of infrapopliteal drug-eluting stents. *Cardiovasc Intervent Radiol* 2013; 36(1): 90–7.

CASE

# 9 Thrombolysis for acute lower limb ischaemia

**Athanasios Diamantopoulos**

**Expert commentary** Panos Gkoutzios

## Case history

A 57-year-old female was admitted to the A&E department suffering from symptoms of acute ischaemia of the left lower limb. More specifically, the patient complained that her left leg felt cold and numb, with moderate motor and sensory loss evident.

> **Learning point**
>
> Acute limb ischaemia (ALI) is defined as a sudden event of perfusion deterioration, occurring less than 14 days from presentation, which may potentially cause limb loss [1,2]. It may be either the result of rapid deterioration in a previously symptomatic patient suffering from peripheral arterial disease (PAD), or an acute event in an asymptomatic patient [2]. Native arterial thrombosis remains the main cause of the disease, accounting for 85% of cases, followed by embolism; less common causes include trauma and acute arterial dissection [3]. Unfortunately, even today ALI is related to high major amputation and mortality rates, mainly because of the presence of multiple comorbidities such as cardiopathy [2,3].

The patient's previous medical history included a right common iliac artery (CIA) to right common femoral artery (CFA) bypass followed by a right CFA to left CFA and a left CFA to left popliteal artery bypass using a synthetic graft a year before admission. Post graft placement she underwent two endovascular procedures in order to deal with distal anastomosis stenotic lesions. The remaining medical history included recurrent episodes of urinary tract infection (UTI), chronic obstructive pulmonary disease (COPD), myocardial infraction (MI) with previous stenting, hypertension, and hepatitis C. The baseline routine blood test results and observations are shown in Table 9.1. Her medications included warfarin, isosorbide dinitrate (20mg twice daily), ranitidine (300mg twice daily), atorvastatin (80mg once daily), bisoprolol fumarate (5mg once daily), nicorandil (10mg twice daily), ramipril (5mg once daily), isosorbide mononitrate (60mg once daily), naproxen (500mg twice daily), aspirin (75mg once daily), calcium 600mg, colecalciferol 400 units chewable tablets (once daily), and mirtazapine (30mg once daily).

**Table 9.1 Baseline routine blood test results and observations**

| | | | |
|---|---|---|---|
| Hb | 10.6g/dl | Potassium | 4.7mmol/L |
| White blood count | $6.9 \times 10^9$ | Creatinine | 52μmol/L |
| Platelets | $397 \times 10^9$ | C-reactive protein | <5mg/L |
| INR | 3.1 ratio | Albumin level | 44g/L |
| Class fibrinogen | 3.35g/L | Blood pressure | 138/82mmHg |
| aPTT | 1.4 ratio | $O_2$ | 99% on air |
| Sodium | 142mmol/L | Temperature | 36.7°C |

Both the vascular surgery team and the interventional radiology team were contacted. In order to decide on the therapeutic plan, baseline imaging with a CTA was ordered. The patient was transferred to the CT department for a contrast-enhanced CT scan which showed that both the right-to-left femoral–femoral and the femoral–popliteal bypass grafts were thrombosed (Figures 9.1a, b) with flow reconstitution at the popliteal artery just above the knee joint (Figure 9.1c). A high-grade calcified stenosis of the proximal anterior tibial artery was also evident.

Based on the CTA findings as well as patient's general health condition and previous medical history the consensus was to proceed with catheter-directed thrombolysis by direct puncture of the fem–fem graft. Other treatment options included surgery and intravenous systemic thrombolysis.

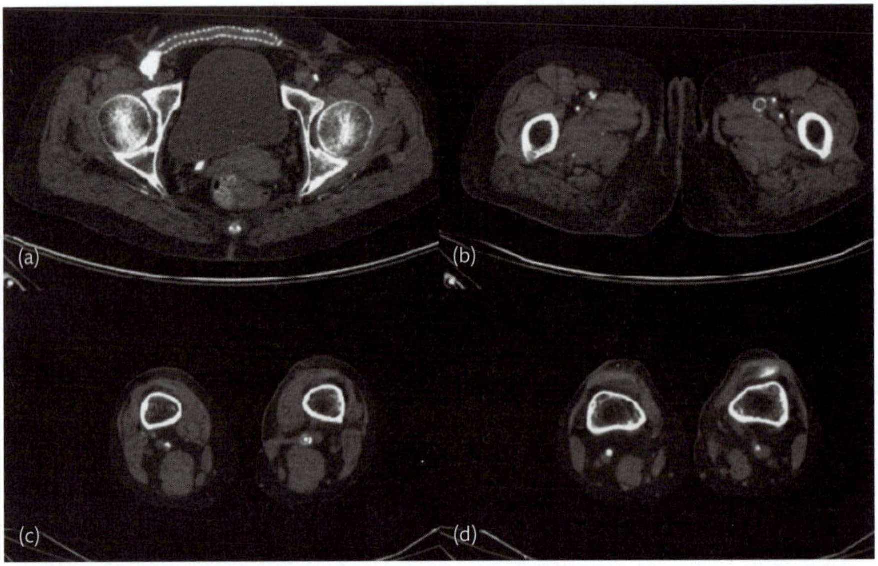


**Figure 9.1** (a) The right-to-left femoral–femoral crossover graft was thrombosed. In addition, (b) the left side femoropopliteal bypass graft was thrombosed and (c, d) there was filling of the above knee popliteal artery.

**Learning point** Treatment options for acute limb ischaemia

Treatment options for ALI include surgery, percutaneous endovascular treatments, and intravenous systemic thrombolysis. More specifically, endovascular options include catheter-directed infusion of pharmacological thrombolysis, mechanical thrombectomy, pharmacomechanical thrombolysis, thrombus aspiration, or a combination of the above [4–8]. Nowadays, thrombolytic catheter-directed treatment of ALI is an established and effective option [9–11].

Pharmacological thrombolysis is defined as thrombus dissolution by selective catheter directed infusion of a thrombolytic agent. The indication for the procedure is the break up of thrombotic occlusions of either native arteries or bypass grafts causing ALI in order to prevent limb loss. Published data suggest significantly better results for thrombolysis than for surgery with respect to limb salvage and mortality rates when the onset of ALI symptoms was less than 14 days previously as well as for recent bypass graft occlusions [12,13].

**Learning point** Contraindications to percutaneous catheter-directed thrombolysis

Absolute contraindications to percutaneous catheter-directed thrombolysis include cases presented with active or recent (within the past 10 days) internal or gastrointestinal bleeding that is not possible to treat, known intracranial tumour, neurosurgery or intracranial trauma within the past three months, a history of recent intracranial haemorrhage, abdominal surgery within the last three weeks, presence or development of compartment syndrome or limb ischaemia associated with tissue loss that may require urgent operation and/or irreversible nerve damage, and finally a known history of a cerebrovascular event within the previous six months including transient ischaemic attacks within the past two months. Relative contraindications include major non-vascular surgery or trauma during the past 10 days, a history of gastrointestinal bleeding, uncontrolled hypertension, puncture of non-compressible vessel, cardiopulmonary resuscitation within the last 10 days, recent eye operation, a history of severe contrast allergy, hepatic failure, especially in cases with coagulopathy, bacterial endocarditis, pregnancy or post-partum stage, diabetic haemorrhagic retinopathy, and life expectancy less than one year [5,7,14].

The patient was informed about both the benefits and the potential risks associated with the procedure and signed a written informed consent form. Under local anaesthesia the right-to-left femoral–femoral graft was single-wall punctured using ultrasound guidance and a 4Fr sheath was antegrade placed. A straight 4Fr catheter with multiple side-holes was carefully advanced just distal to the sheath tip. Both sheath and catheter were secured in place and thrombolysis through the catheter was initiated as per institutional protocol. More specifically, immediately after establishment of safe access 5000IU of heparin was administered followed by 5mg of recombinant tissue plasminogen activator (r-tPA) according to local protocol. A pump infusion of r-tPA at a rate of 1mg/hour for the first six hours followed by 0.5mg/hour for another 18 hours was then initiated. Additionally, infusion of 200IU/hour of heparin was administered through the sheath's side port pump in order to prevent the development of new thrombus around the sheath and the catheter. The patient was then transferred to a high dependency unit where she was closely monitored for 24 hours (blood pressure measurement, heart rate, groin assessment).

**Expert comment**

Thrombolytic or fibrinolytic agents are extensively used for the treatment of ischaemia by enhancing the endogenous thrombolytic system. Several thrombolytic agents are available, including urokinase, natural streptokinase, anistreplase, tissue plasminogen activator (tPA), and recombinant tissue plasminogen activators (r-tPAs) such as alteplase, reteplase, and tenecteplase. The most widely used agents, depending on local protocols, experience, and availability, are urokinase and tPA or r-tPA. Although there are is no available evidence showing the superiority of tPA over urokinase with respect to safety and effectiveness, tPA is preferred because the initial lysis may be more rapid than that of urokinase. Streptokinase is no longer the preferred agent as it has been demonstrated to be less effective and more antigenic [15].

After initiation of the thrombolytic therapy patient must be kept under continuous surveillance in order to detect any adverse events. Vital signs should be closely monitored and laboratory tests, including HCT, Hb, INR, PT, PTT, and serum Cr, should be performed regularly.

Twenty-four hours after initiation of thrombolysis infusion the patient was transfered back to the angiographic suite for a control angiogram. Digital subtraction angiography performed through the sheath demonstrated satisfactory flow of the right-to-left femoral–femoral graft and the left side femoral–popliteal graft with no significant underlying lesions. There was a minor amount of residual thrombus in the proximal segment of the peroneal artery, but the vessel re-formed immediately distally and was patent to the ankle (Figures 9.2 and 9.3). The anterior tibial artery was patent to the foot. The patient regained full motion and sensory feeling in the previously ischaemic limb and the distal foot was significantly warmer than before the procedure. The consensus at that time was to terminate the thrombolysis and start immediate treatment with a therapeutic dose of low-molecular

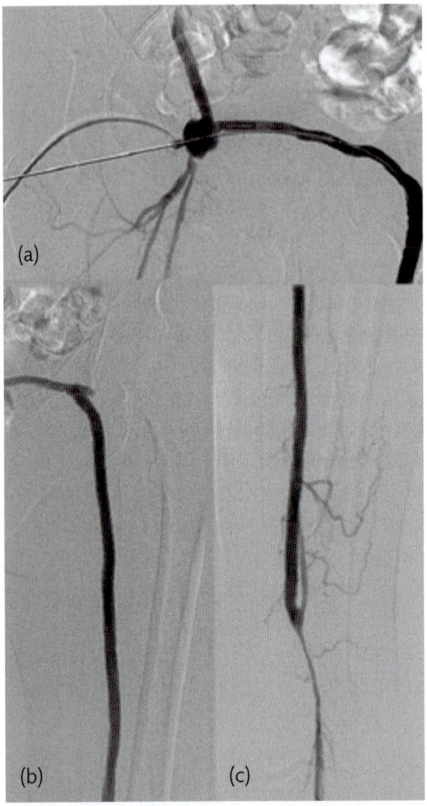


**Figure 9.2** Follow-up DSA showing satisfactory flow in (a) the right-to-left femoral-femoral graft and (b, c) the left side femoral-popliteal graft with no significant underlying lesions being present.

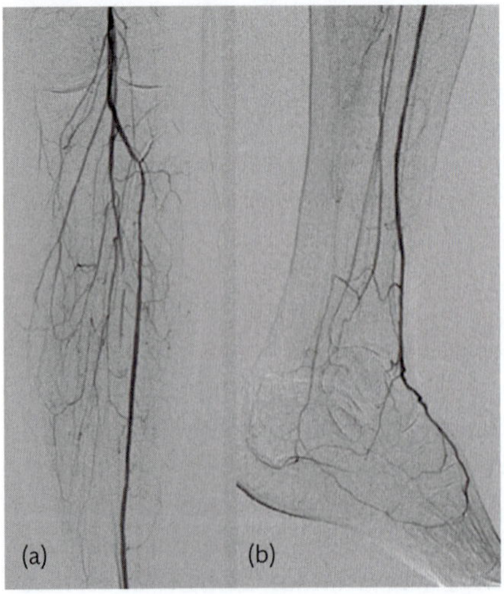


**Figure 9.3** DSA of the outflow vessels showed (a) a small amount of residual thrombus in the proximal segment of the peroneal artery, but the vessel re-formed immediately distally and was patent to the ankle. (a, b) The anterior tibial artery was patent to the foot.

heparin combined with treatment with antiplatelet drugs (clopidogrel 75mg/day). The long term anticoagulation plan was to restart the warfarin that the patient was receiving because of chronic atrial fibrillation. A 6Fr closure device was used to seal the puncture site. No immediate complications were noted and the patient was discharged the following day with instructions to visit the graft surveillance clinic after one month.

**Expert comment**

One of the main advantages of transcatheter thrombolysis is that any underlying lesion can be relatively safely treated. Treatment of such lesions is mandatory considering the superior vessel patency rates at two years when underlying lesions were identified and treated compared with those when this was not the case (79% vs 9.8%) [16]. The treatment of choice in such cases should be primary stenting, if this is possible.

**Evidence base**

The STILE, ROCHESTER, and TOPAS trials are the most important randomized controlled trials comparing catheter-directed thrombolysis with open surgery. These three trials all showed comparable results for limb salvage between surgery and catheter-directed thrombolysis. However, the mortality rates were lower for those cases treated with thrombolysis than for those treated surgically: 16% vs 42% in the ROCHESTER trial [17], 6.5% vs 8.5% in the STILE trial [12], and 13.3% vs 15.7% in the TOPAS trial [18].

A significant conclusion of the STILE trial was that those patients with symptoms for less than 14 days who were treated with catheter-directed thrombolysis had significantly lower amputation rates than those who underwent surgical repair at six months (30% vs 11%) [3,12,18]. Both the TOPAS and the STILE trials showed better outcomes after catheter-directed thrombolysis when ALI occurred in bypass grafts rather in native arteries [12,18].

**Expert comment**

There is enough evidence from RCTs to support the use of catheter-directed thrombolysis in patients presenting with ALI symptoms, especially when for thrombosed bypass grafts. Thrombolysis should be the first-line treatment option, especially as there is published evidence that whenever thrombolysis fails, thrombectomy and/or graft revision are associated with low success rates [16].

**Learning point** Risks of thrombolysis

Mortality, as a result of stroke, major bleeding, and myocardial infarction, is undoubtedly the major risk for ALI patients treated with catheter-directed thrombolysis. More specifically, the incidence of peripheral bleeding ranges from 1% to 25%, and the incidence of intracranial bleeding is between 0% and 2.5% [3]. Less common complications include distal vessel embolization, compartment syndrome, reperfusion syndrome, amputation, puncture site complications (pseudo-aneurysm), and contrast-related complications (renal failure and allergy reactions). Finally, it must be remembered that rarely some thrombolytic agents such as streptokinase may be associated with major allergic reactions.

## Discussion

Since Dotter first introduced catheter-directed thrombolysis, it has become established as an effective treatment option for patients suffering from ALI [9–11]. In view of both the potential benefits and the associated risks of such procedures, only patients with salvageable limbs (i.e. the presence of a venous doppler signal and incomplete motor and sensory loss) should be considered for this treatment [3].

Currently, a number of agents are used, and several administration techniques have been proposed including regional intra-arterial infusion, intra-thrombus infusion, intra-thrombus bolusing, stepwise infusion, continuous infusion, graded infusion, and forced periodic infusion (pulse-spray technique). Regional intra-arterial infusion may be performed with the catheter placed just proximal to the occlusion or with its tip embedded in its most proximal segment. The intra-thrombus technique is characterized by delivery of the lytic agent inside the occlusion. Intra-thrombus bolusing refers to initial administration of concentrated fibrolytic agent in the thrombus. Stepwise infusion involves the initial delivery of the agent in the proximal segment of the thrombus followed by stepwise advancement of the catheter to the distal segment. Continuous infusion is the constant delivery of the agent using a pump. Graded infusion is characterized by time-related delivery of the drug.

Forced periodic infusion or the pulse-spray technique is the forceful infusion of the agent into the thrombus in order to break it up [3].

Intra-thrombus high-dose bolus infusion of a thrombolytic agent, followed by continuous infusion of low doses, is believed to be a less demanding and highly effective technique [6]. The technical or clinical success (defined as symptom relief or decrease in the severity of any subsequent surgical intervention, including amputation) depends on the lytic agent and the technique used [3].

Currently, there is no clear evidence as to whether surgery or catheter-directed thrombolysis provides better immediate and long-term results. Randomized clinical trials suggest that catheter-directed thrombolytic treatment is superior to open surgery when dealing with acute occlusions (symptoms for less than 14 days) in bypass grafts and long-segment lesions with inadequate run-off. In contrast, surgery is superior for subacute or chronic lesions and for occlusions in native arteries.

With regard to the use of different thrombolytic agents, urokinase may be associated with a lower rate of complications than tPA. However, a recent Cochrane systematic review including five randomized control trials concluded that haemorrhagic complications were not statistically significantly higher with tPA than with other agents [15].

## A final word from the expert

Endovascular management of ALI is a highly effective treatment option for disease in both native arteries and bypass grafts, with the latter showing better outcomes. RCTs have shown that although limb salvage rates are not significantly different between catheter-directed thrombolysis and open surgery, mortality rates are significantly lower for the former technique [12,18]. Another significant conclusion of these trials is that thrombolysis outcomes are superior in acute occlusion (symptomatic for less than 14 days) and when the thrombosis affects a bypass graft rather than native artery [12,18].

Before deciding whether thrombolysis should be performed in a specific patient it is important to take into account the presenting symptoms and previous medical history and to evaluate the potential benefits and risks of the planned procedure. All the potential contraindications must be considered, mainly because of the high risk of bleeding associated with the use of lytic agents. Pre-procedure evaluation includes high-quality non-invasive imaging and basic laboratory evaluation.

It should be noted that catheter-directed thrombolysis is not the only endovascular technique that is appropriate for patients presenting with ALI symptoms. Thrombus aspiration, mechanical thrombectomy, and pharmaco-mechanical thrombolysis are alternative endovascular techniques widely used in everyday clinical practice to treat patients suffering from ALI [3].

Thrombus aspiration involves the use of a large-lumen catheter (usually 6–8Fr) connected to a 50–60ml syringe to forcibly aspirate the thrombus from the occluded region and restore blood flow [19,20].

Percutaneous mechanical thrombectomy involves the use of percutaneous thrombectomy devices to break up the thrombus and remove it. The main advantage of the method is that it can be used in cases where thrombolysis is not indicated (e.g. patients suffering from haemorrhagic and/or coagulation disorders). Percutaneous thrombectomy devices are defined according to their mechanism of action including devices that break up the clot mechanically, hydrodynamic/rheolytic catheters, ultrasonic catheters, and combined devices [3].

Finally, pharmaco-mechanical thrombolysis is a combination of mechanical disruption and pharmacological thrombolysis. This results in an increased lytic effect and a reduction in the total time required for the procedure. It is generally in cases of severely ischaemic limbs were time is crucial [3].

Commercially available thrombectomy catheters include the following: Arrow-Trerotola PTD (International Inc., Reading, PA, USA), Castaneda Brush (Micro Therapeutics, Aliso Viego, CA, USA), Cragg Brush (Micro Therapeutics Aliso Viego, CA, USA), Helix (Microvena, White Bear Lake, MN, USA), Roratex/Aspirex catheters (Straub Medical AG, Wang, Switzerland), Gelbfish-Endovac (NeoVascular Technologies, NY, USA), Hydrolyzer (Cordis, Miami, FL, USA), BSIC Oasis system (Boston Scientific, Watertown, MA, USA), veAngioJet (Possis Medical, Minneapolis, MN, USA), ThrombCat thrombectomy catheter system (Kensay Nash Corporation, Exton, PA, USA), Bacchus Trellis (Bacchus Vascular Inc., Santa Clara, CA, USA), OmniSonics Resolution Wire (OmniSonics Medical Technologies Inc, Wilmington, MA, USA), Ekos Lysus system (Ekos Corporation, Bothwell, WA, USA) (see device specifications).

## References


1. Patel N, Sacks D, Patel RI, et al. SIR reporting standards for the treatment of acute limb ischemia with use of transluminal removal of arterial thrombus. Journal of vascular and interventional radiology. *J Vasc Interv Radiol* 2003; 14(9 Pt 2): S453–65.
2. Norgren L, Hiatt WR, Dormandy JA, et al. Inter-Society Consensus for the Management of Peripheral Arterial Disease (TASC II). *Eur J Vasc Endovasc Surg* 2007; 33 (Suppl 1): S1–75.
3. Karnabatidis D, Spiliopoulos S, Tsetis D, Siablis D. Quality improvement guidelines for percutaneous catheter-directed intra-arterial thrombolysis and mechanical thrombectomy for acute lower-limb ischemia. *Cardiovasc Intervent Radiol* 2011; 34(6): 1123–36.
4. Berridge DC, Gregson RH, Hopkinson BR, Makin GS. Randomized trial of intra-arterial recombinant tissue plasminogen activator, intravenous recombinant tissue plasminogen activator and intra-arterial streptokinase in peripheral arterial thrombolysis. *Br J Surg* 1991; 78(8): 988–95.
5. Dormandy JA, Rutherford RB. Management of peripheral arterial disease (PAD). TASC Working Group. TransAtlantic Inter-Society Consensus (TASC). *J Vasc Surg* 2000; 31(1 Pt 2): S1–296.
6. Kessel DO, Berridge DC, Robertson I. Infusion techniques for peripheral arterial thrombolysis. *Cochrane Database Syst Rev* 2004;(1):CD000985.
7. Working Party on Thrombolysis in the Management of Limb Ischemia Party on Thrombolysis in the Management of Limb Ischemia. thrombolysis in the management of lower limb peripheral arterial occlusion-a consensus document. *J Vasc Interv Radiol* 2003; 14(9 Pt 2): S337–49
8. Ouriel K. Endovascular techniques in the treatment of acute limb ischemia: thrombolytic agents, trials, and percutaneous mechanical thrombectomy techniques. *Semin Vasc Surg* 2003; 16(4): 270–9.
9. Bertelsen S, Egeblad K. Experimental thrombolysis by perfusion. I. Reaction of the intestinal wall to plasmin infused intra-arterially. *Acta Chir Scand* 1969; 135(6): 482–5.
10. Dotter CT, Rosch J, Seaman AJ. Selective clot lysis with low-dose streptokinase. *Radiology* 1974; 111(1): 31–7.

11. Timmis GC, Gangadharan V, Hauser AM, et al. Intracoronary streptokinase in clinical practice. *Am Heart J* 1982; 104(4 Pt 2): 925–38.
12. Anon. Results of a prospective randomized trial evaluating surgery versus thrombolysis for ischemia of the lower extremity: the STILE trial. *Ann Surg* 1994; 220(3): 251–8.
13. Comerota AJ, Weaver FA, Hosking JD, et al. Results of a prospective, randomized trial of surgery versus thrombolysis for occluded lower extremity bypass grafts. *Am J Surg* 1996; 172(2): 105–12.
14. Morrison HL. Catheter-directed thrombolysis for acute limb ischemia. *Semin Intervent Radiol* 2006; 23(3): 258–69.
15. Robertson I, Kessel DO, Berridge DC. Fibrinolytic agents for peripheral arterial occlusion. *Cochrane Database Syst Rev.* 2010; (3): CD001099.
16. Sullivan KL, Gardiner GA, Jr, Kandarpa K, et al. Efficacy of thrombolysis in infrainguinal bypass grafts. *Circulation* 1991; 83 (2 Suppl): I99–105
17. Ouriel K, Shortell CK, DeWeese JA, et al. A comparison of thrombolytic therapy with operative revascularization in the initial treatment of acute peripheral arterial ischemia. *J Vasc Surg* 1994; 19(6): 1021–30.
18. Ouriel K, Veith FJ, Sasahara AA. A comparison of recombinant urokinase with vascular surgery as initial treatment for acute arterial occlusion of the legs. Thrombolysis or Peripheral Arterial Surgery (TOPAS) Investigators. *N Engl J Med* 1998; 338(16): 1105–11.
19. Starck EE, McDermott JC, Crummy AB, et al. Percutaneous aspiration thromboembolectomy. *Radiology* 1985; 156(1): 61–6.
20. Sniderman KW, Bodner L, Saddekni S, et al. Percutaneous embolectomy by transcatheter aspiration. Work in progress. *Radiology* 1984; 150(2): 357–61.

CASE

# 10 Renal artery stenosis: angioplasty or stent?

**Shirish Prabhudesai**

**Expert commentary** Narayan Karunanithy

## Case history

A 69-year-old male patient presented to the emergency department with shortness of breath and chest pain. His past medical history included hypertension for which he was on two anti-hypertensive agents. ECG demonstrated ST depression with T-wave inversion and elevated serum troponin levels consistent with non-ST elevation myocardial infarction. Blood results revealed an estimated glomerular filtration rate (eGFR) of 19ml/min (normal range 70–140ml/min), compared with a baseline of 33ml/min one year previously. The chest radiograph revealed evidence of acute pulmonary oedema, and the echocardiogram showed significantly impaired left ventricular function with an estimated ejection fraction of 15–20%. CT coronary angiography revealed focal atheromatous disease in the left anterior descending artery (LAD). He was initially diagnosed with ischaemic cardiomyopathy due to left anterior descending artery (LAD) disease. He underwent percutaneous coronary intervention with placement of a bare metal stent and insertion of a cardiac resynchronization device. Clinical examination also raised suspicion of an abdominal aortic aneurysm (AAA). A CT angiogram of the abdomen confirmed the presence of a 7.2cm infrarenal AAA and high-grade bilateral renal artery stenoses (Figure 10.1).

Despite management of his cardiac disease, he presented on multiple occasions with sudden-onset severe episodes of shortness of breath. Following discussion in the multidisciplinary meeting it was postulated that the patient's renal impairment and repeated presentations with breathlessness might be attributable to flash pulmonary oedema secondary to renal artery stenosis. The decision was made to stent both renal

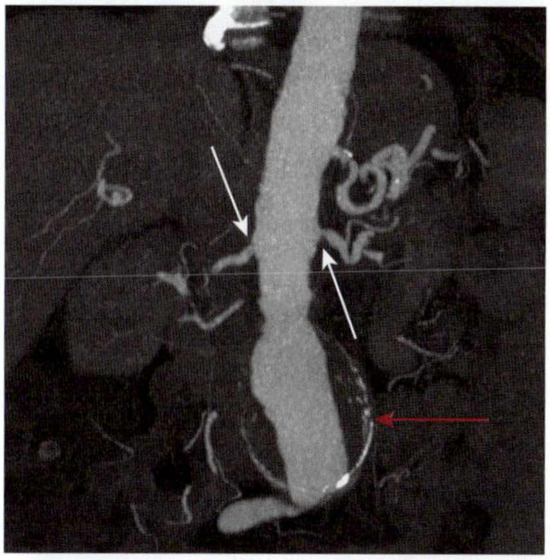

**Figure 10.1** Contrast-enhanced coronal CT (maximal intensity projection) showing bilateral renal artery ostial stenoses (white arrows) and infrarenal AAA (red arrow).

**Learning point**

The clinical presentation of acute shortness of breath associated with rapid accumulation of fluid within the lung's interstitial/alveolar spaces is typical of acute decompensated heart failure (ADHF), the severe form of which is referred to as flash pulmonary oedema. In addition to cardiac causes ADHF can be caused by severe hypertension, renal artery stenosis, severe renal dysfunction, and primary fluid overload [1].

**Clinical tip**

Pre-procedure cross-sectional imaging is extremely valuable for determining the number, location, and orientation of the renal arteries. If the angulation required to view the renal ostium in profile is not achieved, a significant lesion at this site may be missed or underestimated. Also, a highly angulated renal artery may require access from the brachial artery rather than the common femoral artery.

**Clinical tip**

Renal artery stenosis can generallybe crossed with a C2 angulated catheter. For severely angulated and downward-pointing renal arteries, an Sos Omni catheter is used to guide the wire into the distal renal artery. Alternatively, left brachial artery access allows an in-line approach to the renal artery.

**Expert comment**

The distal renal arteries are extremely prone to vasospasm and dissection. Hence, once the ostial lesion is crossed, the hydrophilic guidewire is exchanged for a 0.018 inch guidewire with an atraumatic non-hydrophilic tip. At this stage careful attention to technique to prevent even minimal wire movement and further administration of vasodilators can minimize the incidence of dissection and vasospasm.

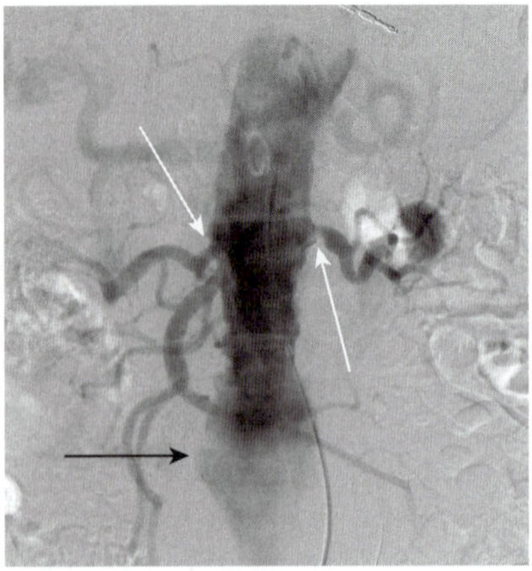

**Figure 10.2** Aortic angiogram obtained via a pigtail catheter showing bilateral renal artery stenoses (white arrows) and infrarenal abdominal aortic aneurysm (black arrow).

arteries, followed by endovascular repair of the infrarenal abdominal aortic aneurysm at a later date. The procedure was performed via right common femoral artery access. An aortogram confirmed high-grade bilateral renal artery stenoses (Figure 10.2).

The sheath was upsized to a 5.5Fr 35cm catheter (Check-Flo; Cook Medical, Bloomington, IN, USA) and 5000 IU heparin was administered intra-arterially as thromboprophylaxis with 500μg isosorbide dinitrate to prevent vasospasm. A 4Fr cobra (C2) catheter (Torcon NB; Cook Medical, Bloomington, IN, USA) and an angled 0.035 hydrophilic guidewire (Glidewire; Terumo, Somerset, NJ, USA) were used to cross the stenotic segment of each renal artery.

The hydrophilic guidewire was exchanged for a 0.018 wire (Thruway; Boston Scientific, Quincy, MA, USA). Primary renal artery stenting was performed with 6mm × 15mm balloon expanded stents (Palmaz Genesis, Cordis, Bridgewater, NJ, USA). Post stent placement angiography demonstrated satisfactory stent placement and patency of both renal arteries (Figure 10.3).

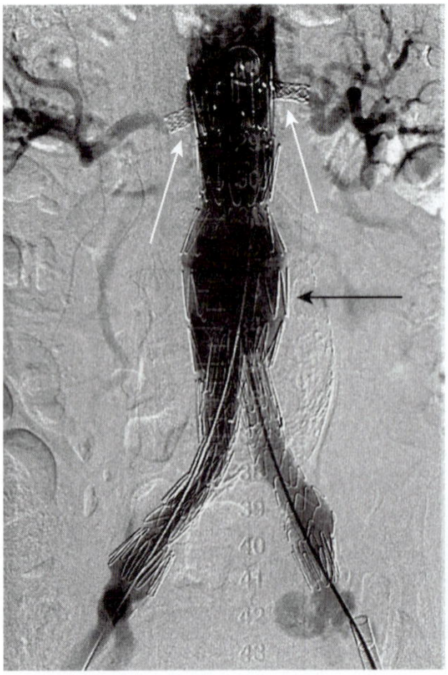

**Figure 10.3** Aortic angiogram obtained during endovascular repair of the aortic aneurysm, showing bilateral renal stents (white arrows) with patent renal arteries and an infrarenal aortic stent graft in situ (black arrow).

A month later the patient underwent uneventful endovascular repair of his infrarenal abdominal aortic aneurysm (Figure 10.3). Twelve months later he remains symptom free with no further presentations of shortness of breath and a significant improvement in renal function (eGFR 39ml/min).

## Discussion

Renal artery stenosis (RAS) is most commonly caused by atherosclerosis (90% of cases) and less commonly by fibromuscular dysplasia (5% of cases) (Table 10.1). RAS impedes blood flow to the kidneys and can result in refractory hypertension, congestive heart failure, and progressively worsening renal function. Atherosclerotic RAS predominantly presents in older patients as part of the systemic atherosclerotic disease process, and usually involves the origin and proximal third of the renal arteries, with disease often present in the adjacent aorta [2]. Fibromuscular dysplasia is a disease of unknown aetiology, predominantly found in young to middle-aged women (15–50 years), and usually affects the distal two-thirds of the renal arteries.

**Learning point**

Differences between RAS due to atherosclerosis and RAS due to fibromuscular dysplasia are shown in Table 10.1.

**Table 10.1 Comparison of RAS due to atherosclerosis and to fibromuscular dysplasia**

| Atherosclerosis | Fibromuscular dysplasia |
| --- | --- |
| Responsible for 90% of RAS | Responsible for 5% of RAS |
| Part of systemic atherosclerotic vascular disease | Commonly affects the renal and carotid arteries, and rarely involves other arteries |
| Presents in older patients | Presents in young to middle-aged women |
| Affects ostial/proximal renal arteries | Affects distal two-thirds of renal arteries |

The true incidence of RAS in the general population is not known. Significant RAS is observed in less than 5% of the hypertensive patient population [3], compared with a prevalence of up to 15% in patients with coronary artery disease undergoing abdominal aortography during cardiac catheterization procedures [4], and 40–45% in patients with lower limb arterial disease [5,6]. The presence of RAS has also been shown to predict other vascular morbidity. The Cardiovascular Health Study demonstrated that patients with atherosclerotic RAS had a higher incidence of hospitalization for angina, myocardial infarction, and coronary revascularization [7].

Percutaneous transluminal angioplasty (PTA) of the renal arteries is well established as an effective treatment for hypertension associated with fibromuscular RAS [8–10]. The optimal treatment for atherosclerotic RAS is less clear. Hypertension and renal dysfunction are initially treated medically with renal artery stenting, which superseded balloon angioplasty [11], and has largely replaced surgical re-vascularization which is reserved for refractory cases [12]. However, given the potential complications of renal artery stenting [13], investigators have sought better evidence for its efficacy and safety. Several randomized controlled trials (RCTs) have examined the role of medical therapy versus renal artery stenting. All trials have randomized patients into two groups: a group for medical treatment plus renal artery stenting versus a group for medical treatment alone.

**Evidence base** STAR trial [14]

- Renal artery stenting with medical therapy versus medical therapy alone in 140 patients with RAS
- Multicentre randomized trial across 10 European centres
- No significant difference in progression of renal failure over two years
- No significant difference in blood pressure control or overall mortality
- Significant complications in stent group: 17% haematoma, 3% mortality
- Authors' conclusion: more harm than apparent benefit from renal stenting
- Limitations:
  (i) Enrolment criteria: resulted in patients with mild RAS being included in stenting group
  (ii) Complications were much higher than in other similar studies

The results of the Stent Placement in Patients with Atherosclerotic Renal Artery Stenosis and Impaired Renal Function (STAR trial) were published in 2009 [14]. This multicentre European RCT recruited 140 patients, who were randomized to either renal artery stenting with medical therapy or medical therapy alone. The selection criteria for patients were (i) renal artery stenosis greater than 50%, (ii) renal impairment (GFR <80ml/min), and (iii) well-controlled blood pressure (<140/90mmHg). The primary endpoint was progression of renal disease defined as 20% or greater decrease in creatinine clearance. Only 46 of the 64 patients (72%) randomized for renal artery stenting actually received a stent. The most common reason for not receiving a stent was insignificant RAS at angiography (stenosis <50%). Overall, 16% of the stent group and 22% of the medical therapy alone group reached the primary endpoint (HR, 0.73; 95% CI, 0.33–1.61) using an intention-to-treat analysis. There were no differences in blood pressure control or overall mortality between the groups. However, complication rates in the stent group were high, and included two deaths (3%) and 11 haematomas (17%). The authors concluded that there was no statistically significant difference in progression of renal failure over two years in the two groups, and that renal stenting caused more harm than apparent benefit. However, they acknowledged that their study was 'underpowered to provide a definitive estimate of efficacy'.

**Evidence base** ASTRAL trial [15]

- Renal artery stenting with medical therapy versus medical therapy alone in 806 patients with RAS
- Multicentre randomized non-blinded trial in Europe and Australia
- No significant difference in blood pressure or adverse renal/cardiovascular events
- Significant complications in stent group: 1.2% toe/limb amputation or death
- Authors' conclusion: renal stenting carries risk of harm and no clinical benefit
- Limitations:
  (i) study design: patients with severe RAS who might benefit most from stenting were excluded
  (ii) poor technical success rate suggests inexperienced operators

The Angioplasty and Stenting for Renal Artery Lesions (ASTRAL) trial [15] was a multicentre randomized trial conducted in Europe and Australia with a design similar to the STAR trial. The inclusion criteria were as follows: (i) patients with hypertension or unexplained renal dysfunction with substantial anatomical atherosclerotic stenosis in at least one renal artery based on imaging studies; (ii) the treating clinician must be uncertain that the patient would benefit from revascularization. Patients were excluded if they were likely to require revascularization within six months. Out of the 806 patients enrolled, only 83% of those randomized to stenting actually underwent the procedure while 6% of the medical arm received renal artery revascularization.

The primary outcome was the change in renal function as assessed by the slope of the reciprocal of serum creatinine level over time. This showed a trend in favour of the stenting group compared with medical therapy during a mean follow-up of 34 months (95% CI, −0.002–0.13; $p = 0.06$). There were no significant differences in blood pressure or adverse renal or cardiovascular events (secondary outcomes) between groups. Five (1.2%) serious complications, including death or amputation, occurred in the stenting group. The authors concluded, similarly to the STAR trial, that renal artery stenting posed substantial risks but no evidence of a worthwhile clinical benefit.

Both the STAR and ASTRAL trials have been criticized for problems with their enrolment criteria, which led to inclusion of patients in the stenting group who were unlikely to benefit from stenting. In the STAR trial this was due to inclusion of patients based on non-invasive assessment of RAS which overestimated the degree of stenosis (19% false-positive rate compared with subsequent angiographic evaluation). As the study was carried out on an intention-to-treat basis, these patients did not receive a stent but were analysed as if they had. In the ASTRAL trial, the stipulation that patient enrolment required physician uncertainty about the benefits of revascularization meant that patients with the most significant disease, who were most likely to benefit from stenting, were excluded. Both trials also demonstrated lower technical success and higher complication rates compared with other renal stenting registries, which called into question the competence and experience of the operators involved in the study. Learning from the shortcomings of these studies, two new randomized controlled trials were initiated.

**Evidence base** CORAL trial [16]–ongoing

- Renal artery stenting with medical therapy versus medical therapy alone in 1080 patients with RAS
- Multicentre international unblinded randomized trial
- Only patients with > 80% stenosis or > 60% stenosis with a significant pressure gradient in addition to hypertension or renal dysfunction are eligible for inclusion
- Primary endpoint: event-free survival from a composite of cardiovascular and renal events
- Aims to determine the value of stenting from the perspectives of quality of life and cost-effectiveness

The Cardiovascular Outcome in Renal Atherosclerotic Lesions (CORAL) trial [17] is an ongoing RCT, the results of which are awaited. The primary entry criteria are (i) an atherosclerotic RAS of at least 60% with a 20mmHg systolic pressure gradient, or at least 80% RAS with no gradient necessary, and (ii) systolic hypertension of at least 155mmHg on at least two antihypertensive medications. The trial will correlate stenosis severity with longitudinal renal function and determine the value of stenting from the perspectives of quality of life and cost-effectiveness. It is hoped that this trial will provide robust evidence to determine which subset of patients may benefit from renal artery stenting.

Although the evidence remains inconclusive, in 2006 the American Heart Association published the following indications for percutaneous revascularization of significant (>50%) atherosclerotic RAS [12].

(i) Hypertension—for patients with accelerated, resistant, or malignant hypertension, or hypertension with an unexplained unilateral small kidney or intolerance to antihypertensive medication.

**Learning points** Indications for renal artery stenting in atherosclerotic RAS

The American Heart Association recommends percutaneous revascularization in atherosclerotic RAS [11] for:

- severe/refractory hypertension
- preservation of renal function
- pulmonary oedema/unstable angina.

(ii) Renal dysfunction—to preserve residual renal function in patients with progressive deterioration in kidney disease.
(iii) Pulmonary oedema—for patients who present with recurrent acute decompensated heart failure and/or unstable angina.

In the case described here, bilateral renal artery stenting helped resolve the patient's episodes of shortness of breath and optimize his renal function, which were both refractory to coronary intervention. While conclusive evidence from randomized trials is still pending, what is clear is the importance of careful patient selection prior to renal artery stenting.

## A final word from the expert

Renal artery stenting is a challenging interventional procedure which requires meticulous preparation and careful attention to detail. The controversy surrounding the results of the published randomized controlled trials has made this an even more difficult area. However, anecdotally there are numerous instances when renal artery stenting has resulted in dramatic clinical improvement.

The emphasis is currently on careful patient selection based on clinical and imaging parameters. Parameters that can accurately predict favourable outcome after renal artery stenting have not been established, which make this an exciting area for clinical research.

## References

1. Ware LB, Matthay MA. Clinical practice. Acute pulmonary edema. *N Engl J Med* 2005; 353(26): 2788–96.
2. Kaatee R, Beek FJ, Verschuyl EJ, et al. Atherosclerotic renal artery stenosis: ostial or truncal? *Radiology* 1996; 199(3): 637–40.
3. Maxwell MH, Bleifer KH, Franklin SS, Varady PD. Cooperative study of renovascular hypertension. Demographic analysis of the study. *JAMA J Am Med Assoc* 1972; 220(9): 1195–1204.
4. Harding MB, Smith LR, Himmelstein SI, et al. Renal artery stenosis: prevalence and associated risk factors in patients undergoing routine cardiac catheterization. *J Am Soc Nephrol* 1992; 2(11): 1608–16.
5. Missouris CG, Buckenham T, Cappuccio FP, MacGregor GA. Renal artery stenosis: a common and important problem in patients with peripheral vascular disease. *Am J Med* 1994; 96(1): 10–14.
6. Olin JW, Melia M, Young JR, et al. Prevalence of atherosclerotic renal artery stenosis in patients with atherosclerosis elsewhere. *Am J Med* 1990; 88(1N): 46N–51N.
7. Edwards MS, Craven TE, Burke GL, et al. Renovascular disease and the risk of adverse coronary events in the elderly: a prospective, population-based study. *Arch Intern Med* 2005 24; 165(2): 207–13.
8. Birrer M, Do DD, Mahler F, et al. Treatment of renal artery fibromuscular dysplasia with balloon angioplasty: a prospective follow-up study. *Eur J Vasc Endovasc Surg* 2002; 23(2): 146–52.
9. Surowiec SM, Sivamurthy N, Rhodes JM, et al. Percutaneous therapy for renal artery fibromuscular dysplasia. *Ann Vasc Surg* 2003; 17(6): 650–5.

10. De Fraissinette B, Garcier JM, Dieu V, et al. Percutaneous transluminal angioplasty of dysplastic stenoses of the renal artery: results on 70 adults. *Cardiovasc Intervent Radiol* 2003; 26(1): 46–51.
11. Leertouwer TC, Gussenhoven EJ, Bosch JL, et al. Stent placement for renal arterial stenosis: where do we stand? A meta-analysis. *Radiology* 2000; 216(1): 78–85.
12. Hirsch AT, Haskal ZJ, Hertzer NR, et al. ACC/AHA 2005 Practice Guidelines for the Management of Patients With Peripheral Arterial Disease (Lower Extremity, Renal, Mesenteric, and Abdominal Aortic). *Circulation* 2006; 113(11): e463–654.
13. Ivanovic V, McKusick MA, Johnson CM 3rd, et al. Renal artery stent placement: complications at a single tertiary care center. *J Vasc Interv Radiol* 2003; 14(2 Pt 1): 217–25.
14. Bax L, Woittiez AJ, Kouwenberg HJ, et al. Stent placement in patients with atherosclerotic renal artery stenosis and impaired renal function: a randomized trial. *Ann Intern Med* 2009; 150(12): 840–8.
15. ASTRAL Investigators: Wheatley K, Ives N, Gray, R., et al. Revascularization versus medical therapy for renal-artery stenosis. *N Engl J Med*. 2009; 361(20): 1953–62.
16. Schwarzwälder U, Hauk M, Zeller T. RADAR—A randomised, multi-centre, prospective study comparing best medical treatment versus best medical treatment plus renal artery stenting in patients with haemodynamically relevant atherosclerotic renal artery stenosis. *Trials* 2009; 10: 60, doi: 10.1186/1745-6215-10-60.
17. Cooper CJ, Murphy TP, Matsumoto A, et al. Stent revascularization for the prevention of cardiovascular and renal events among patients with renal artery stenosis and systolic hypertension: rationale and design of the CORAL trial. *Am Heart J*. 2006; 152(1): 59–66.

CASE

# 11 Below the ankle angioplasty: treatment rationale and access techniques

**Panagiotis Kitrou**

**Expert commentary** Konstantinos Katsanos

## Case history

A 70-year-old female patient underwent an urgent endovascular below-the-knee revascularization procedure. The patient suffered from critical limb ischaemia (CLI) and a previously placed common femoral artery–popliteal artery (CFA–POP) venous bypass graft. The urgent referral form from the vascular surgeons team described the condition as follows: 'Patient with a left CFA–POP vein graft bypass and a single vessel to the foot (peroneal artery). Ulcers don't heal. Please attempt to improve blood flow'.

Physical examination demonstrated an extensive foot ulcer located mainly at the posterior aspect of the distal calf and the calcaneus and the posteromedial aspect of the right foot (tissue loss, Rutherford stage 6). A previous angiogram, performed in the context of an angioplasty for treatment of a proximal bypass juxta-anastomotic stenosis, had shown that only the peroneal artery was patent to the foot. The posterior tibial artery (PTA) was absent and the anterior tibial artery (ATA) was occluded halfway to the foot. The patient was on clopidogrel 75mg/day and aspirin 100mg/day.

Antegrade access to the left groin was achieved with a micropuncture kit (S-MAK™; Merit Medical Systems, South Jordan, UT, USA). Images acquired confirmed that the peroneal artery (PA) was the only patent vessel to the foot (Figures 11.1a, b). Interestingly, a large collateral vessel of the PA was supplying the half-formed plantar arch by interconnecting to the last 2–3mm of the salvaged PTA (Figure 11.1b). At the level of the trifurcation the origin of the PTA was absent (flush occlusion) and the ATA blocked at its proximal third (Figure 11.1c). Antegrade access was established with a standard 4Fr vascular sheath. Although branches of the half-formed plantar artery reached the foot ulcer of interest (Figure 11.1b), blood supply was undoubtedly inadequate. The interventional plan was to re-establish flow to the area of tissue loss through the PTA, which may be the direct line of blood flow in accordance with the angiosome concept [1]. The plan was also to attempt to re-open the ATA, if possible, in order to maximize reperfusion of the pedal arch and the entire foot.

Retrograde access to the inframalleolar PTA was decided as no vessel stump was visible at the tibioperoneal bifurcation (flush occlusion); this technique of a combined antegrade and retrograde approach is often described as the SAFARI angioplasty technique [2].

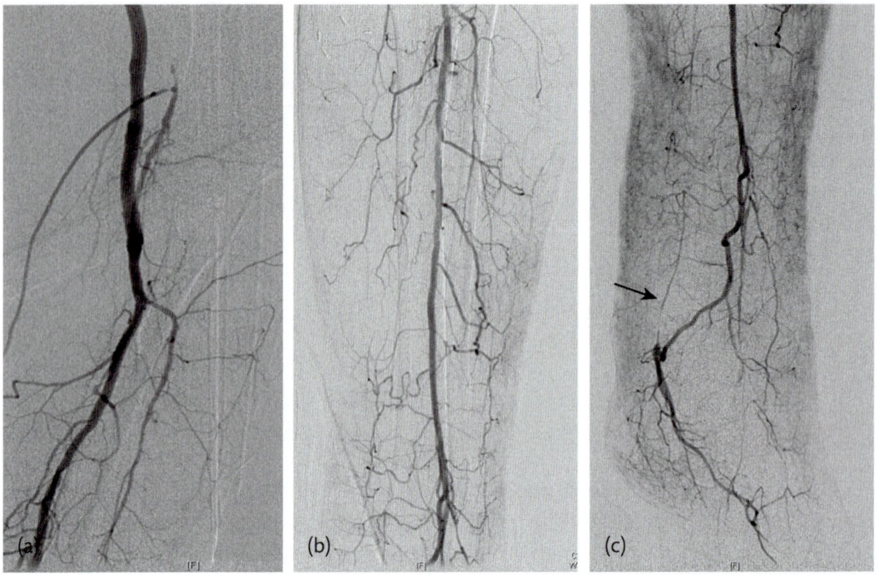


**Figure 11.1** DSA showing the following: (a) the anterior tibial artery is patent to its proximal third; (b) the peroneal artery is the only patent vessel to the foot; (c) a large collateral of the peroneal artery supplies the plantar artery. The black arrow shows the small distal salvaged posterior tibial artery to which the retrograde puncture was performed.

**Learning point** The angiosome concept

The angiosome concept divides the human body into three-dimensional tissue areas, which are supplied with blood by specific arteries and drained by specific veins. Adjacent angiosomes are connected by a mesh of collateral vessels. According to the angiosome concept the foot is divided into five angiosomes supplied by the three tibial vessels.

- Anterior tibial artery: when the ATA reaches the foot it becomes the dorsalis pedis artery (DPA) which supplies the dorsum of the foot.
- Posterior tibial artery (PTA): the PTA supplies the foot via three main branches. The medial calcaneal artery (MCA) supplies the heel, the medial plantar artery (MPA) supplies the medial aspect of the sole with the first toe and its interconnecting space, and the lateral plantar artery (LPA) supplies the remaining, lateral aspect of the sole and the remaining e toes and their interconnecting spaces.
- Peroneal artery: the PA supplies the foot via the lateral calcaneal artery (LCA) which supplies the anterior and lateral part of the ankle and the lateral and plantar aspect of the heel.

The clinical application of the angiosome concept for below the knee disease is an attempt to establish flow to an area of reversible ischaemia (foot ulcer) by direct revascularization of this area via its source feed artery.

**Learning point** Chronic total occlusion (CTO) revascularization techniques to improve below the ankle blood supply

- SAFARI (subintimal arterial flossing with antegrade–retrograde intervention) is a CTO revascularization technique in which a simultaneous antegrade (from above) and retrograde (from below) approach is achieved for tibial and below the ankle vessels. The retrograde approach by cutdown of the pedal arteries was first described by Iyer et al. in 1990 [3]. Access sites are the distal PTA, the ATA, and the pedal and plantar arteries or collaterals as long as the lumen diameter is appropriate. Retrograde puncture is always performed under ultrasound guidance. Usually no

(continued)

sheath is used (sheathless approach) which is why a micropuncture kit may be the best way to do it. A low profile balloon is used to pass through the access and dilate the occlusion. The risks with this technique are vessel perforation during puncture, vessel thrombosis, and inability to cross the lesion retrogradely or even to puncture the vessel of interest. The main risk is damage of the pedal artery, which could be used in the future for a surgical bypass.

- The pedal-plantar loop is the technique by which a loop is created with a guidewire from one tibial artery to the other via collaterals. The lateral plantar artery communicates with the dorsalis pedis artery via the deep perforating artery.
- Once the wire is looped to the contralateral vessel, a catheter is introduced in an antegrade manner, via the same sheath used for the looped wire, towards the contralateral tibial vessel. The catheter does not cross the lesion. The looped wire is directed to the catheter and then pulled with the help of a retrieving device. A balloon can then be forwarded to the lesion in an antegrade manner.

The puncture site had to be located just above the connection of the peroneal collateral to the last part of the PTA shown in Figure 11.1b as this was the only vessel supplying the foot and should not be jeopardized. Ultrasound-guided puncture was performed using a micropuncture kit (S-MAK™; Merit Medical Systems, South Jordan, UT, USA) and access was gained to the residual true lumen of the distal PTA just above the connection with the peroneal collateral (Figure 11.2).

Since no further true lumen was present, a Half Stiff (J-tipped) hydrophilic guidewire (Terumo, Japan) was employed for retrograde subintimal recanalization. Re-entry to the proximal true lumen occurred spontaneously at the tibio-peroneal trunk, and access was secured by further advancing the wire in the distal part

**Expert comment**

The best way to perform a retrograde puncture is with the help of a micropuncture kit with a short needle and a 0.014 inch guidewire. An attempt to puncture the only vessel supplying the foot can have a disastrous result as, if it fails, it may lead to acute limb ischaemia and potential limb loss. A retrograde puncture requires familiarity with ultrasound- and/or fluoroscopic-guided vessel puncture techniques and should generally be reserved for cases with no other option following a failed antegrade attempt at recanalization.

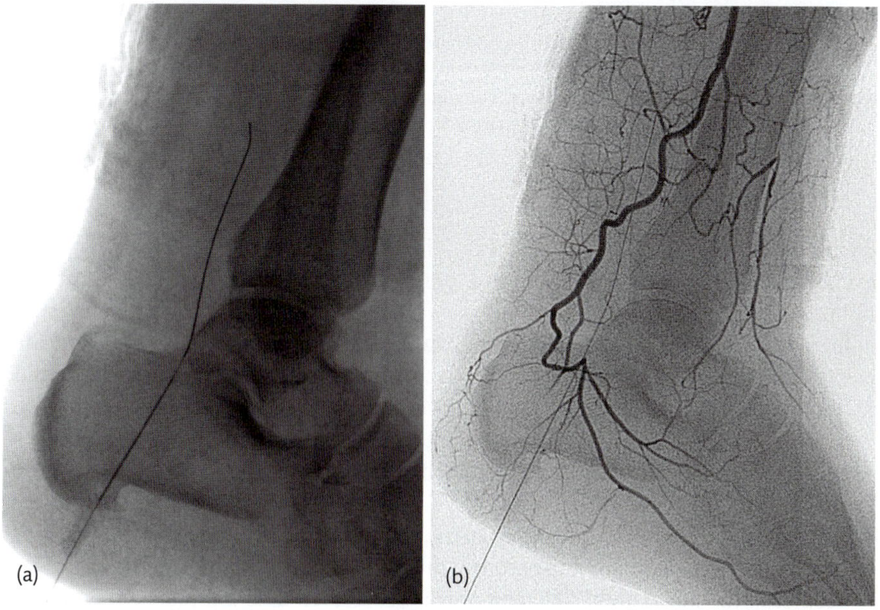


**Figure 11.2** Retrograde puncture of the posterior tibial artery ((a) fluoroscopy; (b) DSA) showing the puncture site as well as the wire being advanced in the subintimal plane along the tract of the posterior tibial artery.

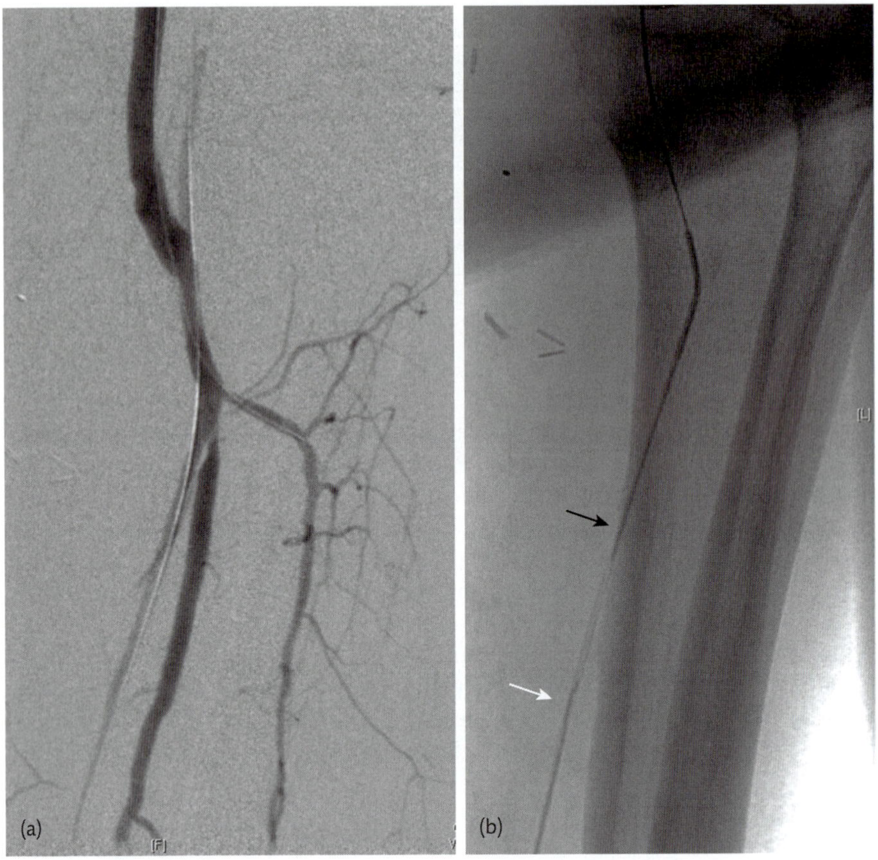


**Figure 11.3** (a) Wire from the retrograde puncture in the true lumen of the PTA and further advanced into the SFA. The other wire from the antegrade puncture is directed to the ATA. (b) The wire from the retrograde puncture (black arrow) is retrieved from the catheter, while the wire from the antegrade puncture (white arrow) is forwarded into the catheter.

of the native superficial femoral artery (Figure 11.3a). A 4Fr straight catheter was exchanged over the wire at the access point and advanced retrogradely up to the tibial trifurcation. The Half Stiff wire was retracted and an 0.014 inch wire from the antegrade access (PT2; Boston Scientific, Natick, MA, USA) was passed into the catheter from above (Figure 11.3b) in order to convert the angioplasty from retrograde to antegrade. The 4Fr catheter was removed and the 0.014 inch wire was advanced into the distal lateral plantar artery. Then the PTA was dilated with a long (3mm × 150mm) low-profile balloon (Coyote; Boston Scientific, Natick, MA, USA) with a very good angiographic result (Figure 11.4).

The completion angiogram shows brisk antegrade flow to the foot supplied from both the posterior tibial and the peroneal artery, and the plantar branches are directly supplying the pedal arch. The patient was prescribed dual antiplatelet therapy for six months. Duplex ultrasound surveillance three months later showed that both vessels were patent without any significant restenosis and there was progressive healing of the wound.

**Expert comment**

Despite the different theories concerning 'the right vessel to treat' when dealing with the healing of an ulcer, a vascular interventionist should always bear in mind the motto 'treat as many vessels as possible and safe to do'.

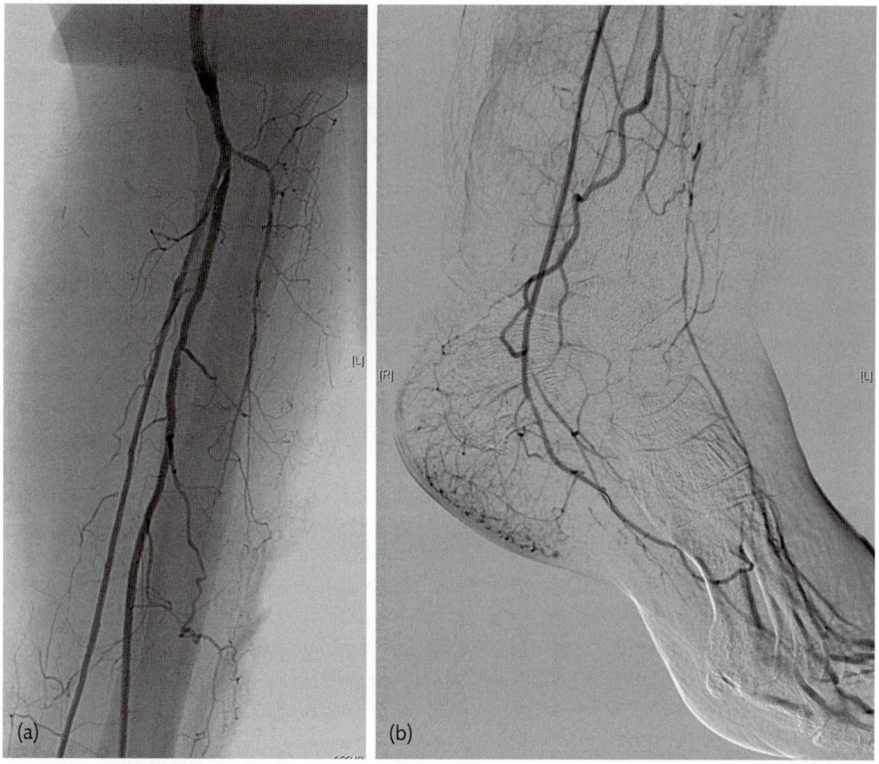


**Figure 11.4** Completion angiogram: posterior tibial artery patent from the bifurcation (a) down to the foot (b).

## Discussion

Infra-popliteal angioplasty is now the method of choice for treating below the knee lesions in CLI patients [4–6]. Furthermore, arterial occlusive disease in the setting of CLI may be multilevel affecting even the distal tibial vessels in the region below the ankle. Of interest, isolated inframalleolar lesions may be present in as many as 5% of the cases [7]. Patency of the superficial femoral artery or proximal tibial vessels may be compromised if treatment of the run-off vessels is not pursued [8]. As the surgical approach to land a distal bypass anastomosis on vessels like the plantar or the dorsalis pedis artery may be challenging, if not impossible, because of the atheromatous nature of these vessels or their complete absence, interventional techniques have been developed to become a valid alternative treatment. However, evidence for that hypothesis is not strong enough as only a small number of studies have been published so far; nonetheless, they demonstrate that interventional treatment, either intraluminal or subintimal, of below the ankle arteries is feasible and safe [7,9–13]. Additionally, the applicability of new technologies such as drug-eluting stents, self-expandable drug-eluting stents, or drug-coated balloons and their possible superiority over 'traditional' angioplasty remains to be investigated and proved.

The calibre of small vessels is the main reason for the delay in focus on the infra-inguinal region, which in turn explains the lack of evidence. So far, below ankle angioplasty has been reserved for the exceptional treatment of complications like distal embolism or dissection [13–15]. Only recently has the introduction of dedicated devices and low-profile balloons allowed infra-malleolar endovascular treatment and the development of new access techniques such as SAFARI, the pedal–plantar loop, and even the trans-collateral retrograde approach provided that the vessel diameter is adequate.

**Expert comment**

When manoeuvring with catheters and wires in the fine vessels of the delicate infra-malleolar region, the operator should be aware of the anatomical changes following foot movement. As the plantar and dorsal flexion of the ankle joint has the ability of angulation of up to 90° the soft tissue anatomical structures and the vessels also comply with this movement. Therefore, as well as fixing the foot in the appropriate anatomical position depending on the vessel treated (i.e. plantar flexion for the dorsalis pedis artery and dorsal flexion for the plantar artery), one should also avoid stenting these areas.

In 1987, Taylor and Palmer [1] published their work on angiosomes (Figure 11.5). Since then, many fields of medicine adapted their treatment strategies by taking this approach into consideration. Nevertheless, there are only few studies investigating whether the angiosome concept is of use when planning the vascular treatment of a foot in order to improve ulcer healing or limb salvage rates [16–21]. The question is whether a direct revascularization, which establishes a straight vascular line to

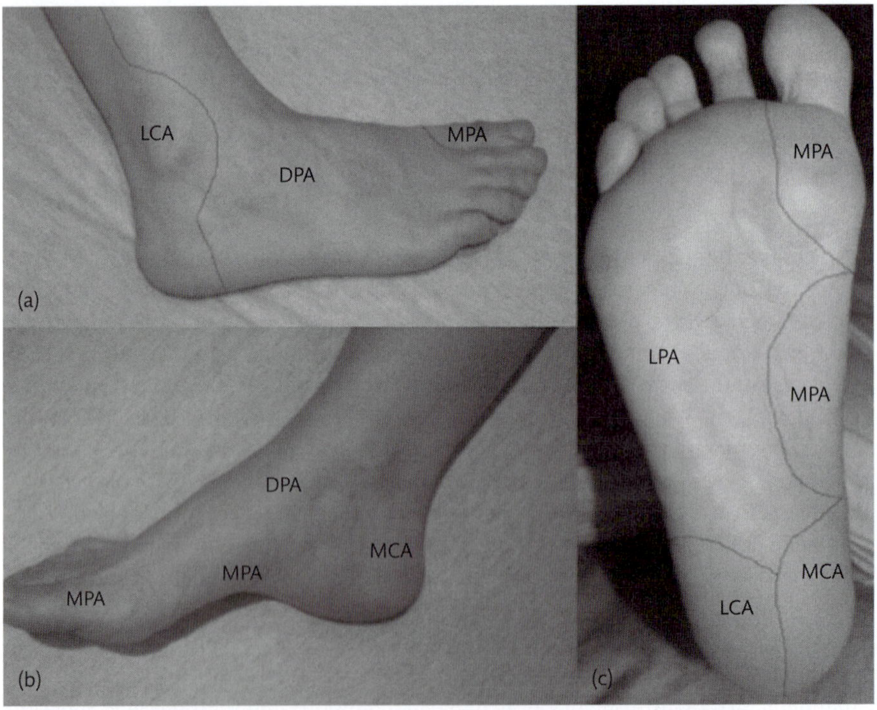


**Figure 11.5** Vascular distribution of the foot according to the angiosome concept: (a) lateral view; (b) medial view; (c) plantar view. LCA, lateral calcaneal artery; DPA, dorsalis pedis artery: MPA, medial plantar artery; MCA, medial calcaneal aretry: LPA, lateral plantar artery.

the ulcer site, would give a higher ulcer healing rate (or lower healing failure) than an indirect revascularization, which treats a tibial vessel that does not supply the angiosome of the ulcer.

## A final word from the expert

In the case presented here, the ulcerated region was fed by collaterals from the PA and not by the main 'direct' feeding vessel of the corresponding angiosome, which is the PTA. The improvement of the ulcer at three months suggests that the angiosome directed healing strategy followed may be beneficial. As noted, support for this theory is based mainly on retrospective data collection. Alternatively, there is evidence of ulcer healing in the presence of a patent arch with functioning collaterals and no patent direct flow line [22–24]. Everyday practice lies between these two theories. The interventionist attempts to improve blood supply to the foot using the maximum number of vessels and in the safest way given the individual circumstances. However, as these patients usually present with only one patent vessel, which is frequently diseased, an attempt to repair even this single vessel may be catastrophic, i.e. in the case of failure acute ischaemia may occur and it may be necessary to amputate the limb Therefore the benefits of such an interventional procedure should be balanced against its high risks and discussed with the patient beforehand. In conclusion, patent infra-malleolar vessels not only establish blood flow to the foot but also improve the patency of treated SFA or tibial vessels. An interventionist should always aim for the maximum number of patent vessels to the foot, ideally including the one supplying the area of tissue loss, provided that it is deemed safe to pursue their recanalization,. The new techniques available for this purpose should be applied wisely and after taking into consideration not only the intended benefits but also the associated risks.

## References


1. Taylor GI, Palmer JH. The vascular territories (angiosomes) of the body: experimental study and clinical applications. *Br J Plast Surg* 1987; 40(2): 113–41.
2. Spinosa DJ, Harthun NL, Bissonette EA, et al., Subintimal arterial flossing with antegrade-retrograde intervention (SAFARI) for subintimal recanalization to treat chronic critical limb ischemia. *J Vasc Interv Radiol* 2005; 16(1): 37–44.
3. Iyer SS, Dorros G, Zaitoun R, Lewin RF. Retrograde recanalization of an occluded posterior tibial artery by using a posterior tibial cutdown: two case reports. Cathet Cardiovasc Diagn 1990; 20: 251–3.
4. Siablis D, Karnabatidis D, Katsanos K, et al. Infrapopliteal application of sirolimus-eluting versus bare metal stents for critical limb ischemia: analysis of long-term angiographic and clinical outcome. *J Vasc Interv Radiol* 2009; 20(9): 1141–50.
5. Hirsch AT, Haskal ZJ, Hertzer NR, et al. ACC/AHA Guidelines for the Management of Patients with Peripheral Arterial Disease (lower extremity, renal, mesenteric, and abdominal aortic) *J Vasc Interv Radiol* 2006; 17(9): 1383–98.
6. Bosiers M, Hart JP, Deloose K, et al. Endovascular therapy as the primary approach for limb salvage in patients with critical limb ischemia: experience with 443 infrapopliteal procedures. *Vascular* 2006; 14(2): 63–9.
7. Katsanos K, Diamantopoulos A, Spiliopoulos S, et al. Below-the-ankle Angioplasty and stenting for limb salvage: anatomical considerations and long-term outcomes. *Cardiovasc Intervent Radiol* 2013; 36(4): 926–35.

8. Hasanadka R, Brown KR, Rilling WS, et al. The extent of lower extremity occlusive disease predicts short- and long-term patency following endovascular infrainguinal arterial intervention. *Am J Surg* 2008; 196(5): 629–33.
9. Zhu YQ, Zhao JG, Li MH, et al. Retrograde transdorsal-to-plantar or transplantar-to-dorsal intraluminal re-entry following unsuccessful subintimal angioplasty for below-the-ankle arterial occlusion. *J Endovasc Ther* 2010; 17(6): 712–21.
10. Zhu YQ, Zhao JG, Liu F, et al. Subintimal angioplasty for below-the-ankle arterial occlusions in diabetic patients with chronic critical limb ischemia. *J Endovasc Ther* 2009; 16(5): 604–12.
11. Abdelhamid MF, Davies RS, Rai S, et al. Below-the-ankle angioplasty is a feasible and effective intervention for critical leg ischaemia. *Eur J Vasc Endovasc Surg* 2010; 39(6): 762–8.
12. Kawarada O, Yokoi Y, Higashimori A, et al. Stent-assisted below-the-ankle angioplasty for limb salvage. *J Endovasc Ther* 2011; 18(1): 32–42.
13. Fusaro M, Tashani A, Mollichelli N, et al., Retrograde pedal artery access for below-the-knee percutaneous revascularisation. *J Cardiovasc Med (Hagerstown)* 2007; 8(3): 216–18.
14. Manzi M, Fusaro M, Ceccacci T, et al. Clinical results of below-the knee intervention using pedal-plantar loop technique for the revascularization of foot arteries. *J Cardiovasc Surg (Torino)* 2009; 50(3): 331–7.
15. Fusaro M, Dalla Paola L, Biondi-Zoccai G. Pedal-plantar loop technique for a challenging below-the-knee chronic total occlusion: a novel approach to percutaneous revascularization in critical lower limb ischemia. *J Invasive Cardiol* 2007. 19(2): E34–7.
16. Iida O, Nanto S, Uematsu M, et al. Importance of the angiosome concept for endovascular therapy in patients with critical limb ischemia. *Catheter Cardiovasc Interv* 2010: 75(6): 830–6.
17. Söderström M, Albäck A, Biancari F, et al. Angiosome-targeted infrapopliteal endovascular revascularization for treatment of diabetic foot ulcers. *J Vasc Surg* 2013; 57(2): 427–35.
18. Hoffmann U, Schulte KL, Heidrich H, et al. Complete ulcer healing as primary endpoint in studies on critical limb ischemia? A critical reappraisal. *Eur J Vasc Endovasc Surg* 2007; 33(3): 311–18.
19. Alexandrescu V, Vincent G, Azdad K. A reliable approach to diabetic neuroischemic foot wounds: below-the-knee angiosome-oriented angioplasty. *J Endovasc Ther* 2011; 18(3): 376–87.
20. Neville RF, Attinger CE, Bulan EJ, et al. Revascularization of a specific angiosome for limb salvage: does the target artery matter? *Ann Vasc Surg* 2009; 23(3): 367–73.
21. Azuma N, Uchida H, Kokubo T, et al. Factors influencing wound healing of critical ischaemic foot after bypass surgery: is the angiosome important in selecting bypass target artery? *Eur J Vasc Endovasc Surg* 2012; 43(3): 322–8.
22. Fossaceca R, Guzzardi G, Cerini P, et al. Endovascular treatment of diabetic foot in a selected population of patients with below-the-knee disease: is the angiosome model effective? *Cardiovasc Intervent Radiol* 2013; 36(3): 637–44.
23. Varela C, Acín F, de Haro J, et al. The role of foot collateral vessels on ulcer healing and limb salvage after successful endovascular and surgical distal procedures according to an angiosome model. *Vasc Endovascular Surg* 2010; 44(8): 654–60.
24. Dosluoglu HH, Cherr GS, Lall P, et al. Peroneal artery-only runoff following endovascular revascularizations is effective for limb salvage in patients with tissue loss. *J Vasc Surg* 2008; 48(1): 137–43.

SECTION 2

# Venous procedures

CASE

# 12 Dialysis access at risk: balloons or stent grafts?

**Stavros Spiliopoulos**

**Expert commentary** Dimitrios Karnabatidis

## Case history

A 34-year-old male was referred to the interventional radiology department with thrombosis of a straight brachiocephalic synthetic (PTFE) haemodialysis graft in the upper-arm. The diagnosis of the thrombotic event was based on clinical evaluation indicating an impalpable graft and inability to perform haemodialysis. The arteriovenous (AV) access had been created two months previously and the referring physician reported increased venous pressure during dialysis, indicating a possible stenosis, during the last two sessions before the thrombotic event. The patient's baseline demographics and dialysis access characteristics are presented in Table 12.1.

**Table 12.1 Patient's baseline demographics and dialysis access circuit characteristics**

| | |
|---|---|
| Gender | Male |
| Age | 34 years |
| Side of dialysis access | Right |
| Body region | Upper arm |
| Configuration of synthetic graft | Straight brachiocephalic |
| Graft age | 2 months |
| Cause of renal failure: | Unknown |

**Learning point**

The term 'graft monitoring' is used to describe the periodic (usually monthly) physical examination performed by a specialized healthcare professional, and the term 'surveillance' indicates the utilization of special instrumentation, such as Doppler ultrasound, for the assessment of dialysis access functionality. Physical examination should include inspection, palpation, and auscultation. Clinical signs of failing dialysis access detected during monitoring or surveillance include arm swelling, increased bleeding time following needle removal, pseudo-aneurysms, development of collateral vein network, altered characteristics of graft pulse or thrill, elevated venous pressure during dialysis, abnormal recirculation value, and intra-access blood flow <600ml/min. If access flow in a graft is <600ml/min, the patient should be referred for a fistulogram [1].

Two days after the thrombotic event the patient underwent a percutaneous dialysis access declotting procedure using a combined technique of trans-catheter thrombolysis with a bolus dose of alteplase 5mg (Actilyse®; Boehringer Ingelheim Ltd, Bracknell, UK) and mechanical thrombectomy using a 6Fr end-hole guide catheter and balloons as described in the literature [2] Following initial thrombectomy/thrombolysis, some remaining thrombus and an underlying stenosis was detected at the venous anastomotic site. Balloon angioplasty with a long (7 × 100mm) high-pressure balloon catheter (Dorado PTA balloon dilatator catheter; Bard Peripheral Vascular, Tempe, AZ, USA) was performed in order to attain both thrombus laceration and treatment of the underlying lesion. The balloon was inflated for three minutes. Final-check DSA following balloon angioplasty demonstrated a satisfactory result with adequate forward flow. Although a remaining stenosis due to elastic recoil was detected, it was appraised as non-significant and no further action was taken (Figure 12.1).

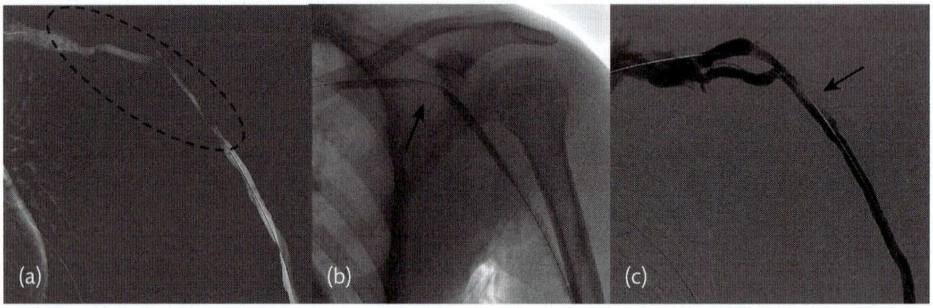


**Figure 12.1** AV graft declotting procedure. (a) Underlying lesion and compromised flow detected at the distal segment of the cephalic vein. (b) Balloon angioplasty with a 7 × 100mm high-pressure balloon catheter. Note that the site of stenosis is depicted during balloon inflation (arrow). (c) Final check DSA demonstrating a satisfactory graft outflow. However, some thrombus is visible within the previously treated cephalic vein segment (arrow).

**Learning point**

Graft thrombosis usually occurs because of an underlying stenosis and/or hypotension during dialysis session. The majority of underlying stenosis occurs at the venous anastomotic site; other stenotic causes are multiple access points at the same graft site leading to the development of fibrotic tissue and/or aneurysmal graft degeneration with concomitant thrombus formation [3]. The main advantage of percutaneous over surgical graft declotting is the ability to treat the underlying lesion, a fact that has been associated with increased access patency [2].

**Learning point**

Suboptimal balloon angioplasty resulting in remaining flow-limiting stenosis or type C flow-limiting dissection and/or rupture are indications for bail-out stenting [4].

The dialysis access was successfully recanalized and a thrill was palpable at the end of the procedure. However, the following day haemodialysis was performed through the jugular catheter as a thrill was no longer palpable. Three days after the declotting procedure the patient returned to the interventional radiology department for a diagnostic fistulogram which revealed a nearly 90% stenosis and intraluminal filling defects attributed to thrombus at the previously treated venous anastomotic site (Figure 12.2a). A 6Fr sheath was positioned, the lesion was crossed using a standard angled catheter, and a straight hydrophilic guidewire and balloon angioplasty was performed, again immediately using a 7 × 80mm high-pressure balloon (Figure 12.2b). However, the angioplasty result was unsatisfactory because of both elastic recoil and remaining thrombus (Figure 12.2c). The suboptimal angioplasty result as well as the fact that clinically significant restenosis occurred within a few days following the first angioplasty were considered as clear indications for the deployment of a covered stent at the point of restenosis. The sheath was subsequently upsized to 9Fr and an 8 × 80mm self-expandable PTFE-covered stent (FLUENCY® Plus vascular stent graft; Bard Peripheral Vascular, Helsingborg, Sweden) was deployed across the restenotic lesion (Figure 12.2d).

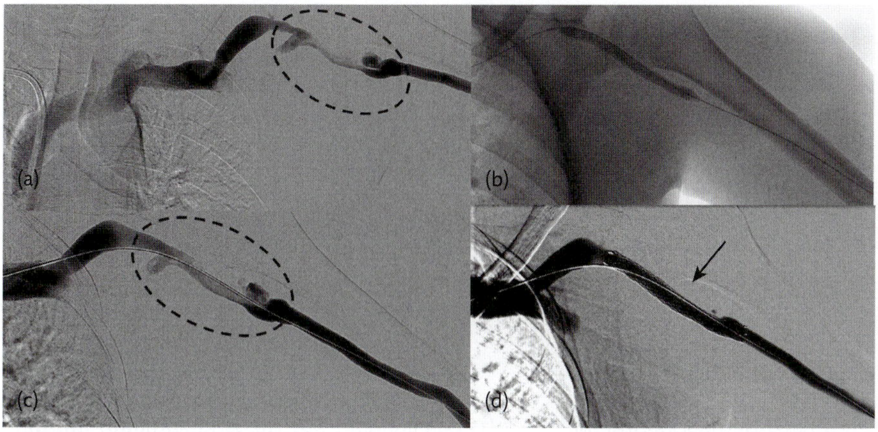


**Figure 12.2** Stenting procedure. (a) Venogram three days after AV graft declotting demonstrating a flow-limiting stenotic lesion and a significant amount of thrombus at the previously treated distal segment of the cephalic vein (dotted area). (b) Balloon angioplasty with a 7 × 80mm high-pressure balloon catheter. (c) Result of suboptimal angioplasty with remaining stenosis and filling defect indicating intraluminal thrombus (dotted area). (d) Final check DSA after the deployment of an 8 × 80mm covered stent across the lesion (arrow). Note that no remaining stenosis or filling defect is evident.

Antiplatelet therapy with clopidogrel 75mg 1 × 1 for life was prescribed and the patient entered in a strict follow-up protocol, which included clinical and imaging co-evaluation of the graft function using regular venograms every three months to assess the clinical importance of a possible stenosis. Check venograms were performed with a standard 23G butterfly needle and a maximum dose of 40ml of non-ionic contrast media. After six months follow-up the dialysis access was fully functional, and there was no angiographic evidence of >30% in-stent or in-graft restenosis (Figure 12.3).

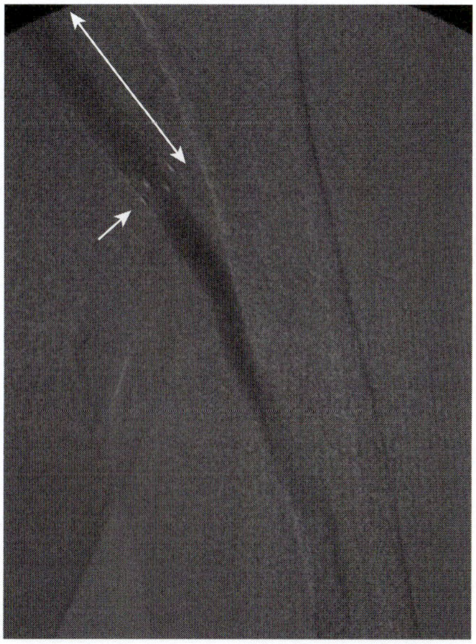

**Figure 12.3** Follow-up. Magnified DSA image at six months follow-up demonstrating the patency of the stent graft with no significant restenosis (double arrow). Note a <30% restenosis at the proximal bare end of the graft (arrow).

**Learning point**

Recent reports, including multicentre randomized trials, have provided high-level scientific evidence regarding the superior patency achieved following the deployment of stent grafts compared with bare metal stents and plain balloon PTA for the management of failing dialysis access [5,6].

**Expert comment**

It has been reported that the majority of restenotic lesions following covered stent deployment take place at the edges of the stent, while most of the late thrombotic events occur where the stent graft was deployed close to a venous valve, probably because of the development of turbulent blood flow [4]. Therefore, it is recommended that the stent graft should completely cover any adjacent venous valve.

**Expert comment**

Regular graft monitoring and surveillance is key to preserving AV access. Although Doppler ultrasound (DU) is considered to be an established method of graft surveillance, clinical experience indicates that in cases of vein stenosis situated more centrally (auxiliary and/or subclavian veins) it has limited diagnostic value. Even high-grade central lesions can remain clinically silent until thrombosis occurs. The fistulogram remains the gold standard for the detection of central stenosis. In addition, it can be performed using a fine 21G needle, which is almost non traumatic and well tolerated by the patients, and the total amount of diluted contrast media needed for the examination should not exceed 60ml. As a result, regular fistulograms performed every two to three months (depending on the case) are recommended as a post-procedural surveillance method, especially when reliable DU is not easily accessible.

## Discussion

Until recently balloon angioplasty was considered to be the gold standard minimal invasive percutaneous endovascular method for the management of failing dialysis access. Its main drawbacks are poor mid- and long-term patency rates [7,8]. The one-year primary patency rate following PTA in synthetic AV grafts is approximately 25% [9]. Several devices, such as cutting balloons, cryoplasty, and plain bare metal stents, have been proposed in the past in order to achieve superior graft patency. However, none of these provided patency rates superior to those obtained with plain balloon angioplasty [10–12]. Recently, novel self-expandable PTFE covered stents were introduced into everyday clinical practice following the superior patency outcomes achieved in a large-scale multicentre controlled trial. Haskal et al. [5] compared plain balloon angioplasty with PTA followed by the insertion of self-expandable covered stent grafts in venous anastomotic site stenosis of failing dialysis access. The six-month primary treatment site patency rate and primary access circuit patency rate were significantly superior (almost double) in the stent-graft group. In agreement with these results, Karnabatidis et al. [4] recently reported significantly superior primary patency rates and a decreased need for repeat procedures following stent-graft placement compared with plain balloon angioplasty (61.4% vs 8.6% at 12 months; $p < 0.0001$) in recurrently failing prosthetic arteriovenous grafts. Initial data reported by Chan et al. [13] following the utilization of a heparin-coated self-expandable stent graft demonstrated significantly superior six-month results compared with conventional stent grafts (57% vs 11%; $p = 0.06$).

**Evidence base** Stent graft versus balloon angioplasty for failing dialysis access grafts [14]

- Multicentre (13 study sites) randomized trial investigating 190 patients
- PTA (93 patients) vs PTA followed by stent-graft deployment (97 patients) at stenosed venous anastomosis sites of failing dialysis access
- At six months follow-up:
  - patency of the treatment area: 51% for grafts versus 23% for PTA ($p < 0.001$)
  - patency of the access circuit: 38% for grafts versus 20% for PTA ($p = 0.008$)
  - freedom from re-intervention: 32% for grafts versus 16% for PTA ($p = 0.03$)
  - binary restenosis: 78% for PTA versus 28% for grafts ($p < 0.001$

In the case reported here of a recently created synthetic AV dialysis graft at risk, the percutaneous declotting procedure was successful and the underlying stenosis at the anastomosis site was treated using high-pressure balloon angioplasty. Although in our department a primary stent-graft stent policy is followed for anastomotic lesions of failing synthetic AV dialysis, in this case, a high-pressure balloon angioplasty was chosen as the first-line treatment as this is a low-cost procedure for restenosis that can be repeated easily and safely. However, a thrill was not palpable 24 hours after declotting and angioplasty and a second balloon angioplasty attempt was not adequate. Based on the superior patency rates reported after covered stent use in stenosis at the anastomotic site of the AV graft, a self-expandable covered stent was deployed. Following covered stent positioning antiplatelet therapy with either clopidogrel 75mg 1 × 1 or aspirin 100mg 1 × 1 should be prescribed. Clopidogrel therapy is preferred in our department [4].

The patient was advised to undergo monthly monitoring and fistulogram surveillance every three months because of the central location of the stenotic lesion. After six months follow-up, only a minor clinically insignificant restenosis (<30%) was detected at the proximal end of the stent. The patient reports very satisfactory haemodialysis sessions and no clinical signs of failing AV access after monitoring for eight months.

**Clinical tip**

Some patients demonstrate resistance to clopidogrel. Moreover, renal failure has been indicated as an independent predictor of increased resistance to clopidogrel. As a result clopidogrel responsiveness should be tested and in cases of resistance to the drug alternative antiplatelet medication should be prescribed.

## A final word from the expert

Recent studies have reported superior patency rates compared with balloon angioplasty following covered stent use mainly in stenosis of the anastomotic site. Therefore the use of bare metal stents in such lesions is not recommended. In this case of a high-grade venous outflow stenosis resulting in thrombosis of the dialysis AV graft access, initial conventional balloon angioplasty following percutaneous declotting procedure was not clinically effective and resulted in immediate restenosis. The subsequent positioning of a self-expandable stent graft in the distal segment of the cephalic vein resulted in a six-month angiographic patency rate and eight-month clinical patency with excellent haemodialysis sessions. Another valid solution would be angioplasty using novel drug-coated balloon catheters, which have recently been reported to achieve significantly superior primary patency rates in venous stenotic lesions of failing dialysis access [14]. Clinical experience and current published data indicate that self-expandable stent grafts are currently the most effective solution to recurrent stenosis jeopardizing dialysis access.

Antiplatelet therapy should be administrated following stent-graft positioning. Frequent monitoring and surveillance are of the outmost importance for the conservation of patent dialysis access. Regular fistulograms are particularly advantageous in detecting central outflow lesions and are recommended as a valid surveillance modality which is safe and easy to perform. Repeat angioplasty procedures should be performed in cases of significant in-stent restenosis, even if clinically silent, as occlusions should be avoided.

## References

1. Rayner HC, Besarab A, Brown WW, et al. Vascular access results from the Dialysis Outcomes and Practice Patterns Study (DOPPS): performance against Kidney Disease Outcomes Quality Initiative (K/DOQI) Clinical Practice Guidelines. *Am J Kidney Dis* 2004; 44: 22–6.
2. Bent CL, Sahni VA, Matson MB. The radiological management of the thrombosed arteriovenous dialysis fistula. *Clin Radiol* 2011; 66(1): 1–12.

3. Kanterman RY, Vesely TM, Pilgram TK, et al. Dialysis access grafts: anatomic location of venous stenosis and results of angioplasty. *Radiology* 1995; 195: 135–9.
4. Karnabatidis D, Kitrou P, Spiliopoulos S, et al. Stent-grafts versus angioplasty and/or bare metal stents for failing arteriovenous grafts: a cross-over longitudinal study. *J Nephrol* 2013; 26(2): 389–95.
5. Haskal ZJ, Trerotola S, Dolmatch B, et al. Stent graft versus balloon angioplasty for failing dialysis-access grafts. *N Engl J Med* 2010; 362: 494–503.
6. Dolmatch BL. Stent graft versus balloon angioplasty for failing dialysis access grafts: a long-awaited advance in the treatment of permanent hemodialysis access. *J Vasc Access* 2010; 11: 89–91.
7. Lilly RZ, Carlton D, Barker J, et al. Predictors of arteriovenous graft patency after radiologic intervention in hemodialysis patients. *Am J Kidney Dis* 2001; 37: 945–53.
8. Asif A. Effectiveness and safety of dialysis vascular access procedures performed by interventional nephrologists. *Kidney Int* 2005; 67: 1634 (author reply).
9. Bittl JA. Catheter interventions for hemodialysis fistulas and grafts. *JACC Cardiovasc Interv* 2010; 3: 1–11.
10. Bakken AM, Protack CD, Saad WE, et al. Long-term outcomes of primary angioplasty and primary stenting of central venous stenosis in hemodialysis patients. *J Vasc Surg* 2007; 45:776–83.
11. Kariya S, Tanigawa N, Kojima H, et al. Percutaneous transluminal cutting-balloon angioplasty for hemodialysis access stenoses resistant to conventional balloon angioplasty. *Acta Radiol* 2006; 47:1017–21.
12. Clark TW. Nitinol stents in hemodialysis access. *J Vasc Interv Radiol* 2004; 15: 1037–40.
13. Chan MG, Miller FJ, Valji K, Kuo MD. Evaluation of expanded polytetrafluoroethylene-covered stents for the treatment of venous outflow stenosis in hemodialysis access grafts. *J Vasc Intervent Radiol* 2011; 22(5): 647–53.
14. Katsanos K, Karnabatidis D, Kitrou P, et al. Paclitaxel-coated balloon angioplasty vs. plain balloon dilation for the treatment of failing dialysis access: 6-month interim results from a prospective randomized controlled trial. *J Endovasc Ther* 2012; 19(2):263–72.

CASE

# 13 Phlegmasia cerulea dolens: percutaneous treatment

**Peter Mezes**

**Expert commentary** Narayan Karunanithy

## Case history

A 45-year-old male patient was transferred from his local A&E department where he had presented with severe pain and swelling of his left leg. His past medical history included type 2 diabetes and hypertension. On examination his leg was markedly oedematous, and cyanotic with multiple bullae around the knee and calf. The femoral arterial pulse was present but the peripheral pulses were not palpable. Venous duplex ultrasound scan of the limb demonstrated fresh occlusive thrombus extending from the central third of the superficial femoral vein to the external iliac vein. A diagnosis of phlegmasia cerulea dolens (PCD) was made. As the circulation to the limb was severely compromised, a multidisciplinary decision was made together with the on-call vascular surgical team to commence catheter-directed thrombolysis.

**Learning point**

Phlegmasia cerulea dolens (PCD) is a rare but severe consequence of lower limb deep vein thrombosis (DVT). It is defined as acute limb ischaemia due to complete obstruction of venous flow caused by extensive proximal, usually iliofemoral, thrombus. The sudden increase in venous pressure leads to translocation of fluid into the extravascular space. The raised intracompartmental pressure results in secondary arteriolar occlusion and venous gangrene. It is associated with a mortality rate of 20–40% and an amputation rate of 20–50% [1].

In PCD, the patient usually complains of unremitting pain and the limb is severely swollen, mottled, and cyanotic. Pulses are not palpable, but arterial flow is detectable by Doppler. As a result of fluid translocation, epidermal bullae can develop. Fluid depletion can be severe, leading to shock. Sensorimotor deficit is usually a sign of iminent gangrene. PCD should be distinguished from phlegmasia alba dolens in which venous collaterals remain patent and provide enough venous return to prevent tissue ischaemia. This is usually a preceding stage to PCD, and the main difference in manifestation is blanching of the limb without cyanosis [1].

After written informed consent had been obtained, the patient was brought to the interventional radiology suite and placed in a prone position. The popliteal fossa was cleaned and draped. An ultrasound scan showed a dilated but patent popliteal vein with markedly reduced flow. Popliteal vein access was gained with a 21G micropuncture needle (Cook Medical, Limerick, Ireland), and a 5Fr sheath (Cordis, Waterloo, Belgium) was introduced using the Seldinger technique. A venogram performed through the sheath confirmed the presence of occlusive thrombus from the superficial femoral vein to the external iliac vein; the common iliac vein and the inferior vena cava (IVC) were patent and thrombus free (Figure 13.1). An

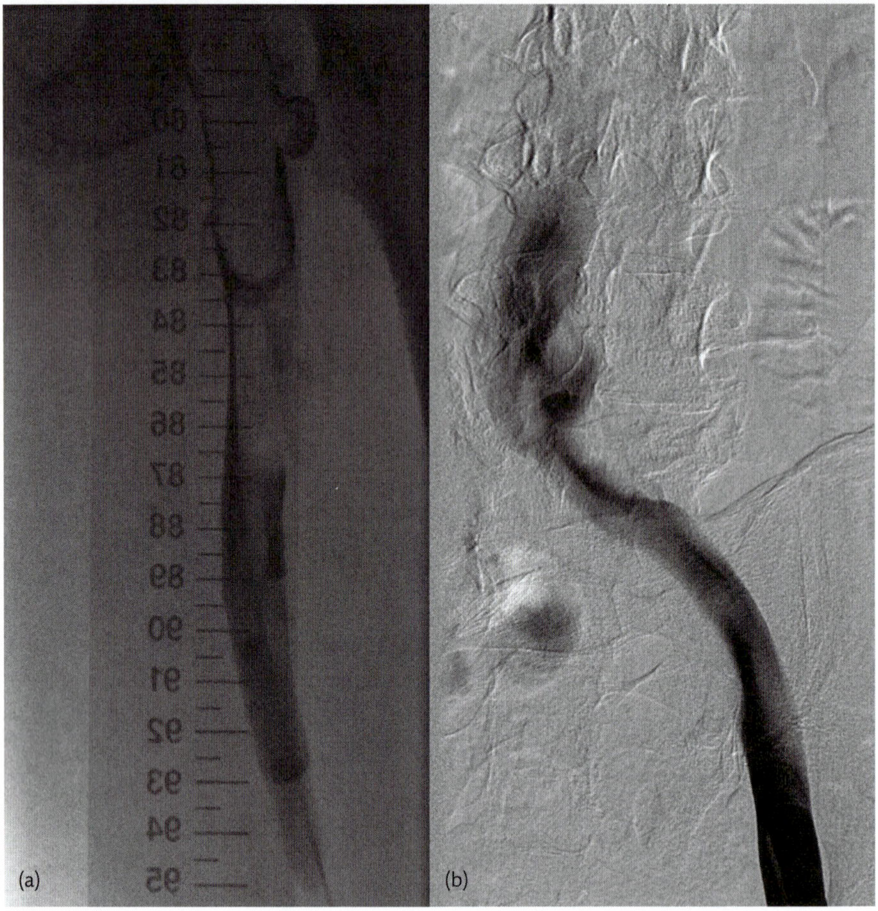


**Figure 13.1** (a) Venogram performed from the catheter in the superficial femoral vein shows occlusive filling defects in keeping with thrombus in the superficial and common femoral veins; (b) the common iliac vein and IVC were clear.

angled hydrophilic guidewire (Terumo UK Ltd, Egham, UK) and a staight 4Fr catheter with side-holes (Cordis, Waterloo, Belgium) were used to cross the thrombosed segment and advanced into the IVC. The thrombosed segment was laced with 5mg rtPA injected whilst withdrawing the catheter. The catheter tip was then placed at the caudal extent of the thrombus and an rtPA infusion was commenced at a rate of 1mg/hour. A heparin infusion was administered at 200IU/h through the 5Fr sheath. The puncture site was covered with sterile dressing and the patient was transferred to the high dependency unit for close observation.

> **Learning point**
>
> Anticoagulation prevents thrombus propagation and lowers the risk of of pulmonary embolism (PE). In patients treated with anticoagulation alone, thrombus resolution occurs through a natural process of organization and vein recanalization. In proximal DVT, particularly when there is large thrombus load, there is a potential for the mechanism of thrombus resolution to be overwhelmed [2].

The patient's symptoms dramatically improved on asessment at three hours, and at the time the check angiogram was performed (12 hours) the leg oedema had markedly reduced and skin colour was noted to be normal. A venogram revealed that inline flow had been restored but significant adherent clot was still present (Figure 13.2). Catheter-directed thrombolysis (CDT) was continued for a further 24 hours but this resulted in no further reduction in thrombus burden. As the patient had become asymptomatic at this stage a decision was made to stop thrombolysis.

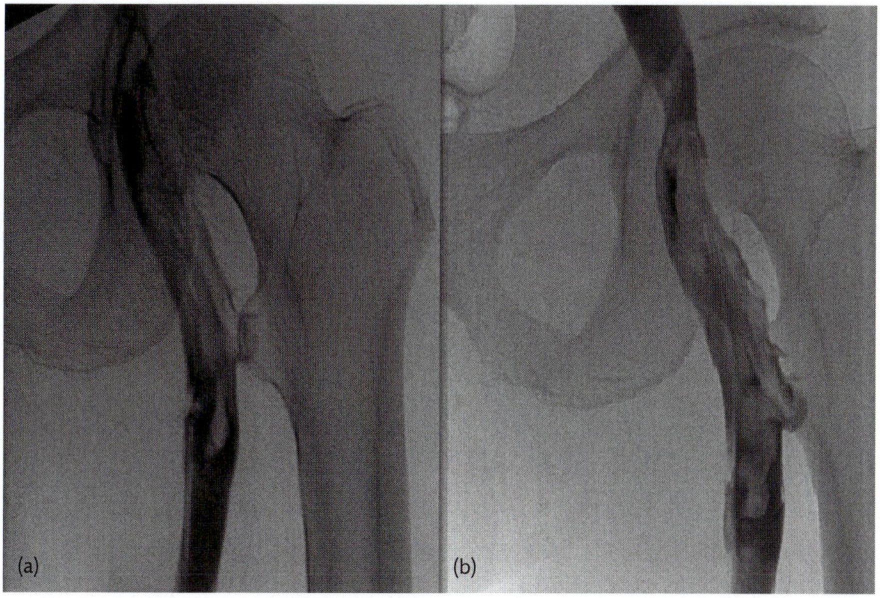


**Figure 13.2** (a) Check angiogram 12 hours after initiation of thrombolysis showed restoration of flow with residual thrombus; (b) angiogram after 36 hours revealed no further improvement.

**Evidence base** Additional catheter-directed thrombolyis versus anticoagulation alone for treatment of iliofemoral DVT

**CaVenT trial [3,4]**

- Open-label prospective randomized control trial
- Anticoagulation only ($n$ = 108) (control) versus CDT plus anticoagulation ($n$ = 101)
- Primary outcomes measured were iliofemoral vein patency at six months and frequency of post thrombotic syndrome (PTS) as assessed by the Villalta score at 24 months
- At six months the iliofemoral vein patency was 65.9% in the CDT group versus 47.4% in the control group ($p$ = 0.012)
- At 24 months the incidence of PTS was 41.1% in the CDT group versus 55.6% in the control group ($p$ = 0.047) which represented an absolute risk reduction of 14.4%
- Twenty bleeding complications related to CDT were reported including three major and five clinically relevant bleeds

**Egypt trial [5]**

- Open-label prospective randomized control trial
- Anticoagulation only ($n$ = 17) versus CDT plus anticoagulation ($n$ = 18)
- Primary outcomes were iliofemoral vein patency and deep venous reflux at six months
- The patency rate was 72% versus 12% in the control group ($p$ < 0.001), and the venous reflux was 11% in the CDT group compared with 41% in the control group ($p$ = 0.04)
- No major bleeding complications and no mortality were reported.

The patient had a full haematological assessment. Thrombophilia screening and search for an occult malignancy were both negative. The patient was anticoagulated and discharged home.

After a symptom-free period of 35 days the patient was readmitted to hospital with recurrent left leg swelling and pain which were less pronounced than on the

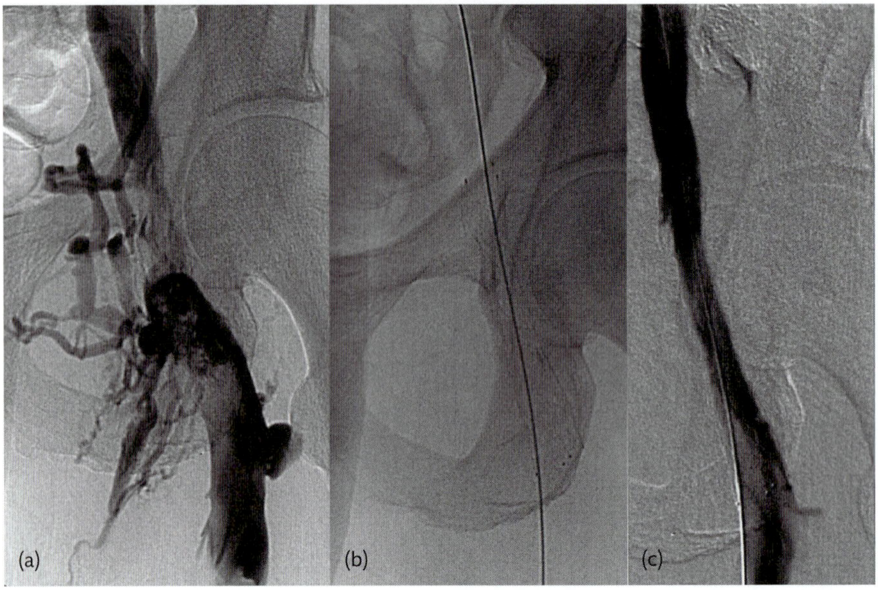


**Figure 13.3** (a) Venogram at time of readmission showed stenosis of the common femoral vein with copious collateral vessel filling. (b) Following pharmacomechanical thrombectomy to remove residual thrombus a self-expanding bare metal stent was inserted and (c) inline flow was established with obliteration of the collateral vessels.

previous admission. Venous duplex ultrasound showed recurrent thrombus occluding the common femoral and external iliac veins. The patient was taken to the interventional radiology suite again, and a venogram performed through the popliteal vein showed occlusion of the common femoral and external iliac veins with numerous collateral vessels (Figure 13.3). Pharmacomechanical thrombectomy was performed to remove the thrombus. Once the thrombus was cleared, an underlying stenosis of the distal external iliac/common femoral veins was revealed. This lesion was treated by placement of a 14mm × 8cm self-expanding bare metal stent (Zilver Vena; Cook Medical, Limerick, Ireland). The completion angiogram showed that unrestricted inline flow had been re-established and the collateral vessels were no longer opacified.

The patient's symptoms improved within hours post procedure and he was restarted on warfarin therapy. During the follow-up of three months the patient remained symptom free and the stent remained patent.

**Expert comment**

In the presence of iliofemoral DVT, there is invariably an underlying lesion in the affected segment of vein. In order to prevent recurrence it is vital that the lesion is identified and treated effectively. In this case it is likely that DVT recurred because the lesion in the external iliac vein had not been effectively treated.

## Discussion

Deep vein thrombosis is a common and potentially lethal disorder which can result in significant long-term morbidity and economic cost. The incidence of DVT is estimated to be 145 per 100,000 population [6]. The early clinical consequences of iliofemoral DVT include pain, swelling, PE, and rarely venous gangrene. In the longer term there is an approximately 25% risk of developing PTS and a 10% risk of venous ulceration [7]. The economic burden to the United Kingdom of treating this condition is estimated to be £640 million per year [6]. It is hoped that early recognition and effective treatment will be able to alleviate the early and late sequelae of this condition.

Anticoagulation alone may not be enough to treat extensive iliofemoral DVT as the body's own mechanisms to resolve thrombus burden may be overwhelmed. Surgical thrombectomy has been shown to improve vein patency and reduce the incidence of PTS [8,9].

**Evidence base** Surgical thrombectomy versus anticoagulation for iliofemoral DVT [8,9]

- Prospective randomized control trial
- Surgical thrombectomy ($n$ = 31) versus anticoagulation only ($n$ = 32)
- Primary outcomes were venous patency at six months and incidence of leg swelling at six months and 10 years
- At six months, the venous patency was 76% in the thrombectomy group compared with 35% in the anticoagulation group ($p < 0.025$), and incidence of leg swelling was 58% in the thrombectomy group compared with 93% in the anticoagulation group
- At 10 years the incidences of leg swelling and ulcers were 46% and 8%, respectively, in the thrombectomy group compared with 71% and 18%, respectively, in the anticoagulation group.

Catheter-directed techniques have recently emerged as a safe and effective alternative to surgical thrombectomy for managing this condition. The CaVenT and Egypt trials have both shown benefits for CDT over anticoagulation alone [4,5]. However, CDT still requires expensive intensive care monitoring for 48–72 hours. Pharmacomechanical thrombectomy (PMT) combines thrombolytic therapy, either catheter directed or administered through the device itself, and mechanical thrombectomy. Various mechanical thrombectomy devices are available and can be categorized based on their mechanism of action. The most popular of these are rheolytic (AngioJet®, MEDRAD, Warrendale, PA, USA), rotational (Trellis™, Covidien, Mansfield, MA, USA) and ultrasound accelerated (EkoSonic®, Ekos Corporation, Bothwell, WA, USA) devices [10].

Two retrospective studies have evaluated PMT as an adjunct to CDT [11,12]. Both studies reported similar clot lysis rates in patients treated with PMT compared with CDT. However the adjunctive use of PMT was associated with significant reduction in treatment time, dose of thrombolytic agent required, intensive treatment unit/hospital stay, and cost. The cost estimates for PMT were \$47,742 ± \$19,247 versus CDT \$85,301 ± \$24,832 ($p < 0.01$). PMT has also been shown to be safe and effective in a study evaluating its use in patients with contraindications to thrombolysis. Currently there are two ongoing randomized controlled trials (ATTRACT and PEARL) that aim to evaluate the early and late outcomes of iliofemoral DVT treated with PMT [13].

The current American College of Chest Physician guidelines recommend PMT in preference to CDT for patients with extensive proximal DVT, good functional status, and low risk of bleeding (Grade 2C). For patients who are at low risk of bleeding, CDT or PMT is preferred to surgical thrombectomy (Grade 2C) [14].

The use of IVC filters in the management of iliofemoral DVT is controversial at present. Whilst there is an increased risk of PE in patients with iliofemoral DVT, treatment with CDT does not appear to increase the risk of symptomatic PE. There may be a higher risk of clot embolism when PMT is employed because of the additional use of the mechanical component for clot dispersion. However the reported incidence of PE with use of the AngioJet® PMT device was 0.3% in the PEARL Registry [15]. Hence the routine use of IVC filters is not recommended. The presence of IVC thrombus, significant PE, and right heart strain at the commencement of treatment are instances when use of a retrievable IVC filter needs to be strongly considered [16]. It is also important that if an IVC filter is placed, it is removed within six weeks.

It is our experience that once the thrombectomy is performed there is invariably an underlying stenotic lesion. Meticulous care needs to be used to identify and treat these lesions. Most lesions are visible on single-projection venography by the presence of luminal narrowing and/or opacification of pelvic collateral vessels. On occasion multiple oblique projections are required to identify the lesion [17]. Intravascular ultrasound (IVUS) has been shown to be a promising technique that is superior to single-plane venography in detection of lesion morphology and degree of stenosis [18]. Because of the high incidence of vessel recoil after plain balloon angioplasty, stenotic lesions are most often treated with large-diameter (14–18mm) self-expanding bare metal stents. The primary, assisted primary, and secondary patency rates at three years for bare metal stents used to treat iliofemoral venous lesions are 75%, 92%, and 93%, respectively [19].

**Clinical tip**

When stenting of the iliofemoral vein segment is performed the following are useful tips.

1. Ensure that large-diameter stents are used, typically 18–24mm in the IVC, 14–18mm in the common iliac vein, and 12–16mm in the external iliac vein.
2. Aim for coverage of the entire lesion with generous upper and lower overlap. Extension of the stent across the confluence of the common iliac veins and into the IVC does not appear to result in adverse outcome and in fact reduces the risk of stent migration resulting in early restenosis [20].
3. If two or more stents are required, deploy the lower stent first and build up to and into the IVC as required. Post dilatation of the first stent deployed prior to placement of the second stent will ensure that foreshortening does not result in under-coverage.

## A final word from the expert

Iliofemoral DVT is a debilitating and often under-treated condition. Advances in endovascular tools and techniques have given us the ability to manage this condition more effectively. Familiarity with the clinical condition, as well as the application of the tools and their potential benefits and drawbacks, needs to be gained.

## References

1. Suwanabol PA, Tefera G, Schwarze ML. Syndromes associated with the deep veins: phlegmasia cerulea dolens, May-Thurner syndrome, and nutcracker syndrome. *Perspect Vasc Surg Endovasc Ther* 2010; 22(4): 223–30.
2. Saha P, Humphries J, Modarai B, et al. Leukocytes and the natural history of deep vein thrombosis: current concepts and future directions. *Arterioscler Thromb Vasc Biol* 2011; 31: 506–512.
3. Enden T, Kløw NE, Sandvik L, et al. Catheter-directed thrombolysis vs. anticoagulant therapy alone in deep vein thrombosis: results of an open randomized, controlled trial reporting on short-term patency. *J Thromb Haemost* 2009; 7(8): 1268–75.

4. Enden T, Haig Y, Kløw NE, et al. Long-term outcome after additional catheter-directed thrombolysis versus standard treatment for acute iliofemoral deep vein thrombosis (the CaVenT study): a randomized controlled trial. *Lancet* 2012; 379(9810): 31–8.
5. Elsharawy M, Elzayat E. Early results of thrombolysis vs anticoagulation in iliofemoral venous thrombosis. A randomised clinical trial. *Eur J Vasc Endovasc Surg* 2002; 24(3): 209–14
6. House of Commons Health Committee. *The Prevention of Venous Thromboembolism in Hospitalised Patients* (London: Stationery Office); 2005.
7. Kearon C. Natural history of venous thromboembolism. *Circulation* 2003; 107(Suppl 1): I22–30
8. Plate G, Einarsson E, Ohlin P, et al. Thrombectomy with temporary arteriovenous fistula: the treatment of choice in acute iliofemoral venous thrombosis. *J Vasc Surg* 1984; 1(6): 867–76.
9. Plate G, Eklöf B, Norgren L, et al. Venous thrombectomy for iliofemoral vein thrombosis-10-year results of a prospective randomised study. *Eur J Vasc Endovasc Surg* 1997; 14(5): 367–74.
10. Karunanithy N, Mezes P, Spiliopoulos S, et al. Acute deep venous thrombosis in the lower limb. In RM Greenhalgh, (ed.), *Vascular and Endovascular Controversies Update* (London: BIBA); 2012: 659–65.
11. Lin PH, Zhou W, Dardik A, et al. Catheter-direct thrombolysis versus pharmacomechanical thrombectomy for treatment of symptomatic lower extremity deep venous thrombosis. *Am J Surg* 2006; 192(6): 782–8.
12. Kim HS, Patra A, Paxton BE, et al. Catheter-directed thrombolysis with percutaneous rheolytic thrombectomy versus thrombolysis alone in upper and lower extremity deep vein thrombosis. *Cardiovasc Intervent Radiol* 2006; 29(6): 1003–7
13. Acute Venous Thrombosis: Thrombus Removal With Adjunctive Catheter-Directed Thrombolysis (ATTRACT): Clinical Trials Identifier NCT00790335.
14. Kearon C, Kahn SR, Agnelli G, et al. Antithrombotic therapy for venous thromboembolic disease: American College of Chest Physicians Evidence-Based Clinical Practice Guidelines (8th edition). *Chest* 2008; 133(6 Suppl): 454S–545S.
15. Lookstein R. Rheolytic thrombectomy for deep vein thrombosis: prospective multi-center registry report. Society of Interventional Radiology; 2012.
16. O'Sullivan GJ. The role of interventional radiology in the management of deep venous thrombosis: advanced therapy. *Cardiovasc Intervent Radiol* 2011; 34(3): 445–61.
17. Neglén P, Raju S. Proximal lower extremity chronic venous outflow obstruction: recognition and treatment. *Semin Vasc Surg* 2002; 15(1): 57–64.
18. Neglén P, Thrasher TL, Raju S. Venous outflow obstruction: an underestimated contributor to chronic venous disease. *J Vasc Surg* 2003; 38(5): 879–85.
19. Neglén P, Hollis KC, Olivier J, et al. Stenting of the venous outflow in chronic venous disease: long-term stent-related outcome, clinical, and hemodynamic result. *J Vasc Surg* 2007; 46(5): 979–90.
20. Vedantham S, Vesely TM, Sicard GA, et al. Pharmacomechanical thrombolysis and early stent placement for iliofemoral deep vein thrombosis. *J Vasc Interv Radiol* 2004; 15(6): 565–74.

CASE

# 14 IVC filters and anticoagulation

**Christopher Burke and Miltiadis Krokidis**

**Expert commentary** Hanno Hoppe

## Case history

A 65-year-old man presented to the A&E department with pleuritic chest pain and dyspnoea over the course of the previous two days. There was a history of a moderate amount of sputum in which he had noticed some intermittent streaks of blood. Two weeks previously he had undergone elective anterior resection for adenocarcinoma of the sigmoid colon and he had only returned home four days ago. He had never experienced such an episode before. Incidentally he had noticed swelling of his left leg over the past two weeks. He denied fevers or chills and otherwise felt well.

There was a history of treated hypertension and hypercholesterolaemia. He was taking bendroflumethiazide (2.5mg once daily) and simvastatin (20mg nocte). He had also suffered a subarachnoid haemorrhage five years previously. This had only required admission for neurological observations, and a small circle of Willis aneurysm was identified on CT angiography. However, no intervention had been performed and he was being managed with regular follow-up and interval imaging. There was a family history of coronary heart disease in his father. He had smoked five to ten cigarettes daily for 30 years but rarely drank alcohol.

In the A&E department he was afebrile and his oxygen saturation was 95%. Arterial blood gas demonstrated a pH of 7.35, $O_2$ of 9.6kPa, $CO_2$ of 4.9kPa, and $HCO_3$ of 24mEq/L. Inflammatory markers were not raised. Blood biochemistry and haematology was unremarkable. ECG demonstrated no acute ischaemia or evidence of right heart strain. Anteroposterior chest radiography demonstrated mild emphysematous changes but did not reveal any focal consolidation or collapse, and the cardiomediastinal contour was within normal limits.

In the clinical decision unit (CDU) the patient was referred for a CT pulmonary angiogram which demonstrated multiple filling defects on the right pulmonary artery consistent with pulmonary embolism (PE) (Figure 14.1). He was admitted and immediately commenced on low molecular weight heparin. Ultrasonography of the lower limbs performed the next day confirmed thrombus within the left common iliac vein. The patient was admitted under the general medical team for management of his acute PE and deep vein thrombosis (DVT). Because of his recent surgery and history of subarachnoid haemorrhage the decision was made not to anticoagulate with warfarin but to continue the low molecular weight heparin and refer to interventional radiology for placement of a retrievable inferior vena cava (IVC) filter.

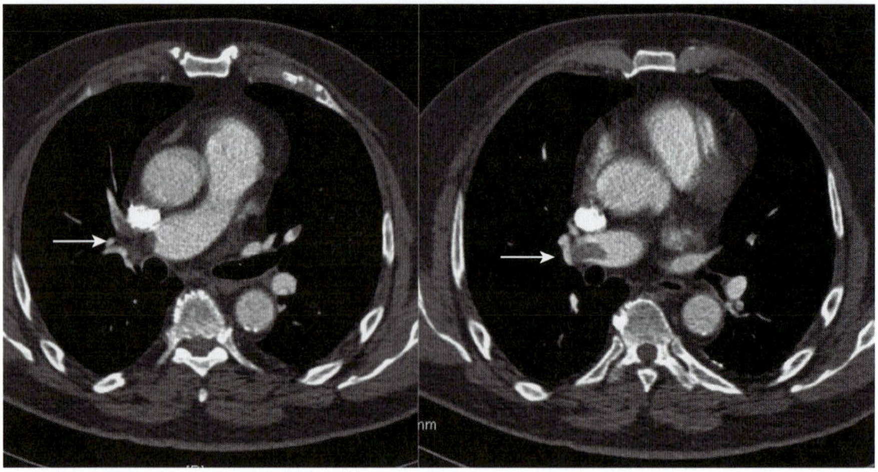

**Figure 14.1** CT scan showing the presence of filling defects in the right pulmonary artery and confirming pulmonary embolism.

**Learning points** Contraindications to oral anticoagulation

- Absolute contraindications:
  - acute intracerebral haemorrhage
  - subarachnoid haemorrhage as a result of intracranial aneurysm
  - haematomyelia
  - current or recent major gastrointestinal haemorrhage
  - structural lesions at high risk of bleeding (e.g. oesophageal varices).
- Relative contraindications:
  - recent (within two weeks) major surgery
  - major trauma including cardiopulmonary resuscitation (CPR)
  - deep biopsy
  - uncontrolled hypertension
  - renal or hepatic disease
  - bleeding diatheses.

Warfarin is contraindicated for anticoagulation in pregnancy because of teratogenicity.

**Expert comment**

In this patient with venous thromboembolism (VTE) a decision was made against oral anticoagulation and for IVC filter placement based on a history of previous major surgery within a two-week interval and remote subarachnoid haemorrhage, which are relative indications for optional IVC filter placement according to current guidelines [1]. In addition, this patient was reported to have proximal DVT of his left common iliac vein, which is also considered a relative indication for IVC filter placement, especially if this thrombus was free floating. In this case, it was reasonable to use an optional IVC filter which can be retrieved once this patient can be fully anticoagulated. Filter retrieval is a minor percutaneous intervention via the internal jugular or femoral vein. It can be performed as outpatient procedure. Filter retrieval has a very low complication rate and should be performed with the patient being fully anticoagulated [2]. An interruption of anticoagulation may put the patient at unnecessary risk of PE, which should be avoided.

The procedure took place in the interventional radiology suite. Local anaesthesia and an aseptic technique were used. The right common femoral vein was checked with ultrasound (US) prior to the procedure to confirm that it was not occluded by thrombus. Access under US guidance was obtained and a 5Fr sheath was inserted. A pigtail catheter was advanced in the lower IVC and a venogram was performed to delineate the level of drainage of the renal veins (Figure 14.2a). A stiff wire was then advanced in the IVC and a filter (Celect; Cook Medical, Limerick, Ireland). was deployed in the portion of the IVC caudal to the insertion of the renal veins (Figure 14.2b).

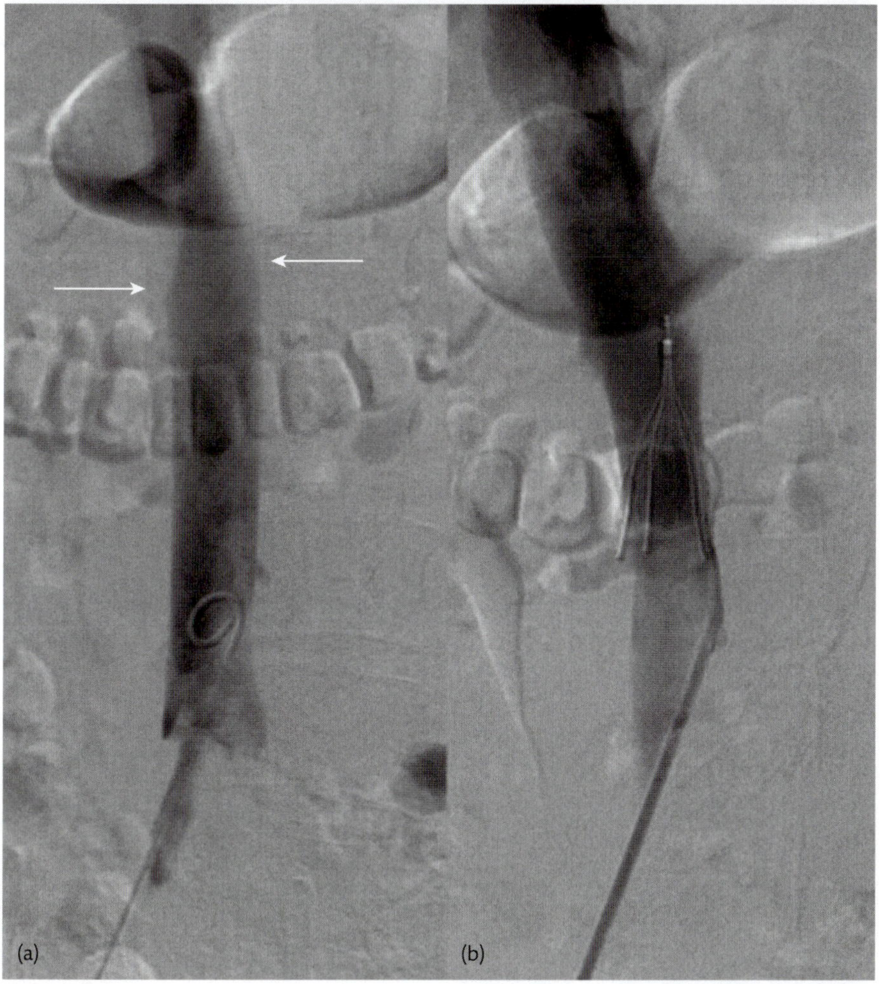


**Figure 14.2** (a) Venogram performed using a pigtail catheter via right common femoral vein access demonstrates patent IVC and location of the renal vein origins (arrows). (b) An IVC filter was deployed caudally to the drainage point of the renal veins.

The patient was kept on low molecular weight heparin for three months and then treatment with warfarin was decided. The filter was no longer necessary and was removed (Figure 14.3).

**Learning point** Cook Celect filter

The Celect IVC filter set consists of a non-magnetic filter (30mm diameter, 48mm long) pre-loaded on a femoral filter introducer, a 7.0Fr coaxial introducer system compatible with a 0.035 inch guidewire, and a hydrophilic-coated dilator. The introducer dilator has eight side-ports and two radio-opaque markers 30mm apart (end to end) to assist in guidance. A jugular introducer is also available in the kit, but the filter needs to be unloaded from the femoral introducer and loaded on the jugular introducer.

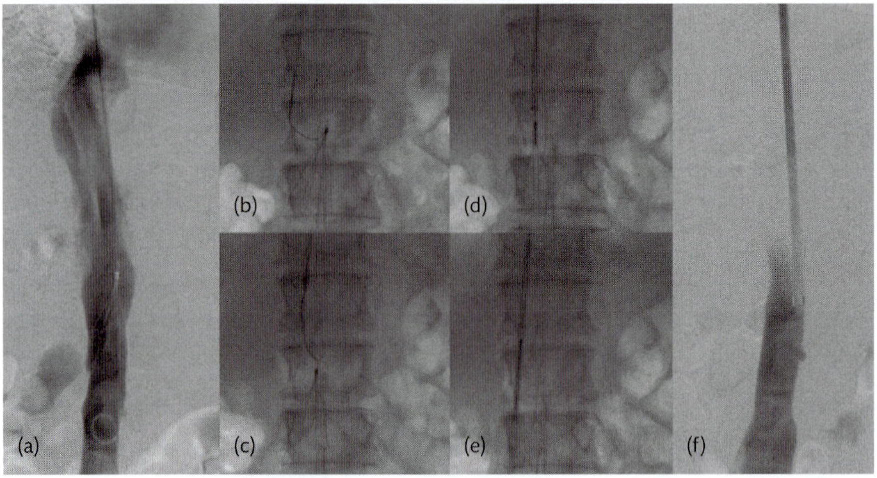


**Figure 14.3** (a) A venogram performed via a pigtail catheter inserted from the right internal jugular vein demonstrates a patent vena cava with no evidence of thrombus prior to removal. (b) A goose-neck snare was advanced within the hook of the device, (c) the snare was straightened without pulling the device cranially, (d) the sheath was slowly advanced forward, and (e) the legs of the filter were collapsed and the filter was successfully retrieved. (f) The post-retrieval venogram confirms that there were no complications.

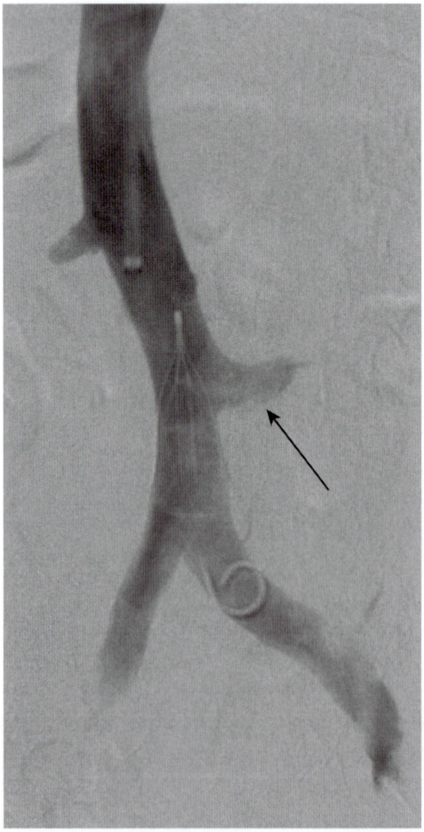

**Figure 14.4** A venogram through a pigtail catheter showing the presence of an anatomical variation of the left renal vein (arrow). An IVC filter was deployed caudally to the drainage point of the left renal vein from a right internal jugular access.

**Learning point**

A catheter-directed central venogram (cavagram) is usually performed prior to filter placement to ensure that the IVC is patent and free from thrombus, identify the origin of renal veins, to measure the caval diameter (ensure that there is no megacava >3cm), or identify any anatomical variants prior to deployment like the example illustrated in Figure 14.4. IVC filters are usually inserted via the right common femoral or right internal jugular routes. The standard placement of an IVC filter is, just below the renal veins to avoid renal vein thrombosis in the event of filter occlusion. The removal of temporary IVC filters differs depending on the brand of filter inserted. A coaxial sheath and a device to snare and grab the top hook are usually used; then the sheath is advanced over the top dome to collapse the legs and the device is retrieved within the sheath.

## Discussion

DVT and PE are major sources of morbidity and mortality, representing the clinical spectrum of VTE. VTE may occur spontaneously or as a common complication during and after hospitalization, as in this case.

The primary therapy for PE as a result of VTE is usually pharmacological, initially instigating subcutaneous low-dose heparin or low molecular weight heparin whilst oral warfarin is commenced and the target INR is reached [1–3]. However, there are contraindications to oral anticoagulation.

IVC filters are metal alloy devices that mechanically trap any fragmented emboli passing from the ileofemoral system through the IVC en route to the pulmonary arterial circulation. Modern devices are usually placed percutaneously via the right internal jugular vein or femoral veins. Several permanent and retrievable devices are commercially available. Filters are designed to be introduced (and in the case of retrievable filters, removed), with relatively low risk to even severely ill patients.

Permanent IVC filters have been available for over 35 years [4], and studies have demonstrated that their use has dramatically increased within the past 20 years [5,6]. Despite this, there is a lack of rigorous clinical studies. The majority of the literature comprises retrospective non-randomized case series.

**Expert comment**

There is a lack of prospectively randomized clinical studies because it would be unethical to allow only a subgroup of patients to have an IVC filter, since we have evidence that IVC filters significantly lower the risk of PE (e.g. the PREPIC study [7]). Angel et al. [8] have performed a systematic review of the use of retrievable IVC filters. Their meta-analysis included 37 studies, of which 11 were prospective, including a total of 6834 patients. They found that IVC filters were effective in preventing PE, but long-term complications (>30 days) were a serious concern (e.g. perforation, migration, filter fracture). According to these findings IVC filter retrieval should be initiated as soon as possible and aggressive follow-up is necessary to ensure that filters are not left in place unnecessarily [9], especially in elderly patients who may be asymptomatic and not understand the reason for IVC filter retrieval [10].

Filters were initially intended for a small group of patients who had VTE and a contraindication to anticoagulation, a complication of anticoagulation, inability to achieve adequate anticoagulation, or recurrent PE despite anticoagulation. The indications have been expanded to include some patients with high VTE risk but no evidence of VTE [5,6]. The availability of retrievable filter designs extends the clinical utility for IVC filters.

Indications now include prophylactic use in patients with major trauma, patients undergoing hip or knee replacement, patients with compromised cardiopulmonary reserve (e.g. cor pulmonale or pulmonary hypertension), burn patients, patients undergoing thrombectomy, embolectomy, or thrombolysis, patients with free-floating iliofemoral thrombus, and pregnant women with DVT (see Table 14.1).

**Table 14.1** **Indications for IVC filtration and recommended filter type [11.12]**

| Indication | Type |
|---|---|
| Unequivocal | |
| • PE with contraindication to anticoagulation | Permanent |
| • Recurrent PE despite adequate anticoagulation | Permanent |
| Relative | |
| • Free-floating ileofemoral/IVC thrombus with high risk of embolization | Retrievable |
| • Patients with PE and severely limited cardiorespiratory reserve | Permanent |
| • Spinal cord injury with paraplegia | Permanent |
| • Severe trauma | Retrievable |
| • Prophylactic—before surgery on patients at high risk of PE/DVT | Retrievable |
| • Pregnant women with DVT pre-delivery | Retrievable |

Source data from Kessel D and Robertson I. Interventional Radiology: A Survival Guide. Churchill Livingstone. Second Edition 2005 and Uberoi R. Interventional Radiology. Oxford Specialist Handbooks in Radiology. Oxford University Press. First Edition 2009.

**Expert comment**

According to the Society of Iinterventional Radiology guidelines, placement of optional filters should be considered if the patient has PE and/or DVT with a transient inability to anticoagulate or for prophylactic prevention of PE in high-risk patients. An optional IVC filter should be used in a patient with a free-floating IVC thrombus, because this thrombus will most likely resolve due to thrombolysis and facilitate future filter retrieval. Even (younger) patients post severe trauma may fully recover and should have their IVC filter retrieved as soon as possible if they are no longer at risk for VTE, so use of an optional filter is recommended in this subgroup of patients .

**Learning point** Types of IVC filter

Permanent and retrievable filter designs are available. There are more extensive data on permanent filter designs, commencing with Greenfield et al. [4] in 1973, covering a total of over 9500 filter placements [13]. Permanent options currently available include the Gianturco Bird's Nest, the titanium and stainless steel Greenfield, Simon Nitinol, Vena Tech, and Trap Ease.

Retrievable designs were originally approved in 2003 and have recommended dwell times ranging from 10 to 100 days. Designs available include the Opt Ease (Cordis, Roden, The Netherlands), Gunther Tulip (Cook, Bloomington, IN, USA), Recovery (Bard Peripheral Vascular, Tempe, AZ, USA) and the ALN filter (ALN Implants Chirurgicaux, Ghisonaccia, France). Although retrieval is associated with relatively low complication rates, longer dwell times decreased the rate of successful retrieval from 100% to as low as 50% with average retrieval rates recently noted at around 22% [11,13, 14]. Thrombus in a retrievable filter may prevent removal until a period of anticoagulation is possible [16]. The successful removal of retrievable filters requires diligent patient follow-up and interdepartmental cooperation, and even so successful removal is not always possible [9].

**Learning point** Superior vena cava filter placement

Filter deployment within the superior vena cava (SVC) has been considered for patients with upper-extremity DVT, although the decision is complicated by the short length of the available SVC and the associated increased risk of problematic migration or thrombosis.

In the PREPIC study published in 1998, 400 patients with iliofemoral DVT at high risk for PE were anticoagulated and assigned to either permanent filter or no filter and checked for PE at two days and again at 8–12 days by ventilation–perfusion scan. Patients receiving filters had fewer pulmonary emboli initially and after two and eight years, but over two years experienced more frequent DVT and no decrease in mortality [17]. It is important to be aware that the PREPIC patients were all anticoagulated, while a typical patient receiving an IVC filter has a contraindication to anticoagulation. Therefore the population of this study was not representative. At eight-year follow up, IVC filters were found to have reduced the risk of PE but increased the risk for DVT, but had no effect on overall survival. Although their use may be beneficial in patients at high risk of PE, systematic use in the general population with venous thromboembolism is not recommended [7].

**Expert comment**

The PREPIC study is one of key studies on permanent IVC filter use, but as correctly mentioned earlier it is not quite representative because all patients received anticoagulation. Furthermore, results may have been different using optional IVC filters, since IVC filter retrieval is believed to reduce long-term complications.

**Evidence base** Eight-year follow-up of patients with permanent vena cava filters in the prevention of pulmonary embolism: the PREPIC (Prevention du Risque d'Embolie Pulmonaire par Interruption Cave) randomized study [7]

- Randomized trial in patients with proximal deep-vein thrombosis: permanent vena cava filters reduced the incidence of PE but increased that of DVT at two years. An eight-year follow-up was performed to assess their very long term effect.
- Four hundred patients with proximal DVT with or without PE were randomized either to receive or not receive a filter in addition to standard anticoagulant treatment for at least three months. Data on vital status, VTE, and post-thrombotic syndrome were obtained once a year for up to eight years. All documented events were reviewed blindly by an independent committee. Outcome data were available for 396 patients (99%). Symptomatic pulmonary embolism occurred in nine patients in the filter group (cumulative rate, 6.2%) and 24 patients (15.1%) in the no-filter group ($p = 0.008$). DVT occurred in 57 patients (35.7%) in the filter group and 41 (27.5%) in the no-filter group ($p = 0.042$). Post-thrombotic syndrome was observed in 109 (70.3%) and 107 (69.7%) patients in the filter and no-filter groups, respectively. At eigh years, 201 (50.3%) patients had died (103 patients in the filter group and 98 in the no-filter group).
- At eight years, vena cava filters reduced the risk of PE but increased that of DVT and had no effect on survival. Although their use may be beneficial in patients at high risk of PE, systematic use in the general population with venous thromboembolism is not recommended.

These studies have emphasized the retrievable filter concept in which the embolic risk appears to be highest early on, while the thrombotic complications, including recurrent DVT and IVC thrombosis, become apparent later.

Cochrane reviews performed in 2007 and 2010 [18,19] examined two controlled clinical trials (CCTs) and randomized controlled trials (RCTs) that investigated the efficacy of filters in preventing PE in a total of 529 patients, but were unable to make any recommendations. One study showed a reduction in PE rates but not mortality, but was subject to significant biases. The PREPIC study lacked statistical power to detect a reduction in PE over shorter and more clinically significant time periods. However, the trial demonstrated that permanent IVC filters were associated with an increased risk of long-term lower limb DVT. The reviews concluded that there was a paucity of outcome evidence for IVC filters when used within currently approved indications and a lack of trials on retrievable filters, and that further trials are needed to assess IVC filter safety and effectiveness.

**Landmark trial** Cochrane Database Review 2010 [19]

- To examine evidence for the effectiveness of IVC filters in preventing PE. Secondary outcomes were mortality, distal (to filter) thrombosis, and filter-related complications.
- The Cochrane Peripheral Vascular Diseases Group searched their Specialized Register (last searched October 2009) and the Cochrane Central Register of Controlled Trials (CENTRAL) in The Cochrane Library 2009, Issue 4, for RCTs or CCTs of IVC filters for the prevention of PE. The authors contacted filter manufacturers for information.
- Selection criteria: CCTs and RCTs that examined the efficacy of filters in preventing PE.

(continued)

- Two authors extracted information independently.
- Two studies were included involving a total of 529 individuals. One open quasi-randomized trial of 129 participants with traumatic hip fractures showed a reduction in PE but not mortality over a 34-day period in the filter group. The PREPIC trial was an open RCT of 400 participants with documented proximal DVT or PE who received concurrent anticoagulation. Permanent IVC filters prevented PE at eight years. No reduction in mortality was seen, but this reflected an older study population; the majority of deaths were due to cancer or cardiovascular causes. There was an increased incidence of DVT in the filter group. Adverse events were not reported.
- No recommendation was made based the two studies. One study demonstrated a reduction in PE rates but not mortality, but was subject to significant bias. The PREPIC study lacked statistical power to detect a reduction in PE over shorter and more clinically significant time periods; however, the trial demonstrated that permanent IVC filters were associated with an increased risk of long-term lower limb DVT. There is a paucity of outcome evidence for IVC filters when used within currently approved indications and a lack of trials on retrievable filters. The authors concluded that further trials are needed to assess IVC filter safety and effectiveness.

Although IVC filters are effective at reducing the incidence of PE, there is a 3–5% recurrence rate. In a 26-year single-institution study of 1765 filters, rates of major complication associated with placement were 0.3%, and rates of post-insertion migration, fracture, and caval perforation ranged from 0.1% to 0.2%. The rate of caval thrombosis was 2.7% (3.2% if the Mobin–Uddin device is included [20]). Other authors cite an IVC thrombosis rate of 2–10%, and up to 30% may thrombose over the long term. Another study shows a complication rate of 4–11%, with insertion and death in 0.12%. As in earlier studies, filters appear to increase incidence of recurrent DVT and have not been shown to increase overall survival in the long term. Anticoagulation, with its associated risks, is recommended for patients with permanent filters in place, although this is controversial. Cross-sectional imaging findings of complications such as maldeployment, malpositioning, tilt, migration, perforation, fragmentation, IVC thrombosis, and recurrent PE are described.

## A final word from the expert

IVC filter insertion is a relatively straightforward procedure that may be used for patients with high risk of pulmonary embolism that cannot be anticoagulated. IVC filters are effective in preventing PE, but their presence might lead to long-term complications (e.g. perforation, migration, filter fracture). Therefore, these devices need to be retrieved whenever the patient may be in a condition to receive therapeutic anticoagulation. Filter retrieval is also straightforward and may be performed as an outpatient appointment. Anticoagulation should not be interrupted for the retrieval of the filter.

## References

1. Caplin DM, Nikolic B, Kalva SP, et al. Quality improvement guidelines for the performance of inferior vena cava filter placement for the prevention of pulmonary embolism. *J Vasc Interv Radiol* 2011; 22(11): 1499–1506.
2. Hoppe H, Kaufman JA, Barton RE, et al. Safety of inferior vena cava filter retrieval in anticoagulated patients. *Chest* 2007; 132(1): 31–6.

3. Kearon C, Kahn SR, Agnelli G, et al. Antithrombotic therapy for venous thromboembolic disease: American College of Chest Physicians Evidence-Based Clinical Practice Guidelines (8th edition). *Chest* 2008; 133(6 Suppl):454S–545S.
4. Greenfield LJ, McCurdy JR, Brown PP, Elkins RC. A new intracaval filter permitting continued flow and resolution of emboli. *Surgery* 1973; 73(4): 599–606.
5. Baadh AS, Zikria JF, Rivoli S, et al. Indications for inferior vena cava filter placement: do physicians comply with guidelines? *J Vasc Interv Radiol* 2012; 23(8): 989–95.
6. Sharifi M, Bay C, Skrocki L, et al. Role of IVC filters in endovenous therapy for deep venous thrombosis: the FILTER-PEVI (filter implantation to lower thromboembolic risk in percutaneous endovenous intervention) trial. *Cardiovasc Intervent Radiol* 2012; 35(6): 1408–13.
7. PREPIC Study Group. Eight-year follow-up of patients with permanent vena cava filters in the prevention of pulmonary embolism: the PREPIC (Prevention du Risque d'Embolie Pulmonaire par Interruption Cave) randomized study. *Circulation* 2005; 112(3): 416–22.
8. Angel LF, Tapson V, Galgon RE, et al. Systematic review of the use of retrievable inferior vena cava filters. *J Vasc Interv Radiol* 2011; 22(11): 1522–30.
9. Lynch FC. A method for following patients with retrievable inferior vena cava filters: results and lessons learned from the first 1,100 patients. *J Vasc Interv Radiol* 201; 22(11): 1507–12.
10. Shaw CM, Scorza LB, Waybill PN, et al. Optional vena cava filter use in the elderly population. *J Vasc Interv Radiol* 2011; 22(6): 824–8.
11. Kessel D and Robertson I. *Interventional Radiology: A Survival Guide* (2nd edn) (Edinburgh: Churchill Livingstone); 2005.
12. Uberoi R. *Interventional Radiology* (Oxford: Oxford University Press); 2009.
13. Berczi V, Bottomley JR, Thomas SM, et al. Long-term retrievability of IVC filters: should we abandon permanent devices? *Cardiovasc Intervent Radiol* 2007; 30(5): 820–7.
14. Rosenthal D, Wellons ED, Hancock SM, Burkett AB. Retrievability of the Günther Tulip vena cava filter after dwell times longer than 180 days in patients with multiple trauma. *J Endovasc Ther* 2007; 14(3): 406–10.
15. Kalina M, Bartley M, Cipolle M, et al. Improved removal rates for retrievable inferior vena cava filters with the use of a 'filter registry'. *Am Surg* 2012; 78(1): 94–7.
16. Teo TK, Angle JF, Shipp JI, et al. Incidence and management of inferior vena cava filter thrombus detected at time of filter retrieval. *J Vasc Interv Radiol* 2011; 22(11): 1514–20.
17. Decousus H, Leizorovicz A, Parent F, et al. A clinical trial of vena caval filters in the prevention of pulmonary embolism in patients with proximal deep-vein thrombosis. Prévention du Risque d'Embolie Pulmonaire par Interruption Cave Study Group. *N Engl J Med* 1998; 338(7): 409–15.
18. Young T, Tang H, Aukes J, Hughes R. Vena caval filters for the prevention of pulmonary embolism. *Cochrane Database Syst Rev* 2007; (4): CD006212.
19. Young T, Tang H, Hughes R. Vena caval filters for the prevention of pulmonary embolism. *Cochrane Database Syst Rev* 2010; (2): CD006212.
20. Athanasoulis CA, Kaufman JA, Halpern EF, et al. Inferior vena caval filters: review of a 26-year single-center clinical experience. *Radiology* 2000; 216(1): 54–66.

CASE

# 15 TIPS and TIPS revision for Budd–Chiari patients

**Vyzantios Pavlidis**

**Expert commentary** Elias Brountzos

## Case history

A 57-year-old female patient presented to the outpatient department with a six-day history of worsening abdominal pain. The patient had a known history of essential thrombocythemia during six years under medical treatment.

Upon admission the patient had a normal heart rate of 75 beats/min and her blood pressure was 172/75mmHg. Physical examination was remarkable for sclera icterus and jaundice of the skin. Further examination of the patient revealed a distended abdomen, which was hard and painful upon palpation, distended superficial abdominal veins, the presence of ascites, and hepatosplenomegaly. The patient had no history of encephalopathy or haematemesis. The electrocardiogram (ECG) and chest X-ray were normal.

The patient was admitted for further evaluation. During hospitalization further physical, laboratory, and imaging exams were performed. Abdominal ultrasonography and duplex ultrasound revealed hepatosplenomegaly, absence of flow in the hepatic veins, and presence of ascites. The portal vein was patent with hepatopetal (towards the liver) flow, intrahepatic collaterals were formed, and the inferior vena cava (IVC) was patent. The findings satisfied the criteria for Budd–Chiari syndrome (BCS).

**Learning point** Essential thrombocythemia (ET) [1,2]

- ET is a myeloproliferative disorder and is mainly identified by a sustained increase in the platelet count (>450 × $10^9$/L) over one month.
- Mean age at diagnosis is 50-60 years.
- Asymptomatic for many years.
- Symptoms are related to arterial or venous thrombosis and gastrointestinal bleeding.
- Risks of thrombosis, transformation to leukaemia, or transformation to idiopathic myelofibrosis at 10 years are 14%, 2.6%, and 3.9–8.3%, respectively.

**Learning point** Ultrasonographic findings for BCS [3,4]

- The liver has a coarse texture. The regenerative nodules found in BCS mimic hepatocellular cancer.
- Hypertrophy of the caudate lobe and caudate vein >3mm.
- Narrowing of the IVC may be due to compression from the hypertrophied caudate lobe or stenosis from an intraluminal thrombus.
- Hepatic veins may or may not be seen. Stenosis is presented with proximal dilatation or, in the case of occlusion, the vein appears as an echogenic band. Colour Doppler depicts flow direction which may be absent, reversed, turbulent, or continuous. Pulse Doppler reveals lack of normal correlation with breathing.
- Portal hypertension is associated with a portal vein diameter >1.3cm, hepatofugal (away from the liver) blood flow, collaterals, and ascites. Reversed blood flow may also exist in splenic and superior mesenteric veins. If thrombosis is present, prognosis is very poor.
- Intrahepatic collaterals with involvement of hepatic venules, caudate lobe, or subcapsular collaterals.
- Extrahepatic collaterals include umbilical vein recanalization, splenorenal shunt, etc.
- Splenomegaly.

Contrast-enhanced abdominal CT (ce-CT) was performed (Figure 15.1). An axial CT scan obtained during the portal phase showed liver of increased size (right lobe craniocaudal diameter ~18cm) that was enhanced in the caudate lobe

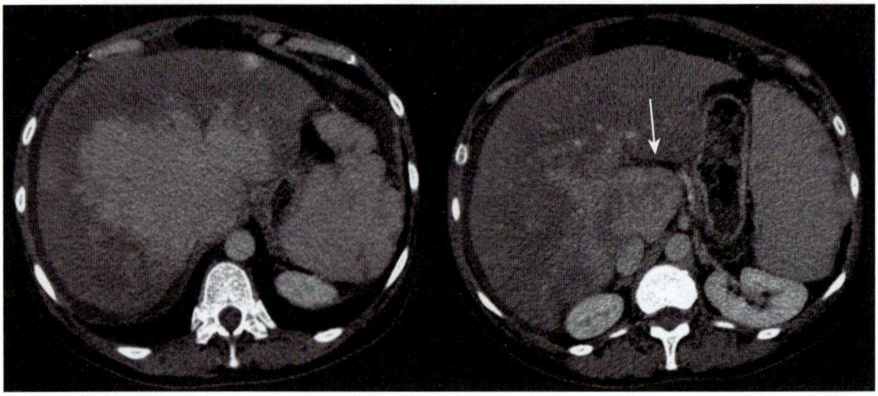

**Figure 15.1** CT scan showing inhomogeneous liver enhancement. Hypodense liver in the periphery is caused by hypoperfusion, while the caudate lobe shows hypertrophy with increased enhancement (arrow) caused by sparing of its venous drainage.

and the central areas and had low or no enhancement in the areas near the capsule. The IVC was compressed by the enlarged caudate lobe. Thrombosis of the left and right hepatic veins was confirmed, with minor enhancement of the middle hepatic vein. The portal vein was patent, and a collateral network was also formed: gastroepiploic, splenogastric, splenorenal. The craniocaudal diameter of the spleen was ~17cm.

**Clinical tip** BCS: ce-CT findings [5]

- Delayed enhancement of the periphery of the liver and around the hepatic veins because of hepatic venous congestion.
- Enlargement of caudate lobe due to drainage maintenance through emissary veins.
- Thrombosis of the portal vein may also be present.
- ce-CT identifies IVC and hepatic vein thrombosis in 18–53% of patients.
- Intrahepatic and portosystemic collaterals.

NB: Hypervascular nodules on ce-CT may comprise normal liver parenchyma.

The clinical, laboratory, and imaging findings were diagnostic for BCS. The patient was referred to the interventional radiology department for treatment by formation of a transjugular intrahepatic portosystemic shunt (TIPS).

**Learning point** Budd–Chiari syndrome [5–7]

- BCS is a rare disorder which is potentially fatal. It occurs most often in the third and fourth decades. It was first described by George Budd in 1845, and Hans Chiari gave the first pathological description in 1899.
- Major causes are disorders with underlying thrombotic diathesis, such as essential thrombocythemia.
- Pathophysiology: obstruction of the hepatic venous outflow leads to hepatic congestion, liver insufficiency, portal hypertension, ascites, and formation of an extensive venous collateral network.
- Common clinical findings: abdominal pain, hepatomegaly, and ascites.
- Patients seek medical care when they have the symptoms and signs of lower extremity oedema, ascites, jaundice, variceal bleeding, or encephalopathy.

**Clinical tip** Hepatic encephalopathy (HE) [8]

- Associated with hepatocellular pathology, portal hypertension, and portosystemic shunts.
- Classification system: West Haven criteria according to one or several neuropsychiatric symptoms.

**Clinical tip** Models for predicting patient outcome after TIPS [9]

- Child–Pugh score: assesses the prognosis of chronic liver disease and predicts mortality during surgery, based on the values for bilirubin, albumin, prothrombin time, ascites, and encephalopathy.
- Meld score: model for endstage liver disease that estimates the patient's mortality rate based on serum bilirubin, INR, and creatinine values.
- Main contraindications to TIPS: right heart failure, severe liver failure, and systemic infection. Encephalopathy, coagulopathy, and portal vein thrombosis are relative contraindications.

**Expert comment**

Pre-interventional ascites evacuation is a standard procedure to create a safer operational environment, minimizing technical failure and avoiding the possibility of bleeding.

**Expert comment**

In the presence of an extensive collateral network, embolization might be necessary to sustain high flow inside the stent graft and eliminate the possibility of shunt dysfunction or even occlusion.

**Learning point** Preparation

Pre-interventional preparation consists of the following.

- Patient's preparation and evaluation from a group of specialists:
  - Detailed briefing and patient's written consent form
  - Ascites evacuation
  - Correction of coagulation deficiencies (INR, PT, aPTT)
  - Correction of abnormal electrolyte and albumin
  - Meld score calculation
  - Availability of packed red cell and free frozen plasma units, in case of intra-procedural bleeding,
  - Anaesthesia pre-operative evaluation—the procedure should preferably be performed under general anaesthesia.
- Procedural planning:
  - Evaluate the following based on the CT scan multiplanar reconstruction (MPR) images:
    - Hepatic anatomy
    - Presence or absence of hepatic veins,
    - Presence of a stump if the main hepatic vein is obstructed
    - Anatomical relationship between hepatic and portal vein,
    - Angles, distance, and course needed to access the branch of the portal vein
    - Presence of collaterals.
  - Have the following devices available:
    - TIPS set
    - Coils, glue, and vascular plug to embolize the collateral network if necessary.

The patient's blood tests showed INR 1.18, creatinine 1.2mg/dl, and total bilirubin 4.11mg/dl. the MELD score was 15. The TIPS procedure was carried out under general anaesthesia. Sterilization of the neck and abdomen was performed and access was obtained via the right internal jugular vein using ultrasound guidance. The small middle hepatic vein was catheterized, and wedged venography showed the spider-web pattern typical of intrahepatic vein obstruction. Using fluoroscopy the 18G needle of a Rösch–Uchida Transjugular Liver Access Set (Cook Medical Europe Ltd) was advanced from the middle hepatic vein into the left portal vein. Entry into the portal vein branch was confirmed by contrast injection, and a guidewire was advanced into the left branch of portal vein and subsequently into the main portal vein. Using the standard technique a pigtail catheter was inserted into the main portal vein and pressure measurement revealed a gradient of 32mmHg. Portography was performed with the calibrated pigtail catheter and the distance between the IVC and the entry site of the left portal vein was measured to select the length of the stent-graft. Following TIPS tract dilatation with an 8mm balloon catheter, two 10 × 60mm Viatorr stent-grafts (W.L. Gore and Associates Inc.) were deployed across the tract. The stent grafts were finally dilated to 10mm to achieve a gradient of 8mmHg (the aim was <12mmHg). Completion portography showed good TIPS patency (Figure 15.2). The patient recovered successfully and was transferred to the ward.

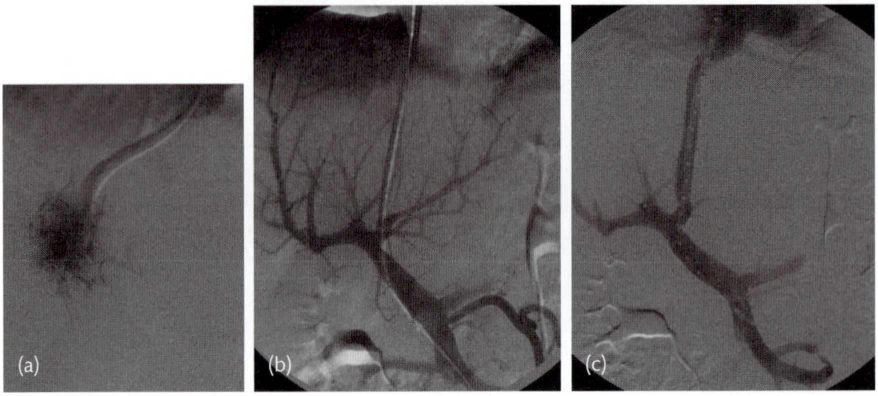


**Figure 15.2** The TIPS procedure: (a) Catheter venography following catheterization of the middle hepatic vein shows the spider-web pattern typical of Budd–Chiari syndrome. (b) Following cannulation of the portal vein, portography was performed via a calibrated catheter to measure the length of the stent graft. (c) Portography following the placement of the stent grafts shows good TIPS patency.

**Expert comment**

The Viatorr stent graft is a self-expanding nitinol stent supporting an expanded polytetrafluoroethylene (ePTFE) graft with a bile-resistant membrane. It consists of two parts: (1) a proximal graft-lined segment, which should be placed in the intrahepatic tract, and (2) a distal bare segment, which should be positioned into the portal vein. The length of the appropriate stent graft can be determined during the intervention, by measuring the distance between the IVC and the entry site into the portal vein using a calibrated catheter.

**Clinical tip**

Main interventional complications:

- Death due to severe haemorrhage (injury to IVC, portal vein, hepatic artery, or hepatic capsule)
- Hepatic haematoma or haemobilia.

Post-interventional management:

- Aims to control haemodynamic changes, preserve shunt patency, and prevent hepatic encephalopathy
- Standard medication consists of antidiuretics, anticoagulants (aiming for an INR of 2.0–3.0) [7], and medications to control post-TIPS encephalopathy.

The response to therapy is based on the elimination of the symptoms.

Three days after the procedure abdominal ultrasound and colour Doppler examination confirmed a patent shunt with complete elimination of the ascites. The patient was discharged with instructions for regular clinical and imaging follow-up with ultrasound.

**Clinical tip** Post-TIPS ultrasound follow-up [10]

- Access standard US findings for BCS, as well as the flow within the shunt.
- Abnormal findings:
  - Stent mean velocity < 50 or >200cm/s
  - Spatial or temporal stent gradients >50cm/s
  - >50% decrease in the shunt flow velocity over time
  - Reversed flow in the portal vein and velocity <30cm/s
  - Occlusion appears as complete absence of flow or pulse within the shunt
  - Stenosis appears as narrowing within the stent and incomplete colour filling of the stent lumen; colour aliasing is caused by turbulent flow.

The patient did not attend her regular follow-up appointments for almost a year. Then she presented to the interventional radiology department with recurrent ascites. Upon admission, Doppler examination demonstrated occlusion of the previous TIPS, but a patent portal venous system. A decision was made to recanalize the occluded TIPS, but all attempts and manoeuvres from both the right jugular and right femoral veins were unsuccessful in catheterizing the occluded shunt (Figure 15.3). Although the recanalization technique seems to be simple it can be technically complex if the shunt thrombosis is chronic. Therefore a decision was made to create a new shunt parallel to the previous one if possible.

The new TIPS procedure was carried out under general anaesthesia, using the procedure described previously. The new access was achieved from a small bulge of

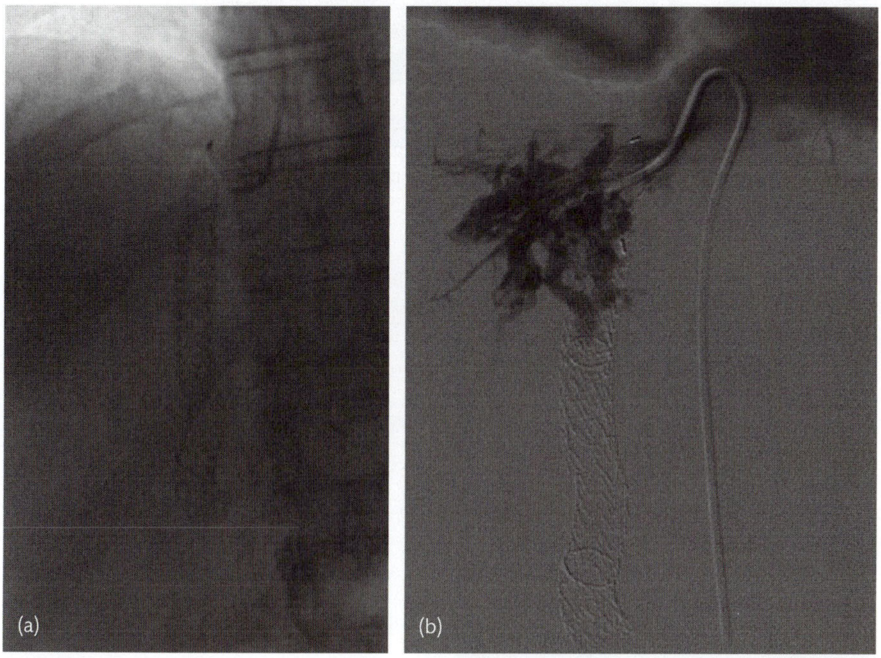


**Figure 15.3** The attempt to reopen the occluded TIPS. (a) Fluoroscopic spot image showing the attempt from the right jugular vein; the catheter could not engage the TIPS stent graft despite numerous attempts. (b) An attempt from the right femoral vein was also unsuccessful. Note the intrahepatic collateral network with a spider-web pattern.

the inferior vena cava (corresponding to the draining site of the right hepatic vein to the IVC) towards the intrahepatic right branch of the portal vein. An angiographic catheter was placed into the splenic vein and direct portography confirmed the patency of the portal vein and primary shunt occlusion. Dilatation of the new intrahepatic parenchymal tract was followed by the placement of two new Viatorr stent grafts (W.L. Gore and Associates Inc.) of dimensions 10 × 80mm and 10 × 60mm. In the final portography picture, patency of the new portosystemic anastomosis was confirmed (Figure 15.4).

The following day the patient was evaluated both with ce-CT and Doppler ultrasound, which confirmed the patency of the second TIPS (Figure 15.5) and regression of the ascites. After two days the patient was discharged and advised to comply with the regular clinical and ultrasound follow-up every three months.

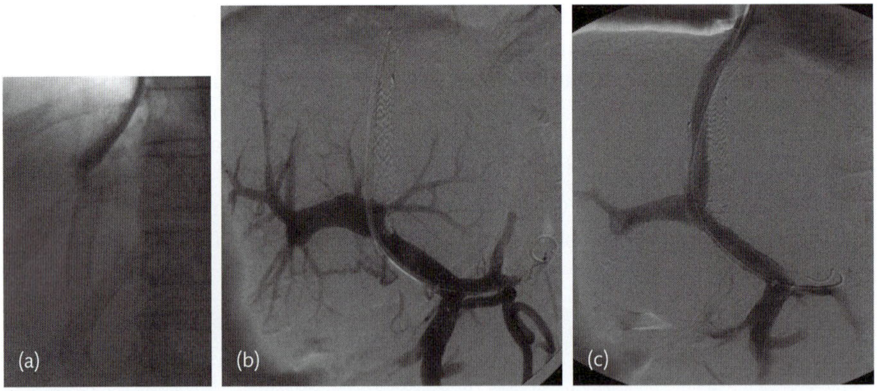


**Figure 15.4** (a) Fluoroscopic image showing the curved cannula wedged into the stump of the right hepatic vein. (b) Direct portography showing the patency of the portal vein. Note the new tract in a parallel course to the occluded TIPS. (c) Final portography showing the patency of the new shunt.

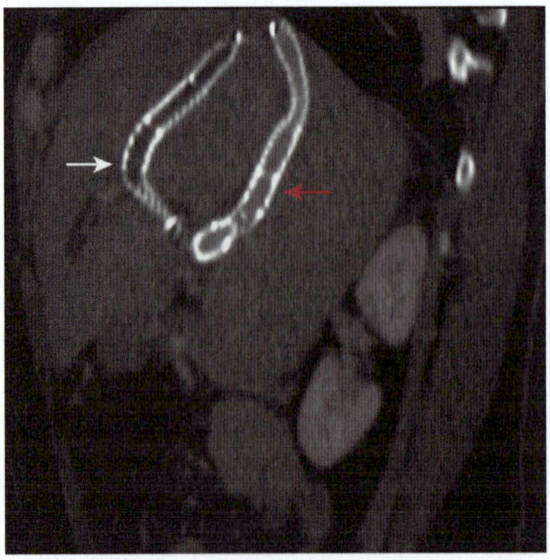

**Figure 15.5** ce-CT para-saggital reconstruction showing the primary occluded TIPS (white arrow) and second patent TIPS (red arrow).

## Discussion

Budd–Chiari syndrome is a life-threatening condition with a mortality rate of 80% [11] in untreated patients. Peltzer et al. [12] first introduced TIPS as a treatment for BCS in 1993, but it was not until 2008 that Garcia-Pagán et al. [13] suggested that TIPS could be the treatment of choice with survival rates of 88%, 78%, and 69% at one, five, and ten years, respectively.

The most challenging step of the procedure is to gain access to the portal vein, because patients with BCS may have either sub-total occlusion of the hepatic veins, with the classic spider-web appearance, or total obstruction of the hepatic veins. In the latter situation the puncture should be performed through the IVC. The puncture is greatly facilitated if a venous stump is present. Several alternative TIPS techniques, using either percutaneous or intravascular US guidance, have been developed to overcome this limitation. Petersen and Binkert [14] proposed a direct intrahepatic portocaval shunt (DIPS) under intravascular US guidance. This procedure proved to be technically feasible and effective for controlling the complications of portal hypertension, but with the additional cost of the intravascular US equipment. However, we have not used this technique in BCS patients.

**Evidence base** TIPS in Budd-Chiari syndrome

Budd–Chiari syndrome used to be treated surgically with portosystemic shunts or liver transplantation. However, in the last decade TIPS has evolved as an alternative treatment when conservative treatment fails and especially when transplantation criteria are not satisfied:

- 10% of patients are controlled with anticoagulation therapy
- 20–30% require anticoagulation in combination with hepatic vein or IVC angioplasty
- 60% require TIPS
- 10–20% are candidates for transplantation [7].

The results of TIPS in BCS are as follows [13,15–17]:

- Technical success, 91–100%
- Five-year transplant-free survival, 77–100%
- 10-year transplant-free survival, 69%
- If anticoagulation is not effective, there is an 80% risk of shunt thrombosis
- 41–85% of patients may need repeated interventional procedures.

A major drawback of TIPS seems to be the underlying thrombotic tendency in BCS patients, although new stents covered with ePTFE membrane show higher primary patency rates that reduce the rate of TIPS occlusion. Interventional recanalization of the shunt is possible but is not always successful, especially in case of total shunt occlusion. The management of such cases may involve the creation of a new shunt.

In our department we perform the TIPS procedure using the Viatorr stent graft under general anaesthesia. The patients are advised to follow anticoagulation therapy, as well as undergoing Doppler ultrasonography monitoring of the shunt patency every three months.

In the case reported here the patient presented with total occlusion of the primary shunt and the treatment options were first an attempt a recanalization of the occlude TIPS, and secondly to create a new shunt if the recanalization attempt was unsuccessful. Performing the second TIPS was a technical challenge. The highlights of the procedure were the small hepatic vein stump, which was the starting point of our transhepatic tract, and the use of the primary shunt as a guide to re-enter into the portal vein.

**Evidence base**

There have been several studies showing a positive outcome of TIPS in patients with BCS, the largest of which was a multicentre multinational study of a series of 124 BCS patients [13].

- Long-term outcome disclosed survival rates free from orthotopic liver transplantation (OLT) of 88%, 78%, and 69% at one, five, and ten years, respectively.
- During follow-up 41% had TIPS dysfunction, 21% developed hepatic encephalopathy, 6.5% required OLT, and 13% died.
- Endpoint: 'TIPS should no longer be considered as a bridge to OLT, but the treatment of choice when medical treatment and hepatic vein recanalization do not succeed'.

## A final word from the expert

- Budd–Chiari syndrome consists of hepatic venous outflow obstruction at any level between the small hepatic veins and the right atrium. Our primary goal is the resolution of hepatic congestion in order to improve liver function.
- Evolution of interventional techniques has made TIPS technically feasible even in challenging cases where there is total occlusion of hepatic veins without a remaining stump. Such techniques are the 'gun-sight' approach or the direct portocaval shunt puncture with percutaneous or intravascular US guidance. In rare cases CT fluoroscopy can help to gain access to the portal vein.
- In the case of TIPS stenosis or occlusion the most commonly applied recanalization technique is transjugular balloon angioplasty with or without stenting. Alternative methods have been described: transjugular stent puncture via a Colapinto or Rösch–Uchida needle, transhepatic stent puncture associated with pull-through technique, or even a more invasive trans-splenic approach. Accessory techniques include thrombolysis and mechanical thrombectomy.
- If the first shunt is occluded and recanalization techniques fail, or if the first shunt fails to decompress the portal system, a new parallel shunt can be created to achieve the desired result.
- Recommendations to maintain long-term patency: (1) use stent grafts because they are associated with a improved patency rate compared with bare stents; (2) post-TIPS start anticoagulation with low molecular weight heparin and change to oral anticoagulants after a few days. Multidisciplinary cooperation with the hepatologists and haematologists is mandatory to address these patients' complex problems.
- Liver biopsies are useful for determining the severity of the disease (congestion, fibrosis, necrosis, regenerative nodules) or post-TIPS liver improvement.
- The primary strategy for BCS patients consists of medical treatment and interventional recanalization of small hepatic vein stenoses. However, there is no evidence that one should wait for the failure of a previous treatment step before creating TIPS in patients with short-length stenoses without, especially since TIPS reduces portal hypertension and improves outcome in all categories of baseline disease severity. The role of liver transplantation (LT) has been revalidated, since post-TIPS LT-free survival rates are comparable with LT survival rates. Thus LT should be reserved as a rescue therapy for patients failing TIPS.
- Advanages of TIPS compared with surgical treatments: (1)TIPs is a minimally invasive technique associated with reduced peri-operational morbidity and mortality rates; (2) TIPS has no negative effects on future LT; (3) TIPS is not associated with risks of long-term immunosuppression; (4) TIPS does not require a liver to be available.

- Treatment strategy is not based on specific timetable criteria according to the progression of the actual disease in the patient. Rather, it is based on failure of previous therapies to control conditions such as ascites and bleeding.
- In my opinion there are three important points to be considered:
  (1) a multidisciplinary team is required because of the multifactorial nature of BCS.
  (2) when an expert interventional experience is available, early TIPS should be considered as a definitive treatment option for improving quality of life.
  (3) patients must be aware of the severity of their disease, of the treatment options and complications, and that long-term cooperation is needed for successful survival.

## References


1. Cervantes F. Management of essential thrombocythemia. *Hematology* 2011; 1: 215–21.
2. Passamonti F, Rumi E, Arcaini L, et al. Prognostic factors for thrombosis, myelofibrosis, and leukemia in essential thrombocythemia: a study of 605 patients. *Haematologica* 2008; 93: 1645–51.
3. Chaubal N, Dighe M, Hanchate V, et al. Sonography in Budd-Chiari syndrome. *J Ultrasound Med* 2006; 25: 373–9.
4. Boozari B, Bahr MJ, Kubicka S, et al. Ultrasonography in patients with Budd-Chiari syndrome: diagnostic signs and prognostic implications. *J Hepatol* 2008; 49: 572–80.
5. Buckley O, O'Brien J, Snow A, et al. Imaging of Budd-Chiari syndrome. *Eur Radiol* 2007; 17: 2071–2078.
6. Cura M, Haskal Z, Lopera J. Diagnostic and interventional radiology for Budd-Chiari syndrome. *Radiographics* 2009; 29: 669–81.
7. Valla DC. Primary Budd-Chiari syndrome. *J Hepatol* 2009; 50 195–203.
8. Cash WJ, McConville P, McDermott E, et al. Current concepts in the assessment and treatment of hepatic encephalopathy. *QJM* 2010; 103: 9–16.
9. Angermayr B, Cejna M, Karnel F, et al. Child-Pugh versus MELD score in predicting survival in patients undergoing transjugular intrahepatic portosystemic shunt. *Gut*. 2003; 52: 879–85.
10. Lee WK, Chang SD, Duddalwar VA, et al. Imaging assessment of congenital and acquired abnormalities of the portal venous system. *Radiographics* 2011; 31: 905–26.
11. Olliff, SP. Transjugular intrahepatic portosystemic shunt in the management of Budd-Chiari syndrome. *Eur J Gastroenterol Hepatol* 2006; 18(11): 1151–4.
12. Peltzer MY, Ring EJ, LaBerge JM, et al. Treatment of Budd-Chiari syndrome with a transjugular intrahepatic portosystemic shunt. *J Vasc Interv Radiol* 1993; 4(2): 263–7.
13. Garcia-Pagán JC, Heydtmann M, Raffa S, et al. TIPS for Budd-Chiari syndrome: long-term results and prognostics factors in 124 patients. *Gastroenterology* 2008; 135: 808–15.
14. Petersen B, Binkert C. Intravascular ultrasound-guided direct intrahepatic portacaval shunt: midterm follow-up. *J Vasc Interv Radiol* 2004; 15(9): 927–38.
15. Molmenti EP, Segev DL, Arepally A, et al. The utility of TIPS in the management of Budd-Chiari syndrome. *Ann Surg* 2005; 241(6): 978–81.
16. Corso R, Intotero M, Solcia M, et al. Treatment of Budd-Chiari syndrome with transjugular intrahepatic portosystemic shunt (TIPS). *Radiol Med* 2008; 113: 727–38.
17. Zahn A, Gotthardt D, Weiss KH, et al. Budd-Chiari syndrome: long term success via hepatic decompression using transjugular intrahepatic porto-systemic shunt. *BMC Gastroenterol* 2010; 10: 25.

SECTION 3

# Embolization

CASE

# 16 Epistaxis: which embolic materials to use?


**Magdalena Jarząbek and Piotr Trojanowski**

**Expert commentary** Małgorzata Szczerbo-Trojanowska


## Case history

A 20-year-old male arrived via ambulance at the A&E Department with severe epistaxis due to maxillofacial trauma following a fall from a height. The patient was conscious. His blood pressure at the time of admission to the hospital was 145/85mmHg, his pulse was 85 beats/min, and an ECG demonstrated normal sinus rhythm. Blood count showed a haemoglobin level of 10.3g/dl. Blood coagulation parameters were within normal limits.

Anterior nasal packing was performed as first-line treatment. Computer tomography of the head revealed a nasal septum fracture as well as blood in the left nasal cavity and within the left maxillary sinus (Figure 16.1).

**Clinical tip**

In patients with massive epistaxis it is essential to localize the origin of the bleeding. Depending to the location of the source of bleeding, epistaxis is classified as anterior or posterior which require different methods of treatment.

Anterior epistaxis from Kiesselbach's plexus (anterior septum) is more frequent, but often less severe. First-line therapies such as vasoconstriction, cautery, or anterior nasal packing are usually sufficient.

Posterior bleeding, which occurs in the posterior superior part of the nasal cavity, is usually caused by major trauma and results from injury to vessels of larger calibre. Blood is often present in the nasopharynx and mouth. Treatment involves posterior packing, surgical or endoscopic artery cauterization, or ligation. Intravascular embolization should also be taken into consideration as an alternative treatment [1–3].

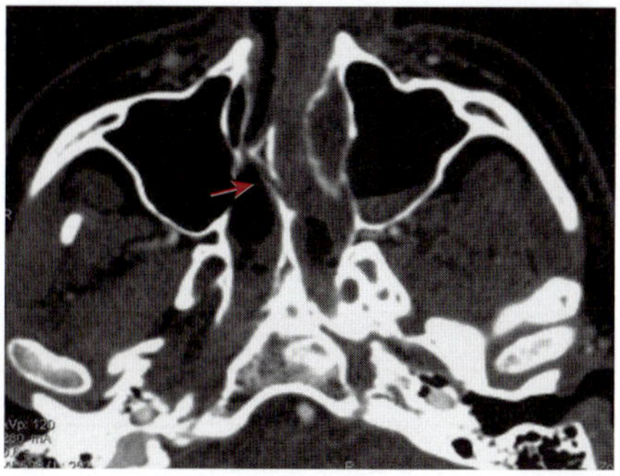

**Figure 16.1** Axial CT scan showing fracture in the posterior part of the nasal septum (arrow), with blood filling the left nasal cavity and present in the left maxillary sinus.

The patient was transferred to the otorhinolaryngology department. Because anterior packing proved to be ineffective, posterior packing was applied. This did not arrest the bleeding, and after 24 hours the haemoglobin level had dropped to 8.6g/dl. Two units of blood were subsequently transfused. The patient's past medical history included hypertension and glucose intolerance.

In addition to nasal packing the patient was treated with tranexamic acid and his hypertension was controlled. Posterior packing was kept in place for 48 hours. At the first attempt at removing the packing, bleeding in the posterior nasal cavity recommenced.

**Learning point**

The Le Fort classification of maxillofacial injuries is shown in Table 16.1 and Figure 16.2. The most common bony fracture after maxillofacial injury is fracture of the nasal bone [4].

**Table 16.1** Le Fort classification of maxillofacial injuries

| Fracture location | Le Fort classification | | |
|---|---|---|---|
| | Type I | Type II | Type III |
| Anterolateral nasal cavity | ✓ | | |
| Maxillary sinuses | ✓ | ✓ | |
| Pterygoid process | ✓ | ✓ | ✓ |
| Inferior orbital rim/wall | | ✓ | |
| Nasal bone | | ✓ | ✓ |
| Lateral orbital wall/rim | | | ✓ |
| Ethmoid or sphenoid sinuses | | | ✓ |
| Zygomatic arch | | | ✓ |

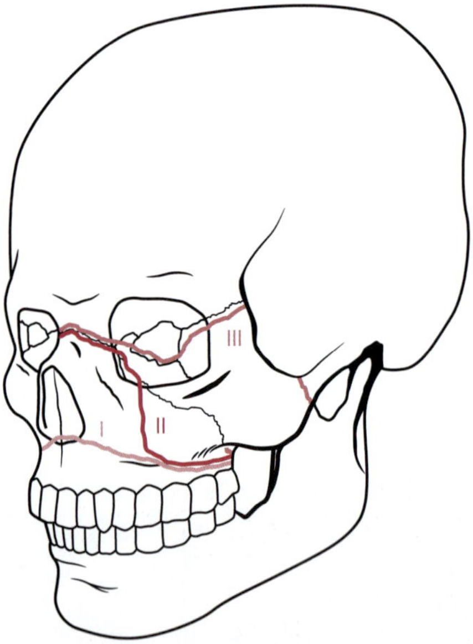


**Figure 16.2** Le Fort classification of maxillofacial injuries

**Expert comment**

The cause of nasal bleeding is not always easy to identify. In this case bleeding was due to trauma. Nevertheless, even in post-traumatic epistaxis it is necessary to exclude other possible causes or predisposing conditions, with injury triggering the bleeding. Medical history is important in making

(continued)

a proper diagnosis. Frequency, severity, duration of previous bleeding episodes, medication, ENT operations, and any coagulopathy symptoms should be taken into account.

Epistaxis can result from various diseases, including systemic illness. In older patients the main causes of nasal bleeds are hypertension and anticoagulation treatment, whereas in younger patients trauma and malignancy are more common (see Table 16.2).

**Learning point**

**Table 16.2 The most common causes of epistaxis in order of incidence [2,5–7]**

| Population | Causes of epistaxis |
|---|---|
| Children | Trauma, tumours, rhinitis, surgery (iatrogenic), systemic coagulopathy |
| Adults | Idiopathic, rhinitis, trauma, tumours, hereditary haemorrhagic telangiectasia (HHT), hepatopathy, aneurysm |
| Elderly | Hypertension, anticoagulation/anti-aggregation treatment, trauma |

Source data from Vaamonde Lago P, Martín Martín C, Lechuga García MR, et al. [Epidemiological notes on nasal bleeding]. [Article in Spanish]. An Otorrinolaringol Ibero Am. 2004; 31(2): 123-32, Pallin DJ, Chng YM, McKay MP, et al. Epidemiology of epistaxis in US emergency departments. Jr. Ann Emerg Med. 2005 Jul; 46(1):77-81. Monjas-Cánovas I, Hernández-García I, Mauri-Barberá J, Sanz-Romero B, Gras-Albert JR. Epidemiology of epistaxes admitted to a tertiary hospital.

Bleeding was still present at removal of the nasal packing so an endoscopy was performed. No obvious bleeding site was detected and posterior packing was reinstated. The patient was then consented for treatment with endovascular arterial embolization.

**Learning point** Vascular anatomy (Figure 16.3) [8]

The arterial supply of the nasal cavity originates from the branches of two main arteries: the external carotid artery (ECA) and the internal carotid artery (ICA). The dominant arteries in the nasal cavity are the posterolateral (conchal) and posteromedial (septal) branches of the sphenopalatine artery, which originate from the pterygopalatine segment of the internal maxillary artery (IMA) (ECA ramification). These branches supply the inferior, middle, and superior turbinates, as well as the nasal septum. The inferior part of the septum is supplied by the greater palatine artery, a branch of the descending palatine artery (IMA ramification). Additional vascularization of the nasal cavity roof comes from branches of the ophthalmic artery (ICA ramification) and the anterior and posterior ethmoidal arteries. The superior labial artery, which is a facial artery branch (ECA ramification), also supplies the floor of the cavity.

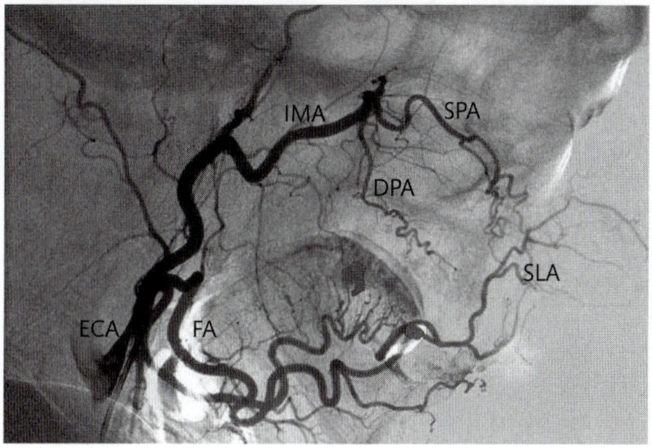


**Figure 16.3** Vascular anatomy of the nasal cavity: ECA, external carotid artery; IMA, internal maxillary artery; FA, facial artery; SPA, sphenopalatine artery, DPA, descending palatine artery; SLA, superior labial artery.

On the third day post admission, the patient underwent angiography to identify the bleeding site and perform embolization. Vascular access was obtained from the right common femoral artery (CFA). Arterial puncture under local anaesthesia and conscious sedation was performed. After introduction of a 5Fr sheath, right and left ICA and ECA diagnostic angiography was performed using a 5Fr cobra catheter. AP and lateral projections were obtained to locate the bleeding site. The angiogram of the left ECA showed signs of bleeding from the left sphenopalatine artery branches (Figure 16.4). The ECA–ICA anastomoses were not visible.

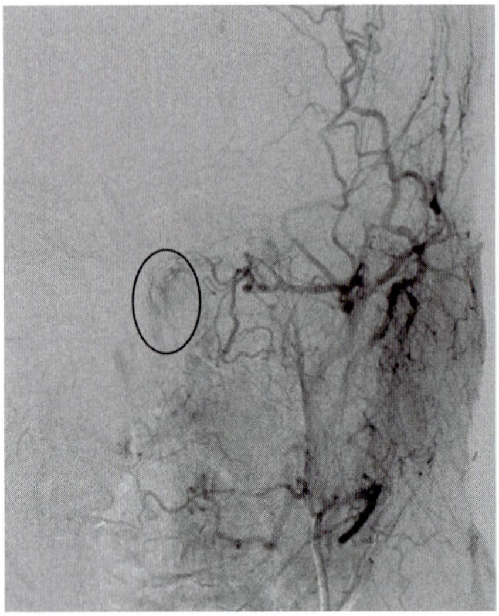

**Figure 16.4** Digital subtraction angiography: the anteroposterior projection of the left ECA shows local hyperaemia in the nasal mucosa vascular network fed by the posterior branches of the left sphenopalatine artery (circled).

Following administration of 3000IU heparin the cobra catheter was introduced to the proximal part of the left IMA and the sphenopalatine artery was approached with a 2.5Fr microcatheter. Embolization was performed using 300–500μm particles (Embosphere; Merit Medical). Control angiography from the cobra catheter showed no flow in the embolized artery and no signs of bleeding (Figure 16.5).

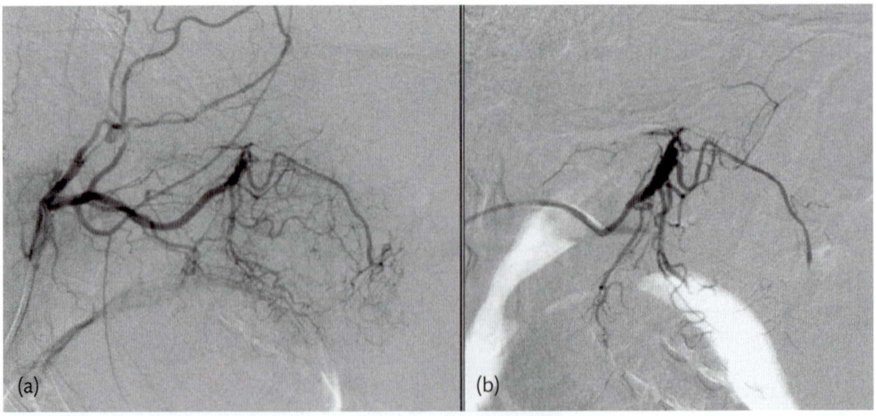


**Figure 16.5** Digital subtraction angiography: (a) lateral projection of the ECA angiogram before the procedure; (b) IMA selective control after embolization shows no flow in the distal part of sphenopalatine artery.

The arterial puncture site was manually pressed for haemostasis. The nasal packing was then removed and there was no bleeding from the nose, indicating that cessation of epistaxis was achieved. There were no post-embolization complications. Dexamethasone 8mg IV and analgesic drugs were administered after the procedure. The patient was discharged in good clinical condition. He was advised to avoid physically strenuous work for a week and to strictly control his blood pressure.

## Discussion

Epistaxis is a common problem with a 60% prevalence of at least one episode a lifetime in the adult population. However, only about 5% originates from the posterior part of the nasal cavity where it is considered to be a major medical problem and first-line treatments such as nasal packing, balloon, or systemic therapy often fail [3]. In post-traumatic patients the injury of vessels, pseudoaneurysm or arteriovenous fistula formation are likely to be the cause of the symptom.

Embolization for bleeding has been a well-recognized procedure for at least three decades. It was first used for epistaxis in the 1970s and is currently a standard procedure when surgery is unsuccessful, contraindicated, or in systemic diseases with multiple bleeding sites [9,10]. Despite increasing acceptance of embolization in head and neck vascular diseases, considering it as an alternative to surgical or endoscopic ligation in epistaxis still remains controversial.

One of the largest studies, conducted by Tseng et al [11], reviewed 107 patients with refractory epistaxis treated with intravascular embolization: 87% of this group suffered idiopathic epistaxis and in the remainder bleeding was post-traumatic or post-surgical. Embolization was performed using a 3Fr microcatheter and 250–700μm polyvinyl alcohol (PVA) particles. In a majority of the patients the ipsilateral IMA branches were embolized. Their five-year experience with 114 embolizations showed that the immediate success rate was 93% with two patients treated twice. In the majority of cases unsuccessful embolization was due to ethmoid arterial involvement, and these patients required ethmoid artery ligation. Long-term follow-up showed a recurrence of 12% from three days to 16 months after treatment. The total rate of complications was 17%; however, the major complication of transient hemiparesis and stroke occurred in only two cases. One of these patients, who suffered a long-term complication of stroke,had undergone extensive bilateral IMA and bilateral facial artery embolization [11]. Complications of embolization in the treatment of epistaxis are shown in Table 16.3.

Other studies based on large groups of patients showed similar results with success rates ranging from 88% to 100% and rare occurrence of major permanent complications in less then 2% of cases [12,13]. The best long-term results were obtained for post-traumatic epistaxis, where definite exclusion of the direct cause of the bleeding can be achieved [14]. The success rate is lower in patients with systemic diseases such as hereditary haemorrhagic telangiectasia [15].

The evidence for superiority of surgical or endovascular treatment lacks randomized controlled trials. A comparison of the treatments was performed by Cullen and Tami [16] and Barlow et al. [17] on groups of 39 and 44 patients, respectively. In both studies the efficacy and complication rates in the surgical and endovascular treatment groups were comparable and there was no significant difference in major complication episodes. The only tendency observed was that complications were more frequent after surgical ligation, but post-embolization complications were more severe. According to the literature, in large studies surgical ligation has proved to be effective in 82–97% of cases of epistaxis treatment [18,19].

**Evidence base** Endovascular embolization techniques

The embolization technique varies depending on the type of disease leading to epistaxis, which could be tumours, vascular malformations, arterial hypertension, telangiectasia, fistulas, aneurysms, or traumatic injury [20].

The main objective of embolization is to place a catheter or a microcatheter in a suitable position for depositing embolic material in the vessels as close to the bleeding site as possible. In maxillary artery embolization, the catheter should be positioned distal to the mandibular part of the IMA, where the origins of the meningeal arteries are located. To ensure effective treatment of patients who have not suffered trauma, especially with multiple sites of bleeding, it is important to embolize selected arteries bilaterally because of frequent side-to-side anastomoses. It is essential to check all the branches of the internal maxillary and facial arteries supplying the nasal cavity, and some authors report greater effectiveness with simultaneous embolization of IMA and FA branches [21].

- Immediate and late clinical success rates in bleeding cessation have been reported to be 88–100% and 71–89%, respectively [11,22,23].
- The risk of major complications has been reported to be 1–6% (see Table 16.3) [12,13,24].
- Recurrence of bleeding is reported in 10–13% of cases [12,22,23].

**Table 16.3** **Complications of embolization in the treatment of epistaxis**

| Severity of complication | Type of complication | Prevalence |
|---|---|---|
| Minor, transient | Pain, oedema, facial numbness paraesthesia, mild ulceration groin haematoma, fever | 25–59% |
| Major, transient | Skin necrosis, hemiparesis, visual field loss, mucosal necrosis | ≤6% |
| Permanent | Scarring after ischaemia, monocular blindness, facial nerve palsy, cerebral infarction, sialadenitis | ≤2% |

**Learning point** Embolic materials

Various occluding materials can be used for the embolization of nasal bleeds. The most commonly used agents are particles, coils, cyanoacrylate glue, Onyx and gel-foam. The technique chosen depends on the primary disease and the angiographic vascular abnormality. However, there are no precise guidelines as to which embolic material should be used for different diseases, and methods are adjusted to each individual case and the experience of the radiologist.

In systemic diseases with a high probability of epistaxis recurrence, such as HHT, the main objective is to stop the bleeding whilst simultaneously maintaining vessel access for future endovascular treatment. Therefore distal and transient embolic materials are preferable: calibrated particles (150–700μm), PVA particles, gelatin sponge, or gel-foam powder [10]. Coiling and permanent vessel occlusion should be avoided [25]. A similar strategy and embolic materials are preferred in idiopathic epistaxis [22,24].

In post-traumatic or iatrogenic bleedings the common angiographic symptoms are extravasation, pseudoaneurysm, or arteriovenous fistula. In cases with visible extravasation, embolization with particles, gel-foam, coils, cyanoacrylate glue, and Onyx are recommended; pseudoaneurysms and fistulas are treated most effectively with covered stents, cyanoacrylate glue, coils, Onyx, detachable balloons, and vascular plugs [14,21,26–28].

In pre-surgical embolization of bleeding from head and neck tumours or in palliative procedures gel-foam, middle and small calibre particles, and coils are used [29–32].

**Evidence base** Therapeutic methods in the treatment of persistent epistaxis.

Persistent epistaxis may be a life-threatening condition. In such cases there are three treatment options: endoscopic electrocautery, endoscopic or surgical vessel ligation, or endovascular embolization.

- There are a few studies comparing embolization and surgical ligation or cauterization [16,17,33,34], but no randomized trials have been reported.
- Most of these studies report similar success rates to those methods with a higher prevalence of minor complications after surgical treatment and rare, but more serious, complications occurring after embolization [16,33–35].
- Hospital stay is shorter after cauterization and embolization than after surgical treatment [34,36].
- Treatment costs for embolization and surgical ligation are similar, although some hospitals report differences [17,34].

## A final word from the expert

In the majority of cases epistaxis is an incidental discomfort which usually resolves without any medical intervention. In cases with trauma or systemic disease involvement, persistent bleeding in 6% of population becomes a health- or life-threatening issue. Depending on the underlying disease pathological angiographic symptoms are hypervascularization, pseudoaneurysms, arteriovenous fistulas, telangiectasias, and hyperaemia. In cases of severe epistaxis, angiographic signs of blood extravasation may be detected. However, there are cases where no vascular abnormality to be found.

Embolization is a rapid and repeatable procedure. In contrast with surgery, it can be performed under local anaesthesia or sedation. It is also a safe method of treatment when good technique is used. It is critical that the interventional radiologist performing embolization is aware of the potentially dangerous anastomoses between branches of the ECA and ICA involving the inferolateral trunk, ethmoidal collaterals, meningohypophyseal arteries, and occipital–vertebral arteries. Therefore vigilance is essential in careful assessment of ECA and ICA angiography for the presence of such anastomoses which may provide a route for embolic material to pass from the extracranial to intracranial circulation, leading to ischaemic complications in the brain, retina, or cranial nerves. To avoid non-target embolization very small particles (<200µm) or gel sponge powder should not be used.

The role of embolization in the management of epistaxis is still debatable. Head and neck surgeons should be able to acquire sufficient knowledge about conventional techniques, but must also be aware of interventional radiology methods in order to recommend the best treatment options to their patients. Frequently, complex medical problems require an individual approach and combined treatment.

## References

1. Corry J, Kucik CJ, Clenney T. Management of epistaxis. *Am Fam Physician* 2005; 71(2): 305–11.
2. Vaamonde Lago P, Martín Martín C, Lechuga García MR, et al. [Epidemiological notes on nasal bleeding]. *An Otorrinolaringol Ibero Am* 2004; 31(2): 123–32 (in Spanish).
3. Viducich RA, Blanda MP, Gerson LW. Posterior epistaxis: clinical features and acute complications. *Ann Emerg Med* 1995; 25(5): 592–6.

4. Hwang K, You SH, Kim SG, et al. Analysis of nasal bone fractures; a six-year study of 503 patients. *J Craniofac Surg* 2006; 17(2): 261–4.
5. Pallin DJ, Chng YM, McKay MP, et al. Epidemiology of epistaxis in US emergency departments. *Ann Emerg Med* 2005; 46(1): 77–81.
6. Monjas-Cánovas I, Hernández-García I, Mauri-Barberá J, et al. Epidemiology of epistaxes admitted to a tertiary hospital. *Acta Otorrinolaringol Esp* 2010; 61(1): 41–7 (in English and Spanish).
7. McIntosh N, Chalmers J. Incidence of oronasal haemorrhage in infancy presenting to general practice in the UK. *Br J Gen Pract* 2008; 58(557): 877–9.
8. Koh E, Frazzini VI, Kagetsu NJ. Epistaxis: vascular anatomy, origins, and endovascular treatment. *AJR Am J Roentgenol* 2000; 174(3): 845–51.
9. Bertrand B, Eloy P, Rombaux P, et al. Guidelines to the management of epistaxis. *B-ENT* 2005; Suppl 1: 27–41.
10. Trojanowski P, Jargiello T, Trojanowska A, Klatka J. Epistaxis in patients with hereditary hemorrhagic telangiectasia treated with selective arterial embolization. *Acta Radiol* 2011; 52(8): 846–9.
11. Tseng EY, Narducci CA, Willing SJ, Sillers MJ. Angiographic embolization for epistaxis: a review of 114 cases. *Laryngoscope* 1998; 108(4 Pt 1): 615–19.
12. Christensen NP, Smith DS, Barnwell SL, Wax MK. Arterial embolization in the management of posterior epistaxis. *Otolaryngol Head Neck Surg* 2005; 133(5): 748–53.
13. Strach K, Schröck A, Wilhelm K, et al. Endovascular treatment of epistaxis: indications, management, and outcome. *Cardiovasc Intervent Radiol* 2011; 34(6): 1190–8.
14. Keeling AN, McGrath FP, Thornton J, et al. Emergency percutaneous transcatheter embolisation of acute arterial haemorrhage. *Ir J Med Sci* 2010; 179(3): 385–91.
15. Elden L, Montanera W, Terbrugge K, et al. Angiographic embolization for the treatment of epistaxis: a review of 108 cases. *Otolaryngol Head Neck Surg* 1994; 111(1): 44–50.
16. Cullen MM, Tami TA. Comparison of internal maxillary artery ligation versus embolization for refractory posterior epistaxis. *Otolaryngol Head Neck Surg* 1998; 118(5): 636–42.
17. Barlow DW, Deleyiannis WB, Pinczower EF. Effectiveness of surgical management of epistaxis at a tertiary care center. *Laryngoscope* 1997; 107(1): 21–4.
18. Soyka MB, Nikolaou G, Rufibach K, Holzmann D. On the effectiveness of treatment options in epistaxis: an analysis of 678 interventions. *Rhinology* 2011; 49(4): 474–8.
19. Howe DJ, Wazir U, Skinner DW. Outcomes of endoscopic sphenopalatine artery ligation for epistaxis: a five-year series from a single institution. *Ear Nose Throat J* 2012; 91(2): 70–2.
20. Broomfield S, Bruce I, Birzgalis A, Herwadkar A. The expanding role of interventional radiology in head and neck surgery. *J R Soc Med* 2009; 102(6): 228–34.
21. Fukutsuji K, Nishiike S, Aihara T, et al. Superselective angiographic embolization for intractable epistaxis. *Acta Otolaryngol* 2008; 128(5): 556–60.
22. Gurney TA, Dowd CF, Murr AH. Embolization for the treatment of idiopathic posterior epistaxis. *Am J Rhinol* 2004; 18(5): 335–9.
23. Elahi MM, Parnes LS, Fox AJ, et al. Therapeutic embolization in the treatment of intractable epistaxis. *Arch Otolaryngol Head Neck Surg* 1995; 121(1): 65–9.
24. Willems PW, Farb RI, Agid R. Endovascular treatment of epistaxis. *AJNR Am J Neuroradiol* 2009; 30(9): 1637–45.
25. Layton KF, Kallmes DF, Gray LA, Cloft HJ. Endovascular treatment of epistaxis in patients with hereditary hemorrhagic telangiectasia. *AJNR Am J Neuroradiol* 2007; 28(5): 885–8.
26. Thiex R, Wu I, Mulliken JB, et al. Safety and clinical efficacy of Onyx for embolization of extracranial head and neck vascular anomalies. *AJNR Am J Neuroradiol* 2011; 32(6): 1082–6.
27. Zhang C, Xie X, You C, et al. Endovascular treatment of traumatic pseudoaneurysm presenting as intractable epistaxis. *Korean J Radiol* 2010; 11(6): 603–11.

28. Remonda L, Schroth G, Caversaccio M, et al. Endovascular treatment of acute and subacute hemorrhage in the head and neck. *Arch Otolaryngol Head Neck Surg* 2000; 126(10): 1255–62.
29. Llorente JL, López F, Suárez V, et al. [Evolution in the treatment of juvenile nasopharyngeal angiofibroma.] *Acta Otorrinolaringol Esp* 2011; 62(4): 279–86 (in Spanish).
30. Giavroglou C, Constantinidis J, Triaridis S, et al. [Angiographic evaluation and embolization of juvenile nasopharyngeal angiofibroma.] *HNO* 2007; 55(1): 36–41.
31. Kakizawa H, Toyota N, Naito A, Ito K. Endovascular therapy for management of oral hemorrhage in malignant head and neck tumors. *Cardiovasc Intervent Radiol* 2005; 28(6): 722–9.
32. Zähringer M, Guntinas-Lichius O, Gossmann A, et al. Percutaneous embolization for cervicofacial neoplasms and hemorrhages. *J Otorhinolaryngol Relat Spec* 2005; 67(6): 348–60.
33. Rudmik L, Smith TL. Management of intractable spontaneous epistaxis. *Am J Rhinol Allergy* 2012; 26(1): 55–60.
34. Strong EB, Bell DA, Johnson LP, Jacobs JM. Intractable epistaxis: transantral ligation vs. embolization: efficacy review and cost analysis. *Otolaryngol Head Neck Surg* 1995; 113(6): 674–8.
35. Holzmann D, Kaufmann T, Pedrini P, Valavanis A. Posterior epistaxis: endonasal exposure and occlusion of the branches of the sphenopalatine artery. *Eur Arch Otorhinolaryngol* 2003; 260(8): 425–8.
36. Frikart L, Agrifoglio A. Endoscopic treatment of posterior epistaxis. *Rhinology* 1998; 36(2): 59–61.

CASE

# 17 Massive haemoptysis: what to embolize?

Kendrick Tang

Expert commentary Philip Kwok

## Case history

A 79-year-old female presented at the A&E department at 5a.m. with haemoptysis. She had a history of right breast carcinoma with mastectomy 18 years previously, and mycobacterium avium-intracellulare (MAI) infection complicated with haemoptysis six years previously. The volume of haemoptysis was estimated to be about 100ml. She was also tachypnoeic with a respiratory rate of 24–28 breaths/minute.

**Learning point** Definition of massive haemoptysis

Massive haemoptysis is commonly defined as the expectoration of an amount of blood ranging from 100ml to more than 1000ml over a period of 24 hours, although no single cut-off volume has been agreed upon in the literature [1].

This is partly due to the fact that sometimes it is not the volume of expectorant seen by the physician which results in significant blood loss and subsequent haemodynamic change; rather, it is the flooding of intra-alveolar space that can only be estimated, with resulting hindrance to the oxygen transfer which causes desaturation and suffocation.

Upon examination, she was afebrile. $SpO_2$ was 88% on 15L oxygen. Her initial chest X-ray in A&E showed consolidation at the right upper lobe with internal cavitations (Figure 17.1a). After admission, she developed further haemoptysis with desaturation and respiratory failure, and was intubated and transferred to the ICU for further care. Fibre-optic bronchoscopy was performed and a large blood clot was found at the right main bronchus with continuous oozing from the right upper lobe. An urgent contrast CT thorax was then requested and showed a large right upper lobe mycetoma (Figure 17.1b) with increased vascularity around the right upper lobe, which were supplied by a tortuous and hypertrophic right intercostal bronchial trunk (ICBT) and right internal mammary artery (IMA) (Figure 17.2). In view of the clinical presentation and the imaging findings, the patient was offered the option of embolization of the abnormal arteries.

**Evidence base** Diagnostic work-up for haemoptysis

Haemoptysis has many different causes, and the prevalence of each of these varies greatly throughout the world. While chronic inflammatory lung diseases and bronchogenic carcinoma remain the most common causes of haemoptysis in western countries, tuberculosis continues to be the leading cause of haemoptysis worldwide [2].

(continued)

**Learning point** Anatomy of the bronchial artery

Cauldwell et al. [4] described four classic bronchial artery branching patterns (Figure 17.3).

- Type I: one right bronchial artery from right intercostobronchial trunk (ICBT), two left bronchial arteries (40.6%).
- Type II: one on the right from ICBT, one on the left (21.3%).
- Type III: two on the right (one from ICBT and one bronchial artery), two on the left (20.6%).
- Type IV: two on the right (one from ICBT and one bronchial artery), one on the left (9.7%).

Traditionally, chest physicians have utilized bronchoscopy as the primary investigation for patients presenting with haemoptysis. It is most useful for localizing the site of haemorrhage and, if a central bronchial lesion is seen, vasoactive medication (e.g. epinephrine) can be applied locally to control bleeding [2]. However, the diagnostic accuracy of bronchoscopy in patients with haemoptysis can be low, and many researchers are currently suggesting that CT should be performed prior to bronchoscopy in all patients with haemoptysis [3]. In addition to localizing the site of bleeding and suggesting the cause of haemorrhage, CT offers the unique advantage of identification of bronchial and non-bronchial systemic feeder vessels, which can be extremely useful if bronchial artery embolization is to be considered.

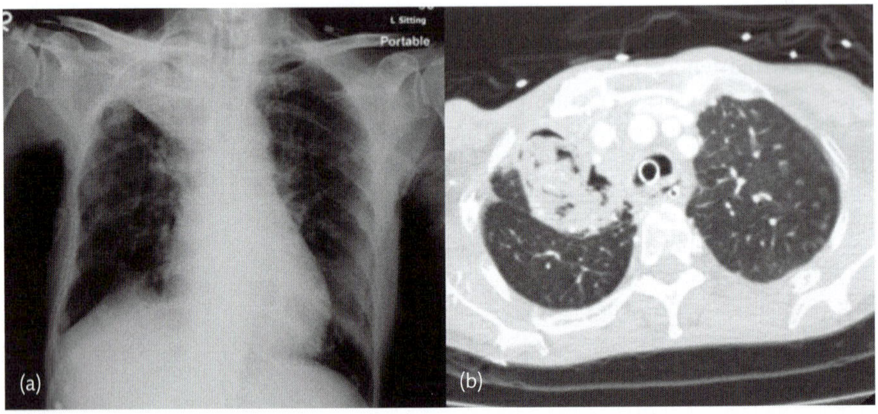


**Figure 17.1** (a) Chest X-ray on admission shows right upper lobe consolidation with internal cavitations. (b) Contrast CT thorax shows cavitating right upper lobe lesion suggestive of mycetoma formation.

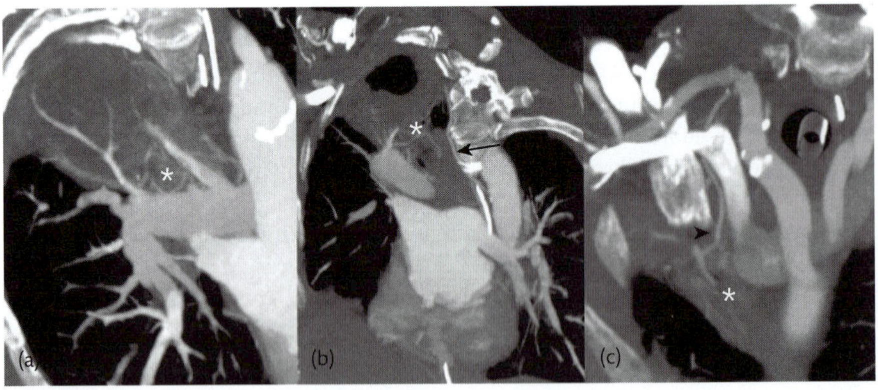


**Figure 17.2** (a)-(c) Contrast CT thorax with re-formation shows increase in vascularity (asterisk) around the right upper lobe supplied by tortuous and hypertrophic branches of right ICBT (arrow in (b)) and right IMA (arrowhead in (c)).

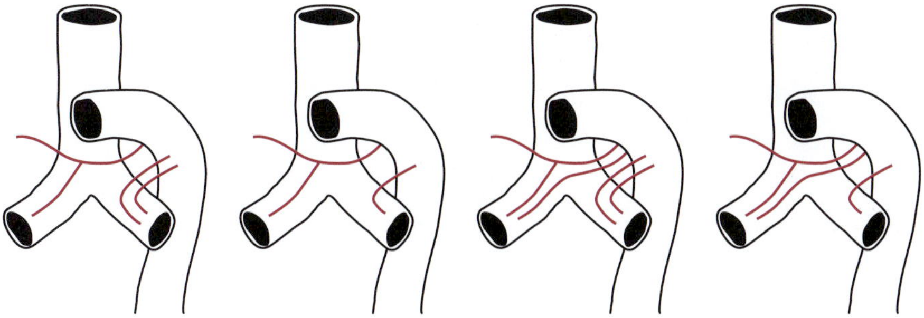


**Figure 17.3** Four main types of bronchial artery anatomy. Type I: one right bronchial artery from right ICBT, two left bronchial arteries (40.6%). Type II: one on the right from ICBT, one on the left (21.3%). Type III: two on the right (one from ICBT and one bronchial artery), two on the left (20.6%). Type IV: two on the right (one from ICBT and one bronchial artery), one on the left (9.7%).

Reprinted with kind permission of Springer Science and Business Media from Chun JY, Morgan R, Belli AM. Radiological management of hemoptysis: a comprehensive review of diagnostic imaging and bronchial arterial embolization. *Cardiovasc Intervent Radiol* 2010 Apr; 33(2):240–50.

**Expert comment** CT angiography versus thoracic aortogram

Before bronchial artery embolization (BAE), we usually perform CTA using multidetector CT (at least 64 slices). The enlarged bronchial arteries or other non-bronchial systemic arteries are shown well. Both axial and sagittal reconstruction can be used to show the take-off of the supplying arteries, and give a better idea of catheter tip orientation during catheterization.

CTA can usually provide adequate information on the enlarged arteries even when the patient is dyspnoeic. It may be difficult to visualize the enlarged bronchial arteries or non-bronchial systemic arteries with a conventional catheter aortogram when the patient is dyspnoeic. A good example is the inferior phrenic artery from the coeliac axis, which is often obscured by the diaphragmatic artefacts in dyspnoeic patients. If CTA is performed immediately before BAE, we can use dimer non-ionic contrast (Visipaque) to reduce the risk of contrast nephropathy.

Diagnostic digital subtraction angiography (DSA) was first performed. It confirmed hypertrophy of the right ICBT with a prominent supply to the right apical mycetoma. The right ICBT was then embolized with 355–500μm PVA particles (Contour; Boston Scientific, Marlborough, MA, USA), which were delivered through a 2.7Fr microcatheter (Progreat; Terumo, Tokyo, Japan) (Figure 17.4).

**Expert comment** Choice of guiding catheter

The enlarged ICBT may arise from the inferior curve of the aortic arch. Judkins left coronary catheter is the catheter of choice. Radiologists may not be familiar with this catheter which is commonly used by cardiologists.

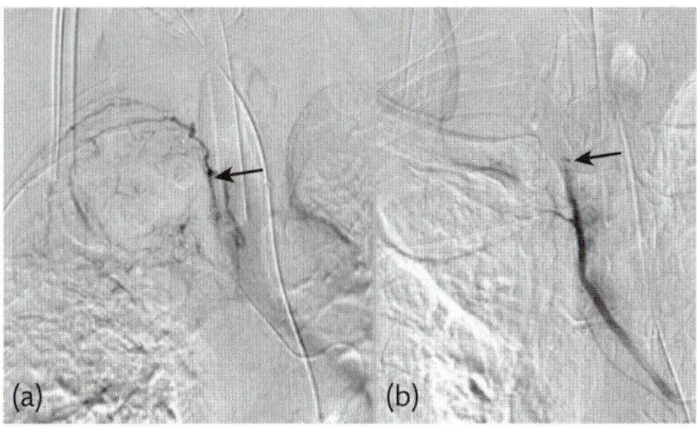


**Figure 17.4** (a) The right ICBT angiogram shows a hypertrophied ICBT (arrow) with prominent supply to the right apical mycetoma. (b) After embolization of the right ICBT with 355–500μm PVA particles, vascularity is markedly reduced (arrow).

**Expert comment** Size of spherical agents

Spherical embolic agents of diameter <700μm can pass through the microcatheter easily, even without flushing with saline between injection. Larger particles (diameter 700–900μm or 900–1200μm) need more dilution and more frequent flushing with saline. Concentrated particles will block the microcatheter.

**Expert comment** n-Butyl cyanoacrylate (NBCA) glue

For patients with a high flow shunt to the pulmonary arteries, 40–50% NBCA glue is useful for shunt blockage.

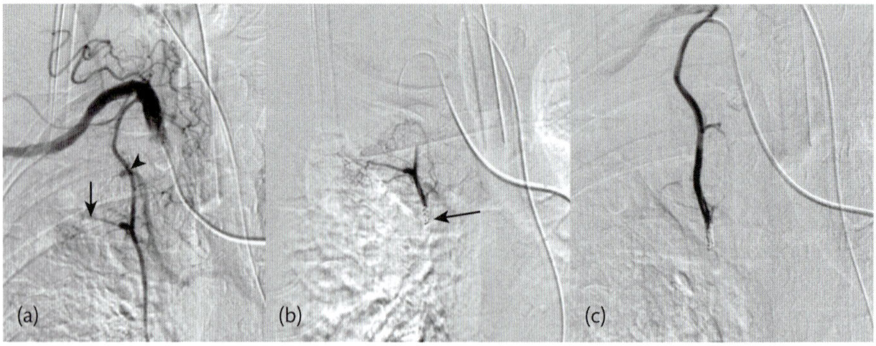


**Figure 17.5** (a) Right subclavian and right IMA angiograms show abnormal transpleural supply (arrow) and a systemic pulmonary shunt (arrowhead) at the right upper zone through the transpleural branches of the right IMA. (b) Microcoils (arrow) are used to occlude the right IMA at the mid-portion for distal flow control. (c) After embolization of the proximal right IMA with 355–500μm PVA particles, vascularity is markedly reduced.

DSA of the right IMA was then performed and showed an abnormal transpleural supply and a systemic pulmonary shunt at the right upper zone through the transpleural branches of the right IMA. Five 2mm/3mm × 22mm microcoils (VortX; Boston Scientific, Marlborough, MA, USA) were used to occlude the right IMA at the mid-portion for distal flow control. Embolization of the proximal right IMA was then performed with 355–500μm PVA particles, again delivered through a 2.7Fr microcatheter (Figure 17.5). Bleeding was successfully controlled and haemoptysis did not recur after the procedure. The patient slowly recovered and was discharged with oral medication to control the fungal infection.

**Expert comment** Other non-bronchial systemic arteries

Fibrosis due to old tuberculosis can often cause pleural thickening and induce non-bronchial systemic supply from branches of the subclavian artery, including the internal mammary arteries, the long thoracic artery, and branches from the costocervical trunk. Systemic heparinization should be used when catheter passes through the subclavian artery, as clots may flow to the vertebral arteries and causes ischaemic stroke. The patient should be warned of this complication and frequently monitored during the procedure.

In patients with a tortuous aortic arch and acute take-off of the supra-aortic branches, a trans-radial or trans-brachial approach can often save a lot of time and reduce complications.

# Discussion

## Bronchial artery and non-bronchial systemic arterial supply: what to embolize?

Percutaneous transcatheter embolization is a safe and effective treatment for patients presenting with life-threatening haemoptysis. In 90% of cases, the source of massive haemoptysis is the bronchial circulation [5]. Previous studies suggest that a reduction of pulmonary circulation in the lesions of inflammatory lung diseases leads to systemic pulmonary anastomosis accompanied by a compensatory increase in systemic circulation, resulting in the rupture of systemic arteries [6].

In a minority of patients, non-bronchial systemic arteries can be the predominant source of massive haemoptysis, especially in those patients with pleural involvement caused by an underlying disease [3]. For example, fibrosis due to old tuberculosis often causes pleural thickening and induces non-bronchial systemic supply. Failure to recognize this alternative supply may result in early recurrence of haemoptysis after apparently successful embolization of the bronchial arteries. These non-bronchial systemic arterial supplies may originate from intercostal artery, the IMA, or other branches of the subclavian artery (such as the long thoracic artery and branches from the costocervical trunk), as well as inferior phrenic artery. As illustrated in the case discussed here, contrast CTA of the thorax is very useful in identifying these arterial supplies, both for planning which vessels to embolize and reducing the risk of early recurrence of haemoptysis which is related to unrecognized abnormal vascular supply.

## Technique of bronchial artery embolization

Conventionally, thoracic aortography is first performed to evaluate the number and sites of origin of the bronchial arteries. It may also detect an anomalous origin of bronchial arteries and the presence of a non-bronchial systemic arterial supply [7]. Alternatively, such information may also be available from contrast CT thorax studies. Standard common femoral arterial access usually suffices, although brachial artery access may occasionally be required to tackle the extraordinarily difficult non-bronchial systemic arterial contributions. However, the latter is believed to be associated with higher morbidity and complication rates [8].

After the abnormal vessels have been identified, they are cannulated with a Simmons catheter or another type of catheter (e.g. Cobra, Shepherd's crook, Mikaelsson, etc.) depending on the anatomical configuration. In many cases, superselection of a more distal branch with the help of a microcatheter is necessary to avoid inadvertent embolization of arteries supplying other normal regions.

## Choice of embolic agents

Various temporary and permanent embolic agents are available. They include Gelfoam, PVA particles, trisacryl gelatin, stainless steel coils, and NBCA.

Gelfoam is a temporary embolic agent. It is cost effective, and the size can be controlled. However, Gelfoam is absorbed spontaneously and recanalization can occur faster than with other permanent embolic agents. Studies have shown that embolization with Gelfoam is associated with a higher rate of recurrence at midterm follow-up compared with other agents such as PVA [9].

The most common practice is to use PVA, which is a permanent embolic agent. PVA particles are available in several size ranges and an appropriate choice must be made. It has been shown that naturally occurring bronchopulmonary arterial anastomoses in the lung can have diameters of up to about 325μm [10]. Therefore PVA particles in the range 355–500μm are chosen, in order to avoid particles that are smaller than the diameter of the bronchopulmonary arterial anastomoses entering the pulmonary circulation and causing pulmonary embolism or infarct.

A disadvantage of PVA particles is that their diameters are non-homogeneous and hence there is an increased risk of obstruction of the catheters, especially if microcatheters are used. Thus, some researchers recommend that spherical agents such as trisacryl gelatin (Embosphere; BioSphere Medical, Rockland, MA, USA) or similar agents such as Bead Block (Terumo, Tokyo, Japan) or Embozene (CeloNova BioSciences, Peachtree City, GA, USA) are preferable for patients in whom microcatheters are used [11].

Stainless steel coils are not recommended for embolization of the bronchial artery, although they can be used for the embolization of the IMA to preserve the normal vascular territory [12].

NBCA is a liquid embolic material. Although initially approved for the embolization of cerebral arteriovenous malformation (AVM), NBCA is now used for the treatment of massive haemoptysis in some institutions. It has several advantages over the other materials: rapid and complete vessel occlusion can be achieved even in patients with coagulopathy, control of embolization by adjusting the polymerization rate, and a relatively short procedure time [13]. However, extreme care is needed when using NBCA because reflux of polymerized NBCA around the microcatheter during injection can adhere to its tip and may be detached during catheter removal, resulting in non-target embolization.

### Reasons for failure

Bronchial artery embolization is a very effective procedure for controlling acute massive haemoptysis. Failure of the procedure or recurrence of haemoptysis can be caused by incomplete embolization, recanalization of embolized vessels, revascularization by collateral circulation, inadequate treatment or progression of the underlying lung disease, or failure to recognize non-bronchial systemic arterial supplies. Careful review of the CT aortogram and conventional thoracic aortogram may show non-bronchial systemic arterial supplies that require embolization. A combination of embolizing agents may sometimes be required for adequate vascular control, as shown in the case described here.

### Complications

Complications can be classified as general (related to vascular intervention) or specific (associated with the embolization procedure). Most of the complications reported are related to the effects of embolization and ischaemia. Chest pain, which is believed to be an ischaemic phenomenon and is usually transient, is the most common complication. Other less common complications include dysphagia, aortic and bronchial necrosis, broncho-oesophageal fistula, pulmonary infarction, and transient cortical blindness. There is also a small risk of subintimal dissection of the arteries during catheter or guidewire manipulation, with a reported prevalence of 1–6.3% [3]. There are usually no symptoms or problems related to the subintimal dissection, and it can be managed conservatively. There is also a case report of iatrogenic rupture of the descending thoracic aorta during bronchial artery embolization which was treated by implantation of an endovascular stent graft in the thoracic aorta [14].One of the most devastating complications of bronchial artery embolization is spinal cord ischaemia due to occlusion of the spinal arteries. This is most likely to occur if the artery of Adamkiewicz is embolized. Therefore, when it is visualized at angiography, embolization should not be performed.

## A final word from the expert

Bronchial artery embolization is an effective treatment for haemoptysis caused by various diseases. Provided that meticulous attention paid to the anatomy and technical details, it is a safe and life-saving procedure for the patient.

# References


1. Ibrahim WH. Massive haemoptysis: the definition should be revised. *Eur Respir J* 2008; 32(4): 1131–2.
2. Jean-Baptiste E. Clinical assessment and management of massive hemoptysis. *Crit Care Med* 2000; 28: 1642–7.
3. Yoon W, Kim JK, Kim YH, et al. Bronchial and nonbronchial systemic artery embolization for life-threatening hemoptysis: a comprehensive review. *Radiographics* 2002; 22(6): 1395–1409.
4. Cauldwell EW, Siekert RG, Lininger RE, Anson BJ. The bronchial arteries: an anatomic study of 105 human cadavers. *Surg Gynecol Obstet* 1948; 86: 395–412.
5. Remy J, Remy-Jardin M, Voisin C. Endovascular management of bronchial bleeding. In J Butler (ed), *The Bronchial Circulation* (New York: Marcel Dekker); 1992: 667–723.
6. Liebow AA, Hales MR, Bloomer WE, et al. Studies on the lung after ligation of the pulmonary artery. II. Anatomic changes. *Am J Pathol* 1950; 26: 177–95.
7. Phillips S, Ruttley MST. Bronchial artery embolization: the importance of preliminary thoracic aortography. *Clin Radiol* 2000; 55: 317–19.
8. Sopko DR, Smith TP. Bronchial artery embolization for hemoptysis. *Semin Intervent Radiol* 2011; 28(1): 48–62.
9. Hahn S, Kim YJ, Kwon W, et al. Comparison of the effectiveness of embolic agents for bronchial artery embolization: Gelfoam versus polyvinyl alcohol. *Korean J Radiol* 2010; 11: 542–6.
10. Pump K. Distribution of bronchial arteries in human lung. *Chest* 1972; 62: 447–51.
11. Ustünsöz B, Bozlar U, Ors F, et al. Bronchial artery embolization: experience with 10 cases. *Diagn Interv Radiol* 2006; 12(1): 43–6.
12. Yoon W. Embolic agents used for bronchial artery embolisation in massive haemoptysis. *Expert Opin Pharmacother* 2004; 5(2): 361–7.
13. Yoo DH, Yoon CJ, Kang SG, et al. Bronchial and nonbronchial systemic artery embolization in patients with major hemoptysis: safety and efficacy of n-butyl cyanoacrylate. *AJR Am J Roentgenol* 2011; 196(2): W199–204.
14. Bautista-Hernandez V, Gutierrez F, Roldan S, et al. Successful stent-grafting for iatrogenic aortic rupture and life-threatening hemoptysis. *Minerva Chir* 2007; 62(5): 425–8.

CASE

# 18 Gastrointestinal bleeding: which embolic material to use?

**Bhaskar Ganai**

**Expert commentary** Michael J Lee

## Case history

A 68-year-old male was admitted via A&E with a two-day history of melaena with fresh blood and clot per rectum (PR). He described mild occasional abdominal discomfort but no significant pain, nausea, vomiting, or weight loss. He maintained a good appetite. He was haemodynamically stable with normal vital signs. Clinical examination was unremarkable. Haemoglobin (Hb) on admission was 10.7g/dl.

Significant past medical history included a traumatic head injury with resultant right hemiparesis and chronic hydrocephalus managed by a ventriculo-peritoneal shunt. The patient had previously undergone a right nephrectomy secondary to staghorn calculus, and had problems with recurrent urinary tract infections (UTIs) and urinary incontinence.

The patient was initially investigated with an upper gastrointestinal (GI) endoscopy, which demonstrated mild duodenitis but no source of upper GI bleeding or stigmata of previous haemorrhage.

**Learning point**

After the patient has been stabilized and resuscitated, upper GI bleeding should initially be investigated with endoscopy. Upper GI bleeding, defined as bleeding proximal to the ligament of Treitz, can present as melaena or, in the case of massive haemorrhage, unaltered blood. On endoscopy, stigmata of previous haemorrhage can manifest as active bleeding, non-bleeding but a visible vessel, fresh blood clot, or black spots [1]. Endoscopy is more often diagnostic in the upper GI tract than in the lower GI tract. For this reason, endoscopy is less often used in the initial approach to lower GI bleeding [2].

Peptic ulcer disease accounts for >80% of upper GI bleeding with varices, Dieulafoy's lesion, Mallory-Weiss tears, inflammation, angiodysplasia, haemosuccus pancreaticus, and malignancy responsible for the remainder [3].

Although the patient remained haemodynamically stable, the Hb dropped to 7.6g/dl and two units of packed red cells were transfused. A colonoscopy was performed to the ascending colon, which confirmed blood within the transverse and ascending colon. However, the bleeding site could not be identified. The patient was transferred to radiology for a contrast-enhanced CT scan which demonstrated an abnormal large arteriovenous (AV) malformation in the jejunum (Figure 18.1). The patient subsequently had a mesenteric angiogram with right AVM coil embolization (Figures 18.2 and 18.3).

**Evidence base**

Upper GI bleeding has a 14% mortality rate [4] and a 20% rebleeding rate [5]. Various endoscopic methods for controlling haemorrhage are available, including local epinephrine injection, thermal coagulation, and mechanical clips, bands, and ligation. The various modalities appear to be equivalent in efficacy for haemostasis, rebleeding rates, and emergency surgery [3], with a combination of two or more therapies giving the best results. Endoscopic therapy is 80–90% effective in non-variceal upper GI bleeding [1].

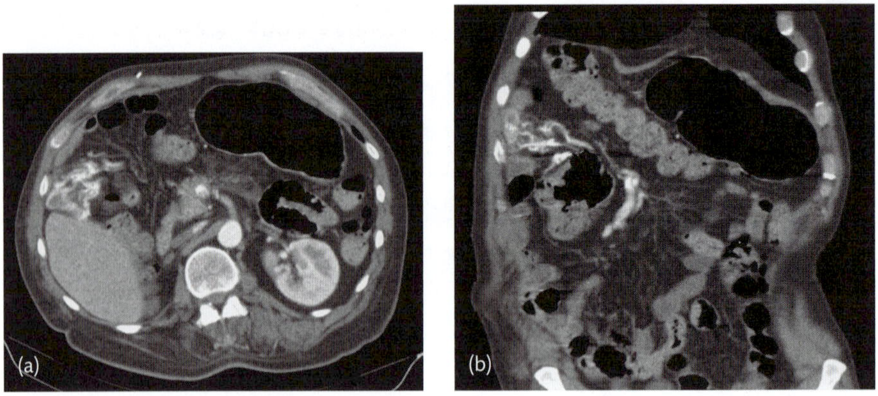


**Figure 18.1** (a) Arterial phase contrast enhanced axial and (b) coronal reformatted CT demonstrating a small bowel AV malformation on the right side of the abdomen.

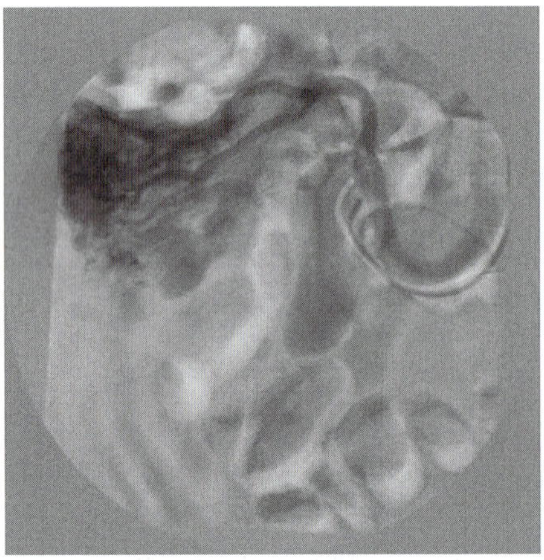

**Figure 18.2** Selective catheter angiography demonstrating AV malformation.

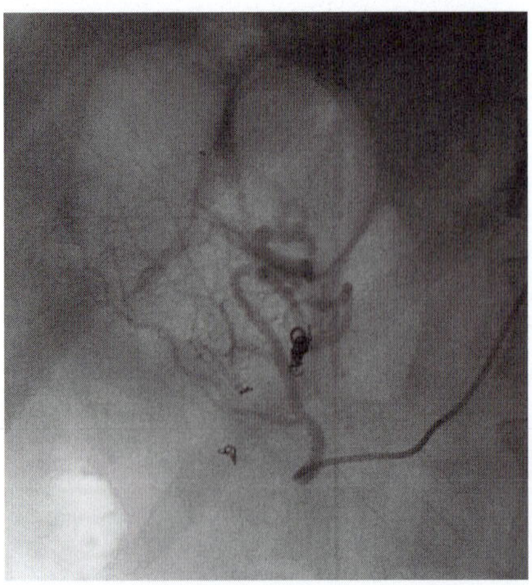

**Figure 18.3** Angiogram following initial coil embolization of AV malformation.

**Evidence base** If endoscopy is unsuccessful, is surgery or embolotherapy more effective?

In a series of 70 patients with refractory upper GI haemorrhage reported by Ripoll et al. [7], 31 underwent embolotherapy with the remaining 39 undergoing surgery. The embolotherapy group were older, had a higher incidence of cardiovascular disease, and were more likely to be anticoagulated. There was no significant difference in rates of rebleeding or death. The patients treated surgically were more likely to require additional surgery, usually for surgical complications rather than rebleeding, although this was not statistically significant (16.1% embolotherapy vs 30.8% surgery).

Defreyne et al. [8] showed that if a bleeding peptic ulcer was unsuccessfully treated at endoscopy, the patient was five times more likely to be referred for surgery rather than embolotherapy.

**Learning point**

Contrast-enhanced multidetector CT is useful in both upper and lower GI bleeding where a source has not been identified endoscopically. It has the advantage of not requiring bowel preparation and is accurate for detection and localization of acute massive GI bleeding [6].

Following embolization there was no further significant bleeding PR. A colonoscopy was performed which was normal to the level of the caecum. The patient remained free from PR bleeding.

However, after almost two years the patient re-presented with melaena. He was haemodynamically stable but anaemic with Hb 8.4g/dl. After transfusion of two units of packed red cells, an angiogram and embolization with 700–900μm Embospheres (BioSphere Medical, Rockland, MA, USA) were performed. The endpoint of embolization was slow flow rather than stasis to avoid ischaemia.

Three months after discharge, the patient was readmitted with PR bleeding. He recovered spontaneously with Hb 9.2g/dl. However, there was continued bleeding with a reduction of Hb to 7.4g/dl. Angiography was performed with further embolization with n-butyl cyanoacrylate (NBCA) glue and lipiodol contrast in a 1:3 ratio. A microcatheter was used to obtain a distal position for embolization (Figure 18.4). A further scheduled embolization with NBCA was performed 6 weeks later. The patient has had no further bleeding.

**Learning point**

Predictors of positive angiography include [9]:

- Clinical signs of bleeding
- Active bleeding on endoscopy
- Bleeding >0.5ml/minute
- Requirement of more than three units of red blood cells within 24 hours
- Underlying vascular abnormality expected
- High shock index (heart rate/systolic BP) [10]

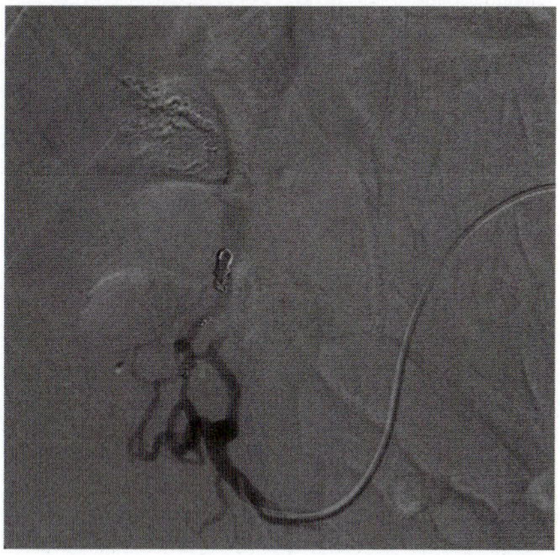

**Figure 18.4** Completion angiogram following glue embolization.

**Evidence base** Which embolic agent should be used?

A large study by Schenker et al. [11] reviewed clinical and technical factors relating to patient outcomes in 163 patients with upper GI haemorrhage. They found no significant difference in outcomes with gelatin sponge, coils, PVA, or a combination of these embolics.

Aina et al. [12] reviewed 75 patients with upper GI haemorrhage who were embolized with coils, NBCA, PVA, Gelfoam, or a combination of these embolics. The use of coils alone was significantly associated with an early rebleeding rate.

Lee et al. [13] reported excellent results with NBCA with almost 90% clinical success, albeit in a small series of 16 patients.

**Expert comment**

Although coils are the mainstay of both upper and lower GI embolization, they may not be suitable for all patients with GI bleeding. In this particular patient, coils were probably not the appropriate choice of embolic agent. Although, the patient had no more GI bleeding for two years, when bleeding did occur, the AV malformation had increased significantly in size making it more difficult to treat. We then tried large particles (700–900μm Embospheres) in an attempt to decrease pulse pressure in the feeding artery, but this did not provide a lasting result. Finally, when the patient bled for the third time a decision was made to use glue. The particular form of glue used was Glubran (Gem Srl, Italy), which is different from the cyanoacrylate Histoacryl (B. Braun) in that it allows much more time before catheters become 'stuck'.

## Discussion

Various embolic agents are available for GI embolization. These can be classified as:

- coils
- particles, including Gelfoam, PVA, and microspheres
- liquid embolics, including glue.

All of these, except Gelfoam, are permanent embolic agents [14].

**Expert comment**

The more dilute the glue solution, the more distally it will embolize. In this patient, a distal embolization was required; therefore, the glue was mixed with lipiodol in a 1:3 ratio. It was planned to perform embolization in two or three sessions to avoid small bowel ischemia, but two sessions were adequate for complete embolization. Onyx is another embolic agent that could have been used with similar results, but it is more expensive and requires DMSO-compatible catheters. Glue is also useful for upper GI embolization if the patient is coagulopathic because coils need clotting factors to induce thrombosis. Similarly, particles may be of use in selected cases of lower GI bleeding where the bleeding site can be seen but a good distal position cannot be reached with a microcatheter. In this situation, it may be reasonable to float PVA particles to the bleeding site to control the bleeding.

There are technical differences in embolization between the upper and lower GI tract. In the upper GI tract, there are arcades and collateral branches, so there is less chance of ischaemia but more chance of persistent bleeding from collateral branches. For this reason both sides of the arcade should be embolized (back-door) and being very selective is not as crucial. This contrasts with lower GI tract, where there are fewer collaterals and a higher probability of ischaemia. This necessitates very selective embolization [9].

In the case of upper GI bleeding, empirical embolization is still worth pursuing if active extravasation is not present on angiography. In a series of 108 patients with acute upper GI bleeding reported by Padia et al. [15], 36 had active contrast extravasation at angiography, whereas active contrast extravasation was not seen in the remaining 72. All were embolized with endoscopy guiding the location of embolization when contrast extravasation was not demonstrated, i.e. proximal stomach bleeding resulted in left gastric artery embolization while distal stomach or duodenal bleeding resulted in gastroduodenal artery, right gastroepiploic, and/or pancreaticoduodenal arcade embolization. The clinical success in the two groups was identical at 44%.

Lower GI embolization is both technically and clinically effective. In a series of 19 patients, d'Othée et al. [16] showed technical success in 89% with full or partial clinical success in 89%. Coil embolization was exclusively used in this study, with two patients requiring colectomy due to ischaemic complications.

Overall, embolotherapy has good technical success but more variable clinical success. There is a suggestion that glue may be a superior embolic agent in upper GI haemorrhage [13], with poorer clinical outcomes in patients with multi-organ failure and coagulopathy (11). Secondary clinical success of arresting haemorrhage after all interventions is high at 85–100%. However, 30 day mortality remains between 9% and 40% [17].

## A final word from the expert

In conclusion, coils remain the embolization material of choice in GI bleeding but it is important to remember that other agents also have a role to play.

## References

1. Lee MJ. Embolotherapy for upper GI bleeding: factors influencing outcome. *GEST 2009*; 2009.
2. Kandarpa K, Machan L. *Handbook of Interventional Radiologic Procedures* (4th edn) (Philadelphia: Lippincott-Williams & Wilkins); 2011.
3. Yuan Y, Wang C, Hunt RH. Endoscopic clipping for acute nonvariceal upper-GI bleeding: a meta-analysis and critical appraisal of randomized controlled trials. *Gastrointest Endosc* 2008; 68(2): 339–51.
4. Rockall TA, Logan RF, Devlin HB, Northfield TC. Incidence of and mortality from acute upper gastrointestinal haemorrhage in the United Kingdom. *BMJ* 1995; 311(6999): 222–6.
5. Martins NB, Wassef W. Upper gastrointestinal bleeding. *Curr Opin Gastroenterol* 2006; 22(6): 612–19.
6. Yoon W, Jeong YY, Shin SS, et al. Acute massive gastrointestinal bleeding: detection and localization with arterial phase multi-detector row helical CT. *Radiology* 2006; 239(1): 160–7.
7. Ripoll C, Bañares R, Beceiro I, et al. Comparison of transcatheter arterial embolization and surgery for treatment of bleeding peptic ulcer after endoscopic treatment failure. *J Vasc Interv Radiol* 2004; 15(5): 447–50.
8. Defreyne L, De Schrijver I, Decruyenaere J, et al. Therapeutic decision-making in endoscopically unmanageable nonvariceal upper gastrointestinal hemorrhage. *Cardiovasc Interv Radiol* 2008; 31(5): 897–905.
9. Van Delden OM. Embolisation (TAE) for arterial hemorrhage of the GI-tract. *ECR 2008*; 2008.
10. Nakasone Y, Ikeda O, Yamashita Y, et al. Shock index correlates with extravasation on angiographs of gastrointestinal hemorrhage: a logistics regression analysis. *Cardiovasc Intervent Radiol* 2007; 30(5): 861–5.
11. Schenker MP, Duszak R, Soulen MC, et al. Upper gastrointestinal hemorrhage and transcatheter embolotherapy: clinical and technical factors impacting success and survival. *J Vasc Interv Radiol* 2001; 12(11): 1263–71.
12. Aina R, Oliva VL, Therasse E, et al. Arterial embolotherapy for upper gastrointestinal hemorrhage: outcome assessment. *J Vasc Interv Radiol* 2001; 12(2): 195–200.
13. Lee C-W., Liu K-L., Wang H-P., et al. Transcatheter arterial embolization of acute upper gastrointestinal tract bleeding with N-butyl-2-cyanoacrylate. *J Vasc Interv Radiol* 2007; 18(2): 209–16.

14. Kessel D, Robertson I. *Interventional Radiology: A Survival Guide* (2nd edn) (Amsterdam:Elsevier); 2005.
15. Padia SA, Geisinger MA, Newman JS, et al. Effectiveness of coil embolization in angiographically detectable versus non-detectable sources of upper gastrointestinal hemorrhage. *J Vasc Interv Radiol* 2009; 20(4): 461–6.
16. d'Othée BJ, Surapaneni P, Rabkin D, et al. Microcoil embolization for acute lower gastrointestinal bleeding. *Cardiovasc Intervent Radiol* 2006; 29(1): 49–58.
17. Lee MJ. Evidence-based review of embolization of upper GIH. *GEST 2007*; 2007.

CASE

# 19 Endovascular approach to the trauma patient

**Athanasios Diamantopoulos**

**Expert commentary** Konstantinos Katsanos

## Case history

A 34-year-old male was admitted to the A&E department 30 minutes after a motorcycle accident. The patient was in a good general state, complaining only of mild left upper quadrant abdominal pain. His blood pressure was 135/70mmHg with a heart rate of 75 beats/minute. The Glasgow coma scale (GCS) was 15/15. His haemoglobin (Hb) count on admission was 13.5g/dl. No relevant past medical history was mentioned by either the patient or his close relatives who escorted him to the hospital. As per institute protocol he underwent focused abdominal ultrasonography (US) (also known as FAST), which at the time showed no signs of intra-abdominal free fluid or site-specific organ injury.

The patient remained in the A&E department under close observation. An hour later he started complaining of worsening abdominal pain on the left side. A second haemoglobin count showed a drop of 2.1g/dl (Hb = 11.4g/dl) although he remained haemodynamically stable. A decision was made to perform a CT scan in order to identify any potential solid organ injury or other source of bleeding. The patient was transferred to the CT department for a contrast-enhanced CT scan in order to identify the cause of the continuing pain. A non-contrast-enhanced CT scan demonstrated a high-density free fluid collection in the lower abdomen and pelvis, suggesting haemorrhage in the abdomen (Figure 19.1a,b). Contrast-enhanced CT scans in both the arterial phase (Figure 19.1c) and the portal venous phase (Figure 19.1d) identified an active bleeding site in the lower pole of the spleen.

**Expert comment**

CT is very useful for assessing trauma patients as it can accurately detect free intra- and retroperitoneal fluid, bone, vascular, and solid organ injuries as well as classify the degree and severity of solid organ injuries, thus altering their clinical management [1]. Contrast-enhanced multidetector CT is very precise for both recognition and localization of acute bleeding, even for bleeding rates as low as 0.02ml/min [2]. However, in acute trauma CT should always follow initial clinical assessment and patient resuscitation, and it may not be appropriate for patients who require immediate lifesaving interventions (e.g. pelvic fixation, surgical laparotomy, etc.).

**Learning point**

Focused abdominal ultrasonography is considered a reliable imaging method for detection of free intra-abdominal fluid in poly-trauma patients. In addition, it is a valid method for assessing possible specific organ injury [1]. However, US may fail to detect injuries within solid organs, and failure to identify free intra-abdominal fluid must not always be assumed to indicate absence of significant organ injury. In cases of uncertainty, clinical observation or a CT of the abdomen is mandatory [1].

Because of the persistence of abdominal pain and the drop in the Hb level a decision was made to immediately transfer the patient to the angiographic suite for embolization in order to control the bleeding. The patient was haemodynamically stable during the whole process, complaining solely of abdominal pain. As expected, selective angiography of the splenic artery verified the presence of

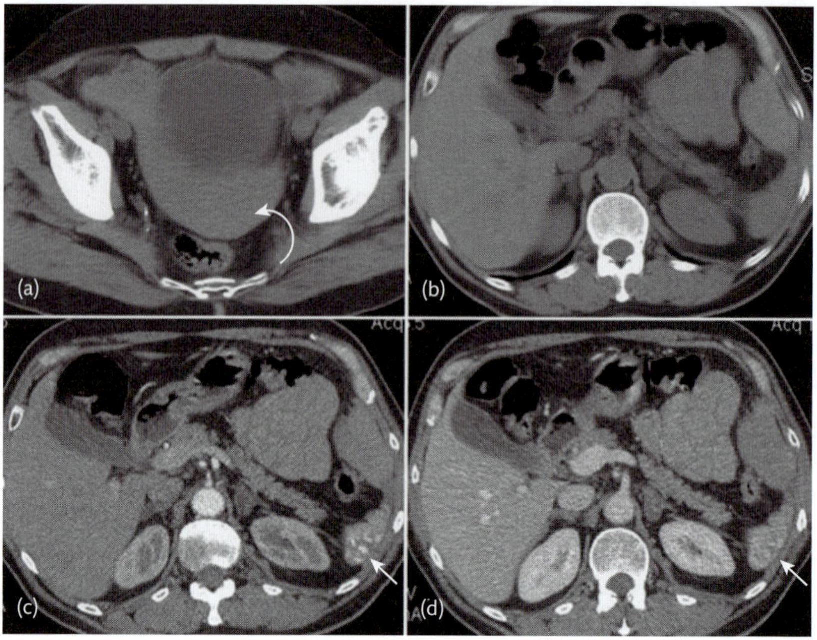


**Figure 19.1** (a, b) Non-contrast-enhanced CT scans show a high-density free fluid collection in the pelvis (curved arrow) with no obvious traumatic injuries in the upper abdominal solid organs. (c, d) Contrast-enhanced arterial and venous phase axial images at the level of the spleen demonstrate a site of intraparenchymal active bleeding from the lower pole of the spleen (straight arrows).

an intraparenchymal active bleeding site (Figure 19.2a). A small peripheral branch of the splenic artery was identified as the culprit-feeding vessel (Figure 19.2b). The branch was selectively catheterized and embolized using a microcatheter and microcoils. Although the final selective angiogram showed effective arrest of bleeding (Figure 19.2c), a second, initially invisible, small peripheral branch contributing to the bleeding was identified on a further angiogram from the origin of the splenic artery (Figure 19.3a). This branch was also superselectively catheterized and embolized with microcoils (Figures 19.3b,c).

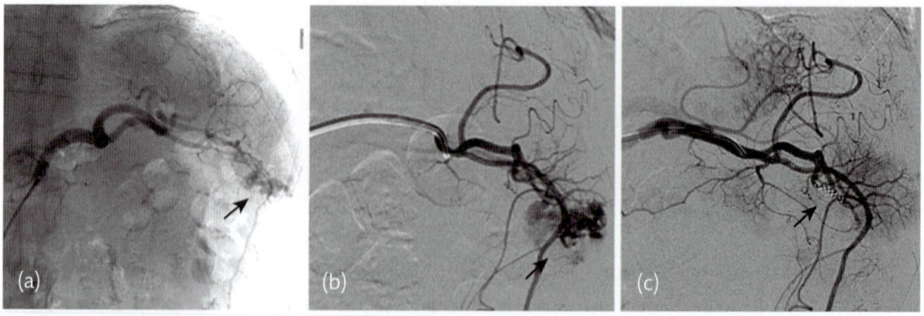


**Figure 19.2** (a) Selective angiography of the splenic artery demonstrating the site of intraparenchymal active bleeding (black arrows). (b,c) The branch was selectively catheterized with a microcatheter and several microcoils were deployed to occlude it as demonstrated on completion angiography.

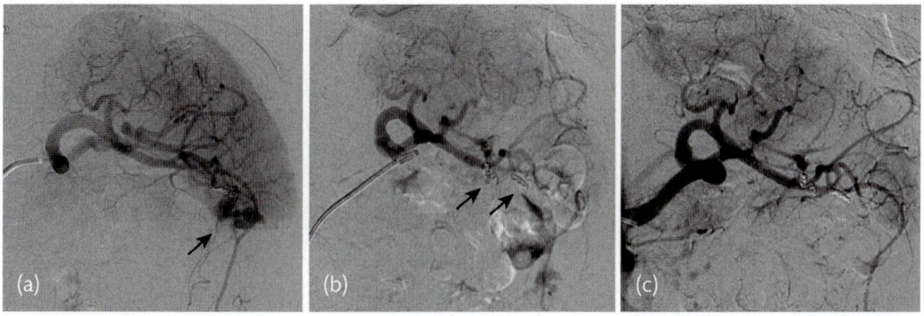


**Figure 19.3** (a) Further angiography from the proximal trunk of the main splenic artery demonstrated active bleeding from another small branch (black arrow). (b,c) The branch was subsequently catheterized and occluded with additional placement of microcoils (black arrows).

**Learning point**

The spleen is the most frequently injured solid organ as a result of either blunt or penetrating trauma [3]. Transcatheter embolization plays an important role in the non-operative management of these cases. Embolization can be performed either proximally or distally. In the case of proximal embolization, coils are usually deployed approximately 2cm distal to the origin of the dorsal pancreatic artery, but ideally proximal to the origin of the pancreatica magna artery [3]. Distal embolization or superselective embolization can be applied when the patient is haemodynamically stable and time allows it, especially if there is a small peripheral vessel or single arterial injury [3]. When superselective embolization is performed, as in the case described here, it is important to remember to obtain a completion angiogram from the proximal splenic artery in order to identify any additional culprit branches that may have been missed on the initial angiograms.

**Expert comment**

Use of endovascular techniques in order to control active haemorrhage originating from the spleen as a consequence of either blunt or penetrating trauma has been a major contributor to the conservative management of allowing preservation of the spleen. The aim of endovascular embolization is to improve the results of the non-operative management of patients with splenic injury and to reduce the rates of splenectomy [4,5]. Splenic vascular trauma management usually consists of proximal embolization of the splenic artery resulting in decreased perfusion of the spleen which controls the bleeding and in addition prevents secondary rupture by reducing the overall pressure. Alternatively, more distal superselective embolization of the suspect arterial branch may be performed. Both management methods are currently considered acceptable [5]. The same principles apply to other solid organs such as liver and kidney. Superselective embolization techniques, if applicable, can be used in order to minimize organ injury and preserve most of the target organ function. Nevertheless, superselective techniques must only be used in cases where the clinical condition of the patient allows sufficient time for this procedure. A proposed principle for trauma patient may be: 'Try to embolize as selectively as time allows'

After the successful embolization procedure the patient was admitted to a surgical ward for observation. There were no further signs of pain or embolization-related complications (post-embolization syndrome). He had an otherwise uneventful recovery and was discharged from hospital three days later.

**Learning point**

Transcatheter embolization to treat splenic arterial injuries is likely to salvage the organ in up to 94% of the cases without the need for any surgical treatment [6,7]. Complications of splenic artery embolization include splenic artery injury, non-targeted embolization, infraction of splenic parenchyma, and most importantly abscess formation and sepsis.

**Expert comment**

The aim of transcatheter embolization for management of splenic artery injuries is to preserve the spleen, which is a key solid organ in the immunological system. Complications of transcatheter embolization can be avoided with experience or, if present, can usually be managed conservatively. Non-target embolization may be the result of improper sizing of the coils or failure to successfully recognize the responsible arterial branch. Abscess formation may occur either immediately after the procedure or in a delayed manner. Abscesses can be managed using standard percutaneous drainage techniques.

## Discussion

Trauma is a major healthcare problem as it is the primary cause of death in young patients. Interventional radiology plays an increasing role in management of trauma patients, especially via percutaneous transcatheter treatment of sites of active haemorrhage that contribute to haemodynamic instability. Patients eligible for endovascular management of traumatic arterial injuries are those who are haemodynamic stable or sufficiently resuscitated to allow enough time for both cross-sectional imaging evaluation and angiographic identification and arrest of the bleeding site.

Endovascular treatment for haemorrhage control was first described in the early 1970s [8]. Since then, the increasing experience of interventional radiologists in the delivery of transcatheter therapies, together with developments in endovascular instruments, has expanded the role of minimally invasive options in the poly-trauma patient. This approach is applicable to almost all vascular territories of the human body that may be injured by either blunt or penetrating trauma, including the thoracic or abdominal aorta, the pelvic and upper or lower extremity arteries, the lumbar arteries, and the major visceral branches feeding the spleen, liver, and kidneys [3,9]. Endovascular techniques can be applied to manage bleeding in all these arterial territories.

The following endovascular options are applicable to the poly-trauma patient: balloon occlusions, embolization using all available embolic agents, and implant of covered metal stents or stent grafts [3,9]. Each of these techniques has its advantages and disadvantages, and the final choice must be individualized based on the specific clinical scenario, availability, and the operator's experience and personal preference. It is essential that the operator involved must have the appropriate catheter skills and knowledge to carry out an effective and safe percutaneous embolization procedure. Knowledge of the arterial anatomy, including the collateral networks, is essential for a successful embolization procedure. The most widely used embolic agents in the trauma setting are coils and Gelfoam [3,9]; coils are more precise but Gelfoam produces quicker arrest of flow.

## A final word from the expert

Over the last few decades the role of endovascular treatment of traumatic arterial injuries has emerged and evolved to allow non operative management of such cases. By using embolic agents, occlusion balloons, and stent grafts radiologists have produced a paradigm shift in the management of such cases. No matter where the injury is located, radiologists can often offer a less invasive therapeutic option. The spleen, which is the most frequently injured solid organ [3], is being preserved in an increasing number of cases (up to 94%) thanks to application of modern imaging and endovascular techniques [6,7]. Liver injuries can involve the hepatic arteries, the portal venous system, or the hepatic veins. Surgical repair of liver injuries can have than mortality rates in excess of 33%, making transcatheter management a more appealing approach [10]. The technical success rate of embolization ranges from 88% to 100% [11,12]. In kidney injuries embolization must be performed as selectively as possible in order to minimize the extent of organ infarction. Gelfoam is preferred because it offers the option of recanalization; however, coils can also be used [3].

Pelvic haemorrhage can be the result of fractured bones or disrupted pelvic veins, and in about 10–20% of cases the source of bleeding is severe arterial injury [13]. Arterial bleeding usually comes from branches of the hypogastric artery. Transcatheter embolization is a highly effective procedure to control bleeding with success rates ranging from 85% to 100%. Nonetheless, corresponding mortality rates are between 17.6% and 47% despite successful transcatheter embolization [14]. Aortic trauma and extremity arterial injuries are also very common. The introduction and widespread use of a variety of endografts and stent grafts have altered the management of such cases, favouring the transcatheter endovascular approach whenever this is possible mainly because of its inherent advantages over open surgery.

## References


1. McGahan JP, Wang L, Richards JR. From the RSNA refresher courses: focused abdominal US for trauma. *Radiographics* 2001; 21(Spec. No.): S191–9.
2. Yoon W, Jeong YY, Shin SS, et al. Acute massive gastrointestinal bleeding: detection and localization with arterial phase multi-detector row helical CT. *Radiology* 2006; 239(1): 160–7.
3. Gould JE, Vedantham S. The role of interventional radiology in trauma. *Semin Intervent Radiol* 2006; 23(3): 270–8.
4. Wahl WL, Ahrns KS, Chen S, et al. Blunt splenic injury: operation versus angiographic embolization. *Surgery* 2004; 136(4): 891–9.
5. Madoff DC, Denys A, Wallace MJ, et al. Splenic arterial interventions: anatomy, indications, technical considerations, and potential complications. *Radiographics* 2005; 25(Suppl 1): S191–211.
6. Sclafani SJ, Shaftan GW, Scalea TM, et al. Nonoperative salvage of computed tomography-diagnosed splenic injuries: utilization of angiography for triage and embolization for hemostasis. *J Trauma* 1995; 39(5): 818–27.
7. Haan J, Scott J, Boyd-Kranis RL, et al. Admission angiography for blunt splenic injury: advantages and pitfalls. *J Trauma* 2001; 51(6): 1161–5.
8. Margolies MN, Ring EJ, Waltman AC, et al. Arteriography in the management of hemorrhage from pelvic fractures. *N Engl J Med* 1972; 287(7): 317–21.
9. Nicholson AA. Vascular radiology in trauma. *Cardiovasc Intervent Radiol* 2004; 27(2): 105–20.
10. Schwartz RA, Teitelbaum GP, Katz MD, Pentecost MJ. Effectiveness of transcatheter embolization in the control of hepatic vascular injuries. *J Vasc Intervent Radiol* 1993; 4(3): 359–65.

11. Hagiwara A, Yukioka T, Ohta S, et al. Nonsurgical management of patients with blunt hepatic injury: efficacy of transcatheter arterial embolization. *AJR Am J Roentgenol* 1997; 169(4): 1151–6.
12. Monnin V, Sengel C, Thony F, et al. Place of arterial embolization in severe blunt hepatic trauma: a multidisciplinary approach. *Cardiovasc Intervent Radiol* 2008; 31(5): 875–82.
13. Hak DJ. The role of pelvic angiography in evaluation and management of pelvic trauma. *Orthop Clin North Am* 2004; 35(4): 439–43.
14. Yoon W, Kim JK, Jeong YY, et al. Pelvic arterial hemorrhage in patients with pelvic fractures: detection with contrast-enhanced CT. *Radiographics* 2004; 24(6): 1591–6.

CASE

# 20 Uterine fibroid embolization: can fertility be preserved?

Leto Maili and Aneeta Parthipun

Expert commentary Irfan Ahmed

## Case history

A 40-year-old woman, who was previously fit and well, presented to her gynaecologist with a long-standing history of menorrhagia and dysmenorrhea. She had a 12-year-old child and was concerned about preserving her fertility. Magnetic resonance imaging (MRI) examination showed a fibroid uterus with multiple intramural and subserosal fibroids. Following contrast administration, there was avid enhancement of the majority of the fibroids (Figure 20.1). There was no endometrial abnormality or additional supply to the uterus via the ovarian arteries.

**Expert comment**

Ideally, all women should have an MRI scan with IV contrast. MRI outperforms transvaginal ultrasound in pre-embolization assessment of the number, size, and location of leiomyomas [1,2] and detection of possible collateral ovarian artery supply to the fibroids. It is also beneficial in predicting the outcome of uterine fibroid embolization (UFE) [3]. For example, leiomyomas with haemorrhagic degeneration have a poor outcome following UFE [4,5]. MRI has the additional benefit of diagnosis of adenomyosis and endometriosis. It is also used to exclude leiomyosarcoma or adnexal malignancy, which are contraindications for UFE [6,7].

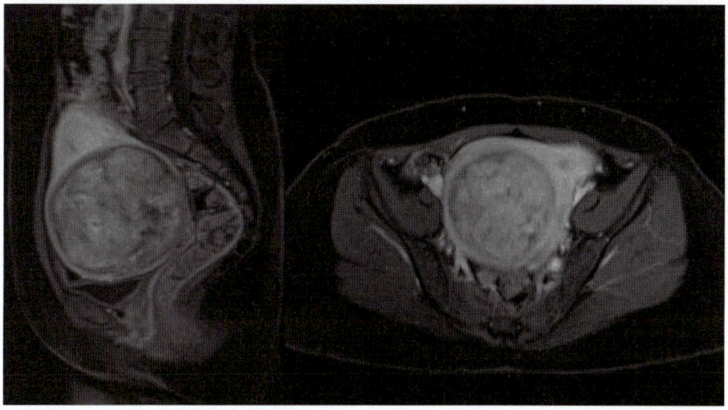

**Figure 20.1** MR sagittal and axial images of the uterus following IV contrast administration reveal large enhancing fibroids.

**Evidence base** HOPEFUL trial [9]: safety and efficacy of UFE

- UK multicentre retrospective cohort trial comparing hysterectomy and UFE for the treatment of symptomatic uterine fibroids.
- UFE ($n = 459$) versus hysterectomy ($n = 649$).
- Average follow-up: 8.6 years for hysterectomy cohort; 8.6 years and 4.6 years in the UFE cohort.
- 85% of UFE patients reported relief from fibroid symptoms versus 95% of hysterectomy patients.
- 23% of UFE patients required further treatment for fibroids.

The interventional radiologist and the gynaecologist both accepted that the patient was a valid candidate for a myomectomy, but also suggested that, because of the presence of multiple fibroids, UFE would be a reasonable alternative. In view of the current literature, the interventional radiologist stated that UFE was an effective form of treatment for symptomatic fibroids. Several studies have also demonstrated that UFE has short-term advantages of UFE over surgery, including less blood loss, shorter hospital stay, and quicker resumption of work [8]. Both the gynaecology and the interventional radiology consultants felt that the patient's preference for a less invasive procedure should be taken into account.

**Evidence base** EMMY trial and REST trial

EMMY Trial [10]:

- Level 1 evidence
- Prospective randomized controlled trial (RCT) ($n = 177$) comparing UFE with hysterectomy
- UFE is an effective alternative to hysterectomy
- Both procedures improved quality of life at two-year follow-up.

REST trial [11]:

- Level 1 evidence
- RCT comparing UFE ($n = 106$) with surgery (hysterectomy ($n = 43$) and myomectomy ($n = 8$))
- 9% of UFE patients required repeat UFE or hysterectomy because of inadequate symptom control
- Symptom scores at one year were better in the surgical group
- Significantly shorter hospital stay and faster return to regular activities in the UFE cohort.

The patient was provided with an information leaflet detailing the procedure and the potential complications. She was also sent for routine blood tests (full blood count, coagulation screen, and renal function tests), which were all normal.

**Learning point** Complications of UFE [12]

- Post-embolization syndrome: this is a common presentation defined by the presence of a low-grade fever, nausea, vomiting, and malaise, which can last for several days after the procedure. It is important that this entity is distinguished from infection.
- Serious infection: a rare complication presenting in 0.5% of UFE patients [13]. It may manifest with pelvic pain, pyrexia, leucocytosis, or vaginal discharge. Risk of hysterectomy is less than 1%.
- Transcervical expulsion of leiomyomas: this is the most common serious complication and is defined as the detachment of fibroid tissue from the uterine wall and subsequent transvaginal passage. The incidence is up to 3% [14–16] and presents with severe menstrual cramps, vaginal discharge, tissue passage, or heavy bleeding. When fibroid impaction occurs in the cervix, gynaecological intervention is mandatory [14].
- Premature ovarian failure: this may occur following UFE and is age dependent. It is estimated that 5% of women over 45 years of age may have temporary or permanent amenorrhea following UFE. The risk decreases to 1% after the age of 40 [17].
- Pulmonary embolism: this is the most common life-threatening complication, with an incidence of around 1 in 400 [18]. Women at significant risk should be anticoagulated; however, there is no indication for routine anticoagulation therapy.

The overall periprocedural complication rate for UFE, including major and minor complications, is 8%. The overall infection rate is 2% [14,19]. Pinto et al. [20] demonstrated that the major complication rate following hysterectomy was 20% compared with 2.5% following UFE.

On the day of the UFE the patient was given a stat dose of diclofenac sodium 100mg PR, metronidazole 500mg IV, morphine sulphate 10mg IM, and ondansetron 4mg IV. This was in accordance with departmental guidelines. A right unilateral common femoral artery approach was performed and a 4Fr sheath was introduced. Both uterine arteries were selectively catheterized with a 4Fr cobra (C2) catheter using a Waltman loop technique [21]. Subsequent embolization was performed using three vials of non-spherical polyvinyl alcohol (PVA) particles of diameter 500–700μm (PVA-500; Cook Medical, Bloomington, IN, USA). The angiographic end-point for embolization was 'almost complete stasis of contrast' in the uterine arteries (Figures 20.2 and 20.3).

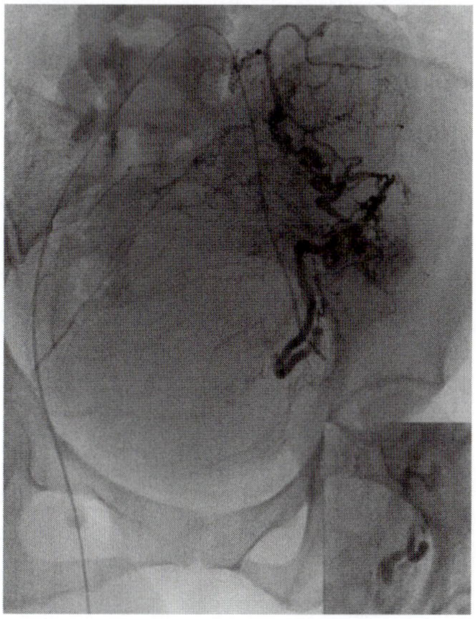

**Figure 20.2** Selective angiogram of the left uterine artery prior to embolization. Inset: Stagnant flow of the left uterine artery with occlusion of its distal branches.

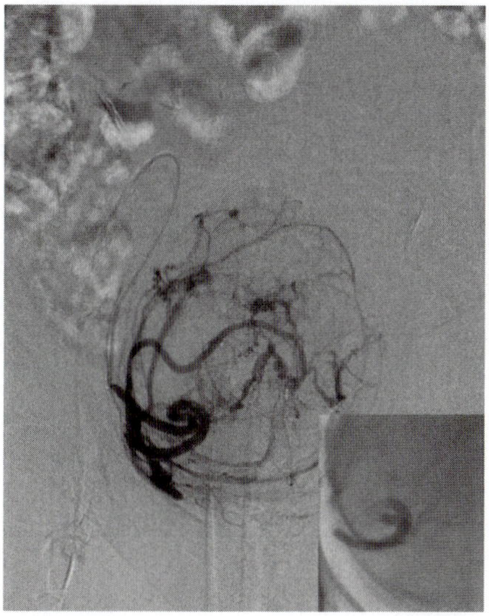

**Figure 20.3** Selective angiogram of the right uterine artery prior to embolization following Waltman loop formation of the catheter. Inset: Stagnant flow of the right uterine artery with occlusion of its distal branches.

**Clinical tip** Unilateral versus bilateral femoral approach

Some interventional radiologists perform bilateral common femoral approaches with two operators as it has been suggested that this reduces radiation exposure [22]. Many, including the authors, use a single 4–5Fr catheter with the Waltman loop technique [21] as this avoids bilateral femoral puncture and the increased complications associated with this. Others prefer the coaxial approach, routinely using a microcatheter to reduce spasm and achieve a more effective flow- directed embolization [13].

The origin and course of the uterine arteries are very variable. Nevertheless the angiographic appearance does not present a problem. Typically they appear symmetrical but sometimes one uterine artery can be absent or much smaller than the other. If there is little vascular supply to the uterus via the uterine artery and the patient has had previous surgery, it is important to consider a possible supply by the ovarian arteries.

At the end of the procedure, the sheath was removed and haemostasis was achieved by manual compression. Pain was controlled with patient-controlled analgesia (PCA) connected to an IV line (administering on demand: 1mg morphine/5min with a maximum dose of 40mg/4h). Because of the risk of respiratory compromise associated with morphine, naloxone was pre-prescribed with a maximum dose of 100μg/2min. If respiratory compromise occurred (<8 breaths/minute) clear instructions were given to stop the PCA immediately and administer the naloxone. Cyclizine 50mg was also pre-prescribed (maximum dose 150mg/24hours) as an antiemetic. The following morning, the patient was reviewed by the interventional radiology team and discharged with oral analgesia (Table 20.1).

**Learning point** Role of ovarian arteries and ovarian-uterine anastomoses [23–25].

- It is important to assess the presence of ovarian collateral supply to the uterus. Ovarian artery collateral supply is recognized as a potential cause of failed UFE.
- The incidence of ovarian collaterals increases with previous pelvic surgery, tubo-ovarian pathology, or large fundal fibroids [23]
- Less than 1% of UFE patients had substantial collateral ovarian artery supply to the uterus. White et al. [24] demonstrated that 17% had at least one visible ovarian artery and 6% had some ovarian collateral supply to uterus.
- Ovarian artery enlargement can be detected on pre-operative magnetic resonance angiography or with the use of aortography during UFE.
- The aortogram is usually obtained after embolization (flow from the ovarian arteries to the uterus detected before embolization requires re-evaluation post-embolization with a second aortogram).
- In some patients, the ovarian and uterine arterial supplies anastomose at the level of the uterus.
- The flow from the ovarian artery aids the carriage of embolic particles to the fibroids.
- Once the UFE is complete, the ovarian arterial flow decreases to near stasis and additional embolization from the ovarian arteries is generally not required.
- To date there are few data about the effectiveness of ovarian embolization as an adjunct to UFE.
- The data available also suggest that menopause is not an associated outcome of the procedure [23,24]
- If a patient wishes to preserve her fertility and undergoes UFE in which the presence of a minor ovarian supply is identified, one option would be to not embolize it and to assess the clinical outcome. If the patient's symptoms persist and MRI follow-up demonstrates residual fibroid perfusion, there should be further discussion of the results with the patient, who can then make an informed decision about the option of ovarian embolization performed as a separate procedure.

**Table 20.1** Medication at discharge as required

| Drug | Dose | Administration |
|---|---|---|
| Paracetamol | 1000mg | Orally 4 times daily |
| Dihydrocodeine | 30mg | Orally 4–6 times daily |
| Ibuprofen | 400mg | Three times daily |
| Senna | 7.5mg | Two tablets orally at night |
| Lactulose (Elixir) | 5–15ml | Orally twice daily |

## Discussion

UFE is a proven and efficacious form of treatment for symptomatic fibroids, but its effects on preserving fertility remain unclear. Currently, myomectomy is considered the only surgical option for women who desire future fertility [25]. This is most appropriate for women with a large solitary fibroid or with a small number of easily accessible fibroids (such as intramural or serosal fibroids).

UFE is more appropriate for patients who have large or multiple fibroids with a history of repeat miscarriages or are subfertile. It is deemed beneficial in such patients on the basis of reducing fibroid volume and therefore increasing the probability of a successful pregnancy. Several studies have demonstrated successful pregnancy following UFE, although the miscarriage rates and incidence of caesarean section may be higher than in an age-matched population without fibroids [9,13,26,27]. However, this may also be true for pregnancies following myomectomy.

There are several studies published on this topic.

**Evidence base** Fertility post UFE versus myomectomy [28]

- Small RCT ($n = 121$; 58 randomized to UFE and 63 to myomectomy of whom 26 were trying to conceive).
- Mean follow-up was 23.9 months.
- Only mid-term results comparing fertility outcomes of UFE with those of myomectomy are available.
- Significant difference in pregnancy rates between the UFE group (pregnancy rate 50%; $n = 13/26$) and the myomectomy group (pregnancy rate 78%; $n = 31/40$).
- Limitations of this study are the small group size, the short follow-up duration, and the high rate of repeat intervention in the UFE group (myomectomy in 32.7%).

In studies such as those of Firouznia et al. [30] and Kim et al. [31] only a small number of the population group tried to conceive post-UFE. In the Firouznia et al. study only 23 of the 102 patients tried to conceive and 14 of this cohort (61%) became pregnant. In the three-year prospective study by Kim et al. only 19 out of the 87 women under 40 years of age undergoing UFE for symptomatic fibroids were trying to conceive; the pregnancy rate was 63% ($n = 12$).

McLucas [32] recently published a retrospective study (covering 14 years) of 40 women less than 40 years old who desired to preserve their fertility. The 48% who were under 40 and desired pregnancies were able to have successful term pregnancies. Unfortunately, this study had a major flaw as it had no active follow-up but instead asked patients to contact the authors if they became pregnant. Thus the percentage of pregnancies may be underestimated as some women may have failed to contact the authors regarding pregnancy.

**Evidence base** Pregnancy rate following UFE [29]

- Prospective study investigating pregnancy rates following UFE ($n = 74$).
- Follow-up over 4.5 years.
- The pregnancy rate was 59.5%. Within this cohort, 84.6% of patients ($n = 39$) completed pregnancies with 33 live births (89.7%) and four spontaneous abortions (10.3%).
- The authors attributed the high number of successful pregnancies to the larger number of younger women (89.7% were <40 years old).

The currently available data demonstrate that more definitive evidence is required to establish a conclusive answer regarding the effect of UFE in patients considering future pregnancies.

One randomized trial [28] has demonstrated that there is a significantly higher probability of a successful pregnancy after myomectomy than after UFE. Other studies have not directly compared pregnancy rates following UFE with surgical options, but nonetheless have shown relatively high pregnancy rates after UFE [29,32]. Studies have demonstrated that the pregnancy rate following UFE varies from 17.5% [33] to 63% [31].

The assessment of fertility following UFE is obfuscated by two major confounding factors—advanced age and the presence of leiomyoma. Two per cent of infertility is caused by fibroids [34] and women with leiomyomas are less likely than control subjects to become pregnant [8]. In addition, female fertility decreased with advanced age and several studies have confirmed the decline in fertility after the mid-thirties [11].

Although the data for fertility following myomectomy are better, it is a more invasive procedure and is technically very difficult when multiple fibroids are present.

## Conclusion

UFE has become a well-established treatment for fibroids worldwide [35] and is associated with shorter hospital stay and faster return to regular activities than surgical treatments, but its effects on future pregnancies remain uncertain. It is apparent that there is a lack of large randomized trials comparing the pregnancy rates following UFE and surgical treatment for women considering future pregnancies.

A definitive answer to this dilemma requires a large RCT with long-term follow-up. In the interim, UFE should be offered to women who desire to preserve fertility where myomectomy, if appropriate, has been discussed but is less appropriate [13]. Patients should be informed of the current trial data and the risks of the procedure (including potential ovarian damage) so that an informed decision can be made. They should be aware of the potential risk of early miscarriage and the risk of post-partum haemorrhage (but the reasons for these remain unclear). Collaborative working with gynaecologists is imperative.

## A final word from the expert

The lack of any robust data directly comparing the impact of myomectomy and uterine fibroid embolization on fertility is disappointing but we eagerly await the findings of the NIHR funded randomized controlled FEMME trial which has recently completed recruitment. In the interim it is imperative that radiologists continue to work closely with gynecologists who are familiar with the issues related to fibroid treatment and the patient if fully acquainted with all the information currently available.

## References

1. Omary RA, Vasireddy S, Chrisman HB, et al. The effect of pelvic MR imaging on the diagnosis and treatment of women with presumed symptomatic uterine fibroids. *J Vasc Intervent. Radiol* 2002; 13: 1149–1153.

2. Dueholm M, Lundorf E, Hansen ES, et al. Accuracy of magnetic resonance imaging and transvaginal ultrasonography in the diagnosis, mapping and measurement of uterine myomas. *Am J Obstet. Gynecol* 2002; 186: 409–415.
3. deSouza NM, Williams AD. Uterine arterial embolization for leiomyomas: perfusion and volume changes at MRI imaging and relation to clinical outcome. *Radiology* 2002; 222: 367–74.
4. Jha RC, Ascher SM, Imaoka I, Spies JB. Symptomatic fibroleiomyomatas: MR imaging of the uterus before and after uterine arterial embolization of uterine arteries. *Radiology* 2000; 214: 729–34.
5. Burn PR, McCall JM, Chinn RJ, et al. Uterine fibroleiomyoma: MR imaging appearances before and after embolization of uterine arteries. *Radiology* 2000; 214: 729–34.
6. Kroencke TJ, Scheurig C, Kluner C, et al. Uterine fibroids: contrast-enhanced MR angiography to predict ovarian artery supply—initial experience. *Radiology* 2006; 241: 181–9.
7. Naguib NN, Nour-Eldin NE, Lehnert T, et al. Uterine artery embolization: optimization with preprocedural prediction of the best tube angle obliquity by using 3D-reconstructed contrast-enhanced MR angiography. *Radiology* 2009; 251: 788–95.
8. van der Kooij SM, Bipat S, Hehenkamp WJ, et al. Uterine artery embolization versus surgery in the treatment of symptomatic fibroids: a systematic review and metaanalysis. *Am J Obstet Gynecol* 2011; 205: 317.e 1–18.
9. Dutton S, Hirst A, McPherson K, et al. A UK multicentre retrospective cohort study comparing hysterectomy and uterine artery embolisation for the treatment of symptomatic uterine fibroids (HOPEFUL study): main results on medium-term safety and efficacy. *Br J Obstet Gynaecol* 2007; 114: 1340–51.
10. Hehenkamp WJ, Volkers NA, Birnie E, et al. Symptomatic uterine fibroids: treatment with uterine artery embolization or hysterectomy—results from the randomized clinical embolisation versus hysterectomy (EMMY) trial. *Radiology* 2008; 246: 823–32.
11. Edwards RD, Moss JG, Lumsden MA, et al. Uterine-artery embolization versus surgery for symptomatic uterine fibroids. *N Engl J Med* 2007; 356: 360–70.
12. Hovsepian DM, Siskin GP, Bonn J, et al. *Quality Improvement Guidelines for Uterine Fibroid Embolization for Symptomatic Leiomyomata*. CIRSE and SIR Standards of Practice Committees; 2004
13. *RCR/RCOG* Report. Clinical Recommendations on the Use of Uterine Artery Embolization in the Management of Fibroids (2nd edn) (London: RCR Press); 2008.
14. Spies JB, Spector A, Roth AR, et al. Complications after uterine artery embolization for leiomyomas. *Obstet Gynecol* 2002; 100: 873–80.
15. Laverge F, D' Angelo A, Davies NJ, et al. Spontaneous expulsion of three large fibroids after uterine artery embolization. *Fertil Steril* 2003; 80: 450–2.
16. Abbara S, Spies JB, Scialli AR, et al. Transcervical expulsion of a fibroid as a result of uterine artery embolization for leiomyomata. *J Vasc Intervent Radiol* 1999; 10: 409–11.
17. Worthington-Kirsch R, Spies J, Myers E, et al. The Fibroids Registry for Outcomes Data (FIBROID) for uterine artery embolization: short term outcomes. *Obstet Gynecol* 2005; 106: 52–59.
18. Czeyda-Pommersheim F, Magee ST, Cooper C, et al. Venous thromboembolism after uterine fibroid embolization. *Cardiovasc Intervent Radiol* 2006; 29: 1136–40.
19. Hovsepian DM, Siskin GP, Bonn J, et al. Quality improvement guidelines for uterine artery embolization for symptomatic leiomyomata. *J Vasc Intervent Radiol* 2001; 12: 1011–20.
20. Pinto I, Chimeno P, Romo A, et al. Uterine fibroids: uterine artery embolization versus abdominal hysterectomy for treatment—a prospective randomized, controlled clinical trial. *Radiology* 2003; 226: 425–31.
21. Pelage JP, Soyer P, Dref OL, et al. Uterine arteries: bilateral catheterisation with a single femoral approach and a single 5F catheter—technical notes. *Radiology* 1999; 210: 573–5.

22. Bratby MJ, Ramachandran N, Sheppard N, et al. Prospective Study of elective bilateral versus unilateral arterial puncture for uterine artery embolization. *Cardiovasc Intervent Radiol* 2007; 30: 1139–43.
23. Pelage JP, Walker WJ, Le Dref O, and Rymer R. Ovarian artery: angiographic appearance, embolization and relevance to uterine fibroid embolization. *Cardiovasc Intervent Radiol* 2003; 26: 227–33.
24. White AM, Banovac F, Yousefi S, et al. Uterine fibroid embolization: the utility of aortography in detecting ovarian collateral supply. *Radiology* 2007; 244: 291–8.
25. Razavi MK, Wolanske KA, Hwang GL, et al. Angiographic classification of ovarian artery-to-uterine artery anastomoses: initial observations in uterine fibroid embolization. *Radiology* 2002; 224: 707–12.
26. Walker WJ, Pelage JP. Uterine artery embolisation for symptomatic fibroids: clinical results in 400 women with imaging follow up. *Br J Obstet Gynaecol* 2002; 109: 1262–72.
27. McLucas B, Goodwin S, Alder L, et al. Pregnancy following uterine fibroid embolization. *Int J Gynaecol Obstet* 2001; 74: 1–7
28. Mara M, Maskova J, Fucikova Z, et al. Midterm clinical and first reproductive results of a randomized controlled trial comparing uterine fibroid embolization and myomectomy. *Cardiovasc Intervent Radiol* 2008; 31: 73–85.
29. Pisco JM, Duarte M, Bilhim T, et al. Pregnancy after uterine artery embolization. *Fertil Steril* 2011; 95: 1121.e 5–8.
30. Firouznia K, Ghanaati H, Sanaati M, et al. Pregnancy after uterine artery embolization for symptomatic fibroids: a series of 15 pregnancies. *AJR Am J Roentgenol* 2009; 192: 1588–92.
31. Kim MD, Kim NK, Kim HJ, Lee MH. Pregnancy following uterine artery embolization with polyvinyl alcohol particles for patients with uterine fibroid or adenomyosis. *Cardiovasc Intervent Radiol* 2005; 28: 611–15
32. McLucas B. Pregnancy following uterine artery embolization: an update. *Minim Invasive Ther Allied Technol* 2012; 22(1): 39–44.
33. Pinto Pabón I, Magret JP, Unzurrunzaga EA, et al. Pregnancy after uterine fibroid embolization: follow-up of 100 patients embolized using tris-acryl gelatin microspheres. *Fertil Steril* 2008; 90: 2356–60.
34. Goodwin SC, Spies JB, Worthington-Kirsch R, et al. Uterine artery embolization for treatment of leiomyomata: long-term outcomes from the FIBROID Registry. *Obstet Gynecol* 2008; 11: 22–33.
35. Ravina J, Herbreteau D, Ciraru-Vigneron N, et al. Arterial embolization to treat uterine myomata. *Lancet* 1995; 346: 671–2.

CASE

# 21 Postpartum haemorrhage: what is the role of occlusion balloons?

**Raj Das**

**Expert commentary** Anna-Maria Belli

## Case history

A 28-year-old female was referred to interventional radiology for elective placement of uterine occlusion balloons for placenta percreta. This was the patient's third pregnancy, following a previous caesarean section. Placenta percreta was diagnosed on antenatal ultrasound and fetal checks were otherwise unremarkable. Elective delivery had been planned at 38 weeks' gestation.

### Procedural details

Pre-procedural blood tests and coagulation were satisfactory. After the anaesthetist had placed an epidural catheter, the patient was transferred to the interventional radiology suite. Under sterile conditions, bilateral arterial access was obtained with retrograde common femoral punctures and insertion of 7Fr arterial sheaths. 4Fr RIM catheters (Rösch-Inferior-Mesenteric (RIM); Cordis, Miami, FL, USA) were inserted bilaterally and across the aortic bifurcation using hydrophilic guidewires to selectively catheterize the anterior divisions of the internal iliac arteries (Figure 21.1).

Once the RIM catheters were positioned in the anterior divisions of the internal iliac arteries, the hydrophilic guidewire was replaced with a 0.035 inch standard wire. Berenstein large lumen occlusion balloon catheters (Boston Scientific, Quincy, MA, USA) were then inserted bilaterally over the wire and positioned within the proximal anterior trunks of the internal iliac arteries. Each balloon was inflated in

**Clinical tip**

Aim to minimize fluoroscopy time by economy of screening, good coning, and minimizing contrast injections. Reduce the fluoroscopy pulse rate to as low a value as possible. In obstetric and gynaecological procedures we use two pulses per second.

**Expert comment**

Avoid entry of the catheter into the uterine artery itself as this may potentially cause arterial spasm and result in fetal compromise.

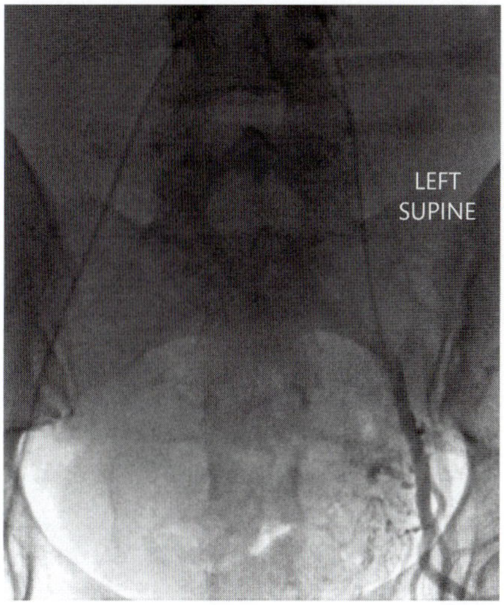


**Figure 21.1** Bilateral internal iliac catheterization performed with low dose fluoroscopy

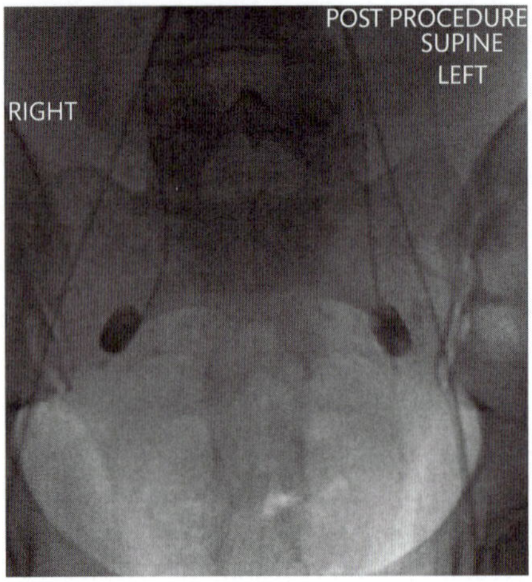


**Figure 21.2** Example of bilateral uterine occlusion balloons in situ with test inflation in the interventional radiology suite.

**Clinical tip**

After balloon test inflation, fill 2ml Luer-lock syringes with the correct volume required for occlusion and attach these to the occlusion balloon catheters. This may be crucially time-saving in an emergency.

the interventional radiology suite with up to 1.5ml of saline/contrast to test its sizing in the relevant artery. The volume required to fill each balloon to occlusion or reduction of flow was noted for use in the operating theatre (Figure 21.2).

The occlusion balloons were then deflated and the sheaths were sutured in position with additional clear adhesive dressings placed over the vascular sheaths and catheters to ensure that the balloon catheters did not become displaced during patient transfer. The patient was then transferred to the obstetric theatre for delivery.

## In the obstetric theatre

Following transfer to the delivery suite, the interventional radiology team attended the patient in the obstetric theatre before the planned caesarean section was started.

Before starting the caesarean section, a mobile image intensifier was used to ensure that the occlusion balloons had not migrated. On this occasion, the right uterine occlusion balloon had migrated from the right internal iliac to the right external iliac artery (Figure 21.3). The balloon was repositioned in the right internal

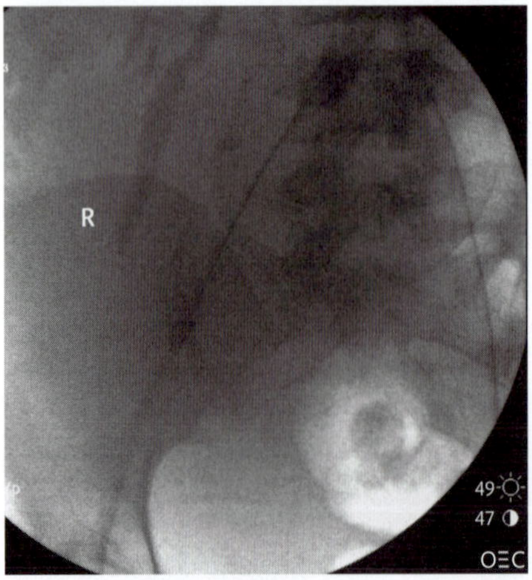


**Figure 21.3** The right uterine occlusion balloon has migrated into the right external iliac artery during transfer of the patient to theatre.

iliac artery. The caesarean section was performed avoiding the placenta (Triple-P technique) [1], the baby was delivered safely, and the umbilical cord was clamped. Following cord clamping both occlusion balloons were inflated.

### Post-delivery

The interventional radiologists were prepared to embolize via the occlusion balloon lumens. Gelfoam and additional embolic agents were taken to the theatre but were not required. Uterine balloons were kept inflated for up to 4 hours after surgical closure of the abdomen. Maternal blood loss was controlled and estimated at 1L.

**Expert comment**

Interventional radiologists should attend the obstetric theatre and be responsible for checking balloon positioning and inflation. Use mobile image intensifiers to verify balloon position. Do not rely on the obstetric or anaesthetic team to supervise balloon positioning or inflation. This is time-consuming but avoids complications.

**Clinical tip**

- If large lumen occlusion balloons (e.g. Berenstein) are used, it is possible to embolize via the balloon lumens to control haemorrhage whilst maintaining proximal control.
- Always have catheters and guidewires ready with embolic agents to perform bilateral uterine artery embolization if there is uncontrolled blood loss. Gelfoam/gelatin sponge is the embolic agent of choice because of its rapid occlusion effects.
- If feasible, the patient should be transferred to the interventional radiology suite for embolization because of its better imaging facilities and access to equipment.

**Clinical tip**

Be prepared to reposition the balloons and have appropriate equipment available (e.g. guidewires, catheters, and iodinated contrast). The balloons should remain inflated during the operation and after the baby is delivered.

Bilateral arterial sheaths were left in situ and secured until the following day in case of delayed haemorrhage. On the following day, arterial closure devices were used (Angioseal™; St Jude Medical) to close the arteriotomies and aid maternal mobilization; 6Fr Angioseal devices are generally sufficient to achieve haemostasis. Maternal haemoglobin was 11.6g/dl before the procedure and 10.0g/dl after the caesarean section, and both mother and baby remained haemodynamically stable throughout.

**Clinical tip**

If embolization is required in the obstetric theatre and large volumes of embolic agents are being injected, exert caution and screen carefully to avoid non-target embolization.

The brief period of uterine balloon catheter malposition was corrected rapidly and no detrimental effect occurred. The patient did not suffer any symptoms of right leg ischaemia, and the right lower limb was neurovascularly intact.

## Discussion

### Pathophysiology of abnormal placentation

Morbidly adherent placenta is a major cause of massive post-partum haemorrhage and is associated with significant maternal morbidity and mortality. Unfortunately, the incidence of morbidly adherent placenta is increasing worldwide and is believed to be associated with a rising prevalence of caesarean sections [2].

The decidua basalis is a natural cleavage plane superior to the placenta which allows appropriate placental separation after delivery. Injury or scarring from previous caesarean section or other trauma is believed to result in damage to the decidua basalis so that it can no longer act as a 'barrier' against deeper trophoblastic invasion. Morbidly adherent placenta, which is also known as abnormal placentation, occurs when a defect within the decidua basalis allows invasion of chorionic villi into the myometrium. It is subdivided depending on the depth of invasion.

Placenta accreta refers to a placenta which is abnormally adherent to, but does not invade, the myometrium. Placenta increta occurs when chorionic villi invade

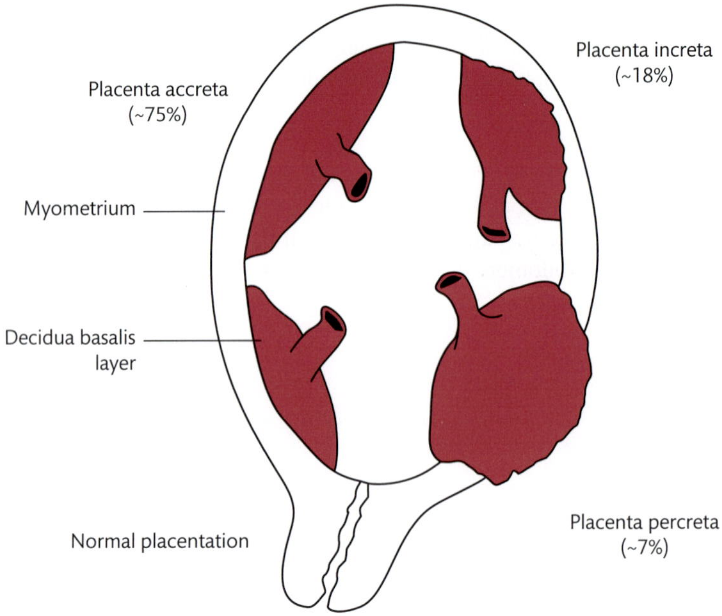


**Figure 21.4** Diagrammatic representation of abnormal placentation

the outer half of the myometrium, and placenta percreta occurs when villi penetrate through the myometrium into the serosa or beyond into surrounding tissues (Figure 21.4). The degree of maternal morbidity is generally related to the extent of placental invasion [3].

The most severe form of placental invasion, placenta percreta, is associated with serious maternal morbidity and mortality as the trophoblasts may invade adjacent organs (the urinary bladder, the colon, or laterally into the broad ligaments and ureters), and may also recruit blood vessels from the arteries supplying these organs. It is reported that 90% of patients with placenta percreta will lose more than 3000ml of blood intra-operatively and will require transfusion [4].

## Surgical and interventional radiology management options

After a caesarean section, there are two main surgical management options. The first is to proceed to total abdominal hysterectomy with no attempt to remove the placenta separately. The emerging approach is to conserve the uterus.

A caesarean hysterectomy may be considered either electively, if the woman has completed her desired family, or as an emergency procedure, when other conservative procedures have failed to control bleeding. However, caesarean hysterectomy itself is associated with significant maternal morbidity and mortality from haemorrhage.

Milder forms of placenta accreta and increta can be managed with multiple haemostatic sutures to the placental bed to arrest bleeding [5]. The use of pelvic arterial embolization (PAE) and internal iliac artery occlusion balloons (IIAOBs) has been outlined in a UK guideline [6].

**Learning point** The Triple-P procedure

The Triple-P procedure for placenta percreta has been developed as a conservative surgical alternative to caesarean hysterectomy [1,5]. Triple-P involves three steps.

1. Peri-operative placental localization using a transabdominal ultrasound scan on the operation table to delineate the upper border of the placenta with delivery of the fetus through a superior uterine incision.
2. Pelvic devascularization immediately after delivery of the fetus by inflation of preinserted uterine artery occlusion balloons, followed by placental non-separation and myometrial excision (to avoid separation of the morbidly adherent placenta from the underlying myometrial bed) with reconstruction of the uterine wall.
3. Avoidance of placental incision by delineating the upper border of the placenta immediately prior to caesarean section and immediate pelvic devascularization prior to myometrial excision helps minimize blood loss.

## The concept of uterine balloon occlusion

Balloon occlusion of the internal iliac arteries cannot completely block the whole blood supply to the pelvic organs because of the existence of a vast network of collateral arteries in the region. The obturator artery provides an important means of communication between the external and internal iliac arteries, as well as the lumbar, sacral, rectal, and femoral branches [7,8] Nevertheless, occlusion reduces perfusion pressure distal to the site of the balloon and minimizes blood loss during surgery. The alternative approach of surgical ligation of the internal iliac arteries is feasible, but the success rate is reported as <50% in the control of haemorrhage in obstetric patients [9,10].

## Technique of pelvic arterial embolization in obstetric haemorrhage

If bleeding is uncontrolled by balloon inflation, or in standard cases of post-partum haemorrhage (without prior knowledge of abnormal placentation), pelvic arterial embolization may be required.

With specific uterine occlusion balloons in situ, it is possible to perform uterine artery embolization via the balloon catheters. Alternatively, the balloons can be rapidly exchanged over the aortic bifurcation for standard 4Fr or 5Fr catheters and microcatheters if necessary.

A knowledge of potential collateral arterial supply is essential to demonstrate anatomy and may reveal active haemorrhage or a cause of haemorrhage, such as a pseudo-aneurysm. Active extravasation of contrast is a relatively infrequent finding, with detection rates of 20–50% reported.

Absence of extravasation of contrast is particularly common in the presence of uterine atony. This is likely to be due to diffuse bleeding from the uterine bed, with no focus of haemorrhage exceeding the rate required for angiographic detection [11]. Low rates of identification of contrast extravasation may be explained by intermittent bleeding or severe spasm of the uterine arteries. Arterial spasm often accompanies post-partum haemorrhage, especially in haemodynamically compromised patients receiving vasopressors.

If a bleeding point is identified, superselective embolization of the appropriate artery can be performed. If no angiographic bleeding site is identified and there is haemodynamic instability or clinical evidence of bleeding, bilateral uterine artery embolization or the anterior division of the internal iliac artery should be performed regardless.

The embolic agent of choice is gelatin sponge, which provides rapid occlusion and cessation of haemorrhage. Small embolic particles (150–250μm) should be avoided because of the increased risk of ischaemic complications [12]. Coils are rarely used because they occlude proximally, allowing ongoing bleeding from collateral vessels, and also impede further attempts at embolization [11]. If there is disseminated intravascular coagulopathy (DIC), there may be a need for other embolic agents, including glue and coils.

## Complications arising secondary to interventional radiology in post-partum haemorrhage

Most complications are minor and common to all procedures involving arterial puncture, including groin haematoma or pseudo-aneurysm. Severe complications can arise from arterial balloon occlusion and embolization, but the incidence is low.

As described in the case reported here, migration of the uterine occlusion balloons can occur and the operator must be vigilant. Additionally, attention should be paid to pericatheter thrombosis, as there are relatively long periods (>24 hours) with the intravascular balloons or sheaths in situ during these procedures. Regular flushing of the catheters and sheaths is recommended. If thrombus forms within the external iliac arteries, or if the balloon migrates for a significant period of time whilst inflated, there is potential for leg ischaemia which may require further vascular intervention.

Pelvic ischaemic complications associated with embolization are rare but have been reported. They may include uterine, vaginal, buttock, and bladder necroses [12,13]. Caution must be exercised if large amounts of embolic agents are used without significant reduction in flow, with care taken to avoid non-target embolization. Post-embolization syndrome is common and includes fever, leucocytosis, nausea, and abdominal pain.

## Fetal complications from interventional radiology in post-partum haemorrhage

Direct rates of fetal complication are difficult to assess, as there are a number of adverse factors that are already present in the context of major peri-partum haemorrhage. We advocate avoidance of catheter placement within the uterine arteries during balloon positioning, as arterial spasm may occur and result in fetal ischaemia or fetal bradycardia.

Fetal radiation exposure should be minimized with strict coning and reduction of fluoroscopy pulse rates. The fetal radiation dose has been estimated at 0.03–0.06 Gray (Gy) [14,15] which theoretically may convey a 0.25% risk of developing a childhood cancer. However no fetal abnormality or subsequent malignancy has yet been associated with IIAOB placement.

**Evidence base**

A small number of comparative studies have been performed demonstrating a mixed outcome/benefit from using uterine artery occlusion balloons. Outcome measures of intra-operative blood loss, transfusion requirements, and mortality have been used but trial methodologies are variable.

A systematic review published in 2012 [16] summarized several major studies [14,15,17] demonstrating inconclusive results with occlusion balloons, but these were used with caesarean

(continued)

hysterectomy rather than uterine conservation. However, more recent publications have reported beneficial effects of occlusion balloons with Caesarean hysterectomy [7].

Our experience is mainly with uterine conserving techniques and we have found great benefit in using IIAOBs. Trends are emerging to conserve the uterus with excellent results. The use of prophylactic balloons will allow a uterus preserving operation to be performed rather than a caesarean hysterectomy. Uterine occlusion balloons are intuitively of great benefit and their use is increasing.

## A final word from the expert

- Meticulous technique must be employed to ensure minimal maternal and fetal morbidity in the peri-partum period.
- It is essential for the interventional radiologist to attend the obstetric theatre and supervise balloon inflation, with preparation for pelvic arterial embolization in case of uncontrolled bleeding.
- Always avoid direct catheterization of the uterine arteries during balloon placement, as there is the potential for fetal compromise if there is arterial spasm.
- Internal iliac artery occlusion balloons are principally reserved for placenta percreta, but this is not always clear from antenatal imaging and as long as the technique of occlusion balloon placement is demonstrated to be safe for mother and baby, it can be also be used safely in placenta increta. Trends to conserve the uterus are now emerging and the recognition of the role of occlusion balloons means that their use is increasing.

## References

1. Chandraharan E. Should the Triple-P procedure be used as an alternative to peripartum hysterectomy in the surgical treatment of placenta percreta? *Womens Health (Lond Engl)* 2012; 8(4): 351–3.
2. Wu S, Kocherginsky M, Hibbard JU. Abnormal placentation: twenty-year analysis. *Am J Obstet Gynecol* 2005; 192(5), 1458–61
3. Miller DA, Chollet JA, Murphy TM. Clinical risk factors for placenta previa-placenta accreta. *Am J Obstet Gynecol* 1997; 177: 210–14
4. Hudon L, Belfort MA, Broome DR. Diagnosis and management of placenta percreta: a review. *Obstet Gynecol Surv* 1998; 53(8): 509–17.
5. Chandraharan E, Rao S, Belli AM, Arulkumaran S. The Triple-P procedure as a conservative surgical alternative to peripartum hysterectomy for placenta percreta. *Int J Gynaecol Obstet* 2012; 117(2): 191–4.
6. Royal College of Obstetricians and Gynaecologists. The role of emergency and elective interventional radiology in postpartum hemorrhage. *Good Practice Guideline No. 6*, Royal College of Obstetricians and Gynaecologists, London; 2007.
7. Carnevale FC, Kondo MM, de Oliveira Sousa W, et al. Perioperative temporary occlusion of the internal iliac arteries as prophylaxis in cesarean section at risk of hemorrhage in placenta accreta. *Cardiovasc Intervent Radiol* 2011; 34(4): 758–64.
8. Hansch E, Chitkara U, McAlpine J, et al. Pelvic arterial embolization for control of obstetric hemorrhage: a five-year experience. *Am J Obstet Gynecol* 1999; 180: 1454–60.
9. Kidney DD, Nguyen AM, Ahdoot D, et al. Prophylactic perioperative hypogastric artery balloon occlusion in abnormal placentation. *AJR Am J Roentgenol* 2001; 176: 1521–4.

10. Evans S, McShane P. The efficacy of internal iliac artery ligation in obstetric hemorrhage. *Surg Gynecol Obstet* 1985; 160: 250–3.
11. Gonsalves M, Belli A. The role of interventional radiology in obstetric hemorrhage. *Cardiovasc Intervent Radiol* 2010; 33(5): 887–95
12. Cottier JP, Fignon A, Tranquart F, et al. Uterine necrosis after arterial embolization for postpartum hemorrhage. *Obstet Gynecol* 2002; 100: 1074–7
13. Ornan D, White R, Pollak J, et al. Pelvic embolization for intractable postpartum hemorrhage: long-term follow-up and implications for fertility. *Obstet Gynecol* 2003; 102: 904–10.
14. Levine AB, Kulhman K, Bonn J. Placenta accreta: comparison of cases managed with and without pelvic artery balloon catheters. *J Matern Fetal Med* 1999; 8: 173–6.
15. Bodner LJ, Nosher JL, Gribbin C, et al. Balloon-assisted occlusion of the internal iliac arteries in patients with placenta accreta/percreta. *Cardiovasc Intervent Radiol* 2006; 29(3): 354–61.
16. Dilauro MD, Dason S, Athreya S. Prophylactic balloon occlusion of internal iliac arteries in women with placenta accreta: literature review and analysis. *Clin Radiol* 2012; 67(6): 515–20.
17. Shrivastava V, Nageotte M, Major C, et al. Case-control comparison of cesarean hysterectomy with and without prophylactic placement of intravascular balloon catheters for placenta accreta. *Am J Obstet Gynecol* 2007; 197(4): 402.e 1–5.

CASE

# 22 Percutaneous varicelectomy: coils or sclerosant agents?

**Piero Venetucci and Miltiadis Krokidis**

**Expert commentary** Vittorio Iaccarino

## Case history

A 19-year-old male with a previous history of surgical treatment of varicocele of the left side presented two years after his initial operation with signs of recurrence. His general practitioner referred him directly to interventional radiology.

**Learning point** varicocele

Varicocele formation is based on the pathological dilatation of the pampiniform plexus (PP) as a consequence of increased venous pressure at the level of the renal vein [1–3]. The incidence of varicocele in young males varies between 8% and 23% [4,5]; it affects the left side most frequently because of the anatomy of the left spermatic vein, but it may also present bilaterally as reported in various series (0–23%) [4,6]. The presence of varicocele may be clinically expressed with pain and/or weight sensation and may also be linked to male infertility.

Meticulous knowledge of the anatomy and physiology of the venous circulation in the renal vein, the spermatic vein, and the PP is of paramount importance for understanding and planning endovascular treatment in order to offer a permanent solution without recurrence. The internal spermatic vein (ISV) is a venous plexus and not a single vein and needs to be treated as such. The angiographic evaluation of the ISV always confirms the presence of a dominant branch, but also indicates the presence of other smaller branches that are not dilated but may be the cause of recurrence if there is surgical or percutaneous obliteration of the single dominant branch. The ISV plexus is connected with the PP at the level of the inguinal canal.

The patient was examined in an outpatient setting and an accurate clinical history was obtained using a questionnaire in order to exclude other potential causes of infertility. A physical examination was performed in both the recumbent and erect positions and confirmed the presence of a left side varicocele and the suspicion of a right side varicocele.

**Learning point** Questionnaire and physical examination

It is important for the interventional radiologist to perform a meticulous physical examination of the patient after the exclusion of other causes of infertility. These include the following: alcohol abuse; prolonged drug therapy with antiepileptics or neuroleptics, antibiotics, or steroids; exposure to toxic substances such as heavy metals, pesticides, paint fumes, or hazardous substances [7]; metabolic and hereditary diseases such as cystic fibrosis or Klinefelter syndrome; previous obesity; scrotal dermatoses; surgically corrected hypospadia, cryptorchidism, hydrocele, or haematocele; infected prostate/urethritis due to *Chlamydia trachomatis*, post-pubertal mumps, or orchiepididymitis.

The physical examination needs to be performed in both the recumbent and erect positions in order to exclude hydrocele, inguinal hernias, edpidydimal cysts, haemangiomas, vascular malformation, haematoma, and testicular cancer. A varicocele present in the recumbent position is considered as secondary to other causes and is not the first problem to treat [8–11].

**Evidence base** Varicocele and male infertility

Varicocele is the most common treatable cause of male infertility. The exact link between the two is not completely clear, but approximately 20–40% of patients affected with varicocele have a reduced reproductive ability [12]. Numerous explanations for this connection have been proposed. The most important factor appears to be the increase in the scrotal temperature [6,13–16]. This hypothesis is supported by the fact that the testicles that are extensively retained in an intra-abdominal position are usually hypoplastic. Telethermography can be used to identify patients who may potentially become infertile and may benefit from treatment of the varicocele. A large varicocele of the left side may cause an increase in temperature that may also affect the contralateral side because of haemodynamic overload over the right plexus.

A colour Doppler ultrasound (CDU) scan was performed and confirmed the presence of a large left-side varicocele (Sarteschi grade 5). US measurement of the testicular volume confirmed a relative reduction of the volume on the left side (11.8ml on the left and 17ml on the right). Laboratory evaluation of the seminal liquid of the patient revealed severe oligospermia (1.4 milion/ml) which appeared to have reduced compared with the value prior to the surgical treatment.

**Evidence base**

Varicocele is classified on the basis of colour Doppler ultrasound of the scrotum. The most widely used classification is that of Sarteschi [17] which defines five grades.

1. A prolonged reflux is detected in vessels in the inguinal channel only during Valsalva's manoeuvre. Scrotal varicosity is not evident in a grey-scale study.
2. A small posterior varicosity that reaches the superior pole of the testis and whose diameter increases after Valsalva's manoeuvre is present. The CDU evaluation clearly demonstrates the presence of a venous reflux in the supratesticular region only during Valsalva's manoeuvre
3. Vessels in the inferior pole of the testis appear enlarged when the patient is evaluated in a standing position,but no ectasia is detected if the examination is performed in the recumbent position. CDU demonstrates a clear reflux only under Valsalva's manoeuvre
4. The vessels appear enlarged, even if the patient is examined in the recumbent position; dilatation increases in the upright position and during Valsalva's manoeuvre. Enhancement of the venous reflux after Valsalva's manoeuvre is the criterion that allow the distinction os this grade from grades 3 and 5. Hypotrophy of the testis is common in this stage.
5. There is an evident venous ectasia even in the upright position. CDU demonstrates the presence of a marked basal venous reflux that does not increase after Valsalva's manoeuvre

This classification is simple and easily reproducible. It is very important to evaluate the testicular volume [18] because in the case of significant volume reduction no treatment may be of any use, particularly for paediatric patients where a seminal liquid examination may not be possible.

A CT venogram (Figure 22.1) was performed to evaluate the level of the surgical clips. The scan revealed the presence of previous surgical clips in the left iliac fossa and a stenosis of the left renal vein caused by external compression from the aortomesenteric axis and subsequent dilatation of the ipsilateral venous plexus.

**Learning point** Imaging

In order to obtain a definitive cure for recurrent or persistent varicocele it is of paramount importance to understand the previous treatment approach. CT and MRI are important for this purpose [19–22] because they can demonstrate the level of the surgical clips, coils, or glue used and offer a complete venous map in order to plan a retrograde or an antegrade approach. If the antegrade approach is the treatment of choice a non-invasive venogram of the non-occluded venous pathways through the anterior PP is required.

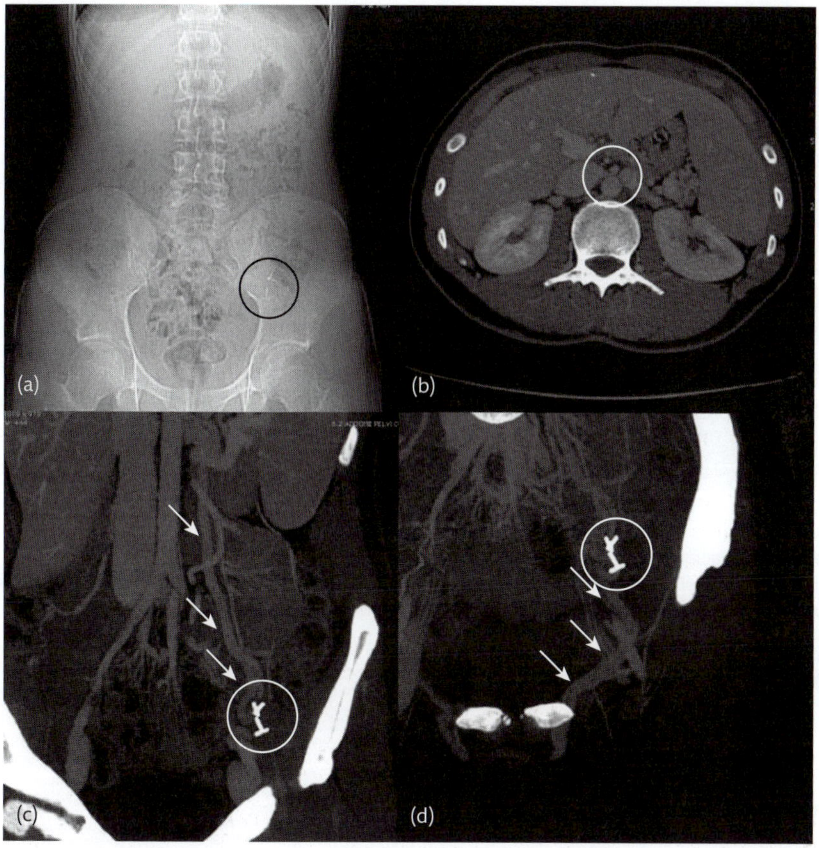


**Figure 22.1** (a) CT scan confirming the presence of metallic clips in the left iliac fossa (black circle). (b) CT axial slice showing stenosis of the left renal vein from the aortomesenteric axis (white circle). (c), (d) reconstructed CT images in an oblique coronal plain showing extensive dilatation of the left internal spermatic vein and the PP (white arrows) and confirming the presence of the metallic clips (white circle) at the level of some of the veins of the internal spermatic plexus.

After evaluation of the CT we decided to treat the patient with percutaneous retrograde approach through access from the common right common femoral vein (Figure 22.2). First, a hydrophilic cobra type catheter was used in conjunction with a hydrophilic guidewire in order to catheterize the left internal spermatic vein up to the level of the pre-existing surgical clips. The catheter was then changed to a vertebral type (Slip-Cath Beacon) for the distal catheterization of the PP. When the PP was catheterized occlusion of the distal vessels with 'scrotal barrage' was performed using an externally applied elastic band. After venographic confirmation that no reflux was present, sclerotherapy was performed 8ml of sodium tetradecyl sulphate 3%.

**Learning point** Sclerotherapy

Our preference for sclerotherapy alone is based not only on our expertise but also on physiopathological considerations. Since varicocele is expressed as a dilatation of the PPA it is essential to block all the plexus and not just the single spermatic vein, and sclerotherapy is the only technique that allows us to do this safely. The use of coils and surgical ligation is limited because only blockage of the ISV occurs.

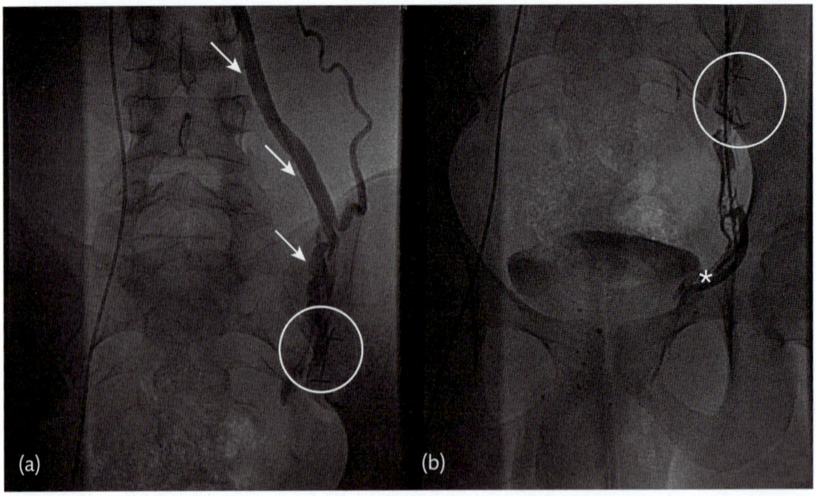


**Figure 22.2** (a) Venogram of the internal spermatic vein of the left side from a retrograde access confirmed that there is dilatation of the main venous branch of the internal spermatic vein (white arrows). The flow is occluded at the level of the surgical clips (white circle). (b) Catheterization of the plexus distally to the surgical clips (white circle) and venogram of the anterior PP. Sclerotherapy from this position followed (asterisk).

**Evidence base** Treatment of varicocele

A variety of surgical and percutaneous techniques to treat left-side varicocele. The most common surgical techniques are as follows.

- Open varicocelectomy and ligation of the internal spermatic vein at various levels:
  - high retropetitoneal ligation—the 'Palomo technique' [23]
  - inguinal, in which the incision is performed at the external inguinal ring
  - subinguinal.
- Laparoscopic vericocelectomy which is generally performed via a transperitoneal shunt [24,25].
- Microsurgical subinguinal varicocelectomy [26,27]. This is the most advanced and most successful surgical technique with the lowest complication rate.

The first step in any percutaneous technique is catheterization of the spermatic vein. In most the cases this access through the right femoral vein is feasible, but in cases of anatomical variants or when the left renal vein has a caudal direction the preferred access is from the brachial vein or the internal jugular vein [28]. The embolization of the ISV can be performed using a variety of techniques and embolic agents.

- Coils are the most common embolic agent and are used by the majority of operators. Coils have evolved significantly over the the years, and those currently used are detachable, permitting a controlled and more precise release. The coating is more thrombogenic but this technology has increased the cost [29].
- Acrylic glue is mainly used in the cases of post-surgical recurrence [30]. However, it is not easy to control and complications may be severe.
- Retrograde sclerotherapy is a very effective technique. Occlusion of the PP with an elastic band is of paramount importance in order to avoid complications, but otherwise it is very safe [31]. Distal catheterization of the ISV (to the ischiopubic level) and the use of a hydrophilic catheter are also required.
- Antegrade sclerotherapy is performed when the retrograde approach is not feasible [32]. Surgical access under local anesthesia, either from the groin or from a subinguinal position, and catheterization of one of the veins of the PP with a 23–25G needle is required,. An elastic band is applied distally to the access site and a venogram is performed to confirm the position. Then injection of the sclerosant follows under Valsalva's manoeuvre [33]. The initial venogram is of paramount importance to avoid serious complications.

Three months later CDU confirmed successful treatment with no residual flow in the anterior PP. The veins of the medial and posterior part of the plexus were patent without evidence of reflux during Valsalva's manoeuvre. The patient remained free of symptoms.

## Discussion

The percentage of varicocele recurrence or persistence varies significantly (2–45%) depending on the technique used for varcicocelectomy. It is not always easy to explain the cause of recurrence or persistence; in the case described here the CT scan revealed the presence of the ISV even though ligation of some of the branches was performed. The ISV plexus was maintained patent because of the high pressure in the circuit between the ISV and the left renal vein. Sclerotherapy through retrograde catheterization of the distal segment of the ISV and 'barrage' of the PP with an externally applied elastic band allows occlusion of all the vessels in the anterior PP at the level of the inguinal canal, excluding the formation of collaterals and therefore the likelihood of recurrence. However, the procedure still does not address the cause of the problem, which is the high pressure in the circuit between the left renal vein and the ISV. Therefore the patients may complain of pain in the initial post-treatment phase. Nevertheless, in the long term the procedure offers a definitive treatment and in our view should be the preferred option for the percutaneous treatment of varicocele.

## A final word from the expert

Varicocele is a very common pathology that affects approximately 15% of young males; in 40% of the cases it is linked with male infertility and therefore treatment is required. The follow-up and treatment of patients with varicocele requires the collaboration between a number of specialties. The role of interventional radiology is crucial in the treatment not only of primary varicocele, but also of recurrence (in my personal 40 years of experience I have had to treat a patient after the recurrence of three surgical interventions and one percutaneous intervention). In the treatment of recurrence a detailed description of the number and type of previous interventions is highly desirable in order to plan access (antegrade or retrograde).

The initial approach is via percutaneous retrograde sclerotherapy, even in the treatment of recurrence, because this is a simple, cheap, quick, and reliable technique. However, the vast majority of patients with varicocele are treated surgically and the recurrence rate is still very high. The role of the interventional radiologist is to make an accurate patient selection after clinical evaluation. Follow-up at three to six months is also required.

## References

1. Morvay Z, Nagy E. The diagnosis and treatment of intratesticular varicocele. *Cardiovasc Intervent Radiol* 1998; 21(1): 76–8.
2. van der Sluiszen PL, Leguit P, Sanders FB. Subcutaneous varices of the scrotum: a possible presentation of varicocele. *Eur J Radiol* 1990; 10(3): 198–200.

3. Weiss AJ, Kellman GM, Middleton WD, Kirkemo A. Intratesticular varicocele: sonographic findings in two patients. *AJR Am J Roentgenol* 1992; 158(5): 1061–3.
4. Meacham RB, Townsend RR, Rademacher D, Drose JA. The incidence of varicoceles in the general population when evaluated by physical examination, gray scale sonography and color Doppler sonography. *J Urol*. 1994; 151(6): 1535–8.
5. Steeno O, Knops J, Declerck L, et al. Prevention of fertility disorders by detection and treatment of varicocele at school and college age. *Andrologia* 1976; 8(1): 47–53.
6. Turner TT. Varicocele: still an enigma. *J Urol* 1983; 129(4): 695–9.
7. Gorelick JI, Goldstein M. Loss of fertility in men with varicocele. *Fertil Steril* 1993; 59(3): 613–16.
8. Ali JI, Weaver DJ, Weinstein SH, Grimes EM. Scrotal temperature and semen quality in men with and without varicocele. *Arch Androl* 1990; 24(2): 215–19.
9. Charny CW. Effect of varicocele on fertility. Results of varicocelectomy. *Fertil Steril* 1962; 13: 47–56.
10. Takihara H, Sakatoku J, Cockett AT. The pathophysiology of varicocele in male infertility. *Fertil Steril* 1991; 55(5): 861–8.
11. Zorgniotti AW, Macleod J. Studies in temperature, human semen quality, and varicocele. *Fertil Steril* 1973; 24(11): 854–63.
12. Mattison DR, Plowchalk DR, Meadows MJ, et al. Reproductive toxicity: male and female reproductive systems as targets for chemical injury. *Med Clin North Am*. 1990; 74(2): 391–411.
13. Roy CR 2nd, Wilson T, Raife M, Horne D. Varicocele as the presenting sign of an abdominal mass. *J Urol* 1989; 141(3): 597–9.
14. Dogra VS, Gottlieb RH, Oka M, Rubens DJ. Sonography of the scrotum. *Radiology* 2003; 227(1): 18–36.
15. Corlett MP, Gwynn BR, Hamer JD. Right-sided varicocele caused by false aneurysm from aortic graft. *Br J Urol* 1992; 70(2): 204–5.
16. Linsell JC, Rowe PH, Owen WJ. Rupture an aortic aneurysm in the renal vein presenting as a left-sided varicocele. Case report. *Acta Chir Scand* 1987; 153: 477–8.
17. Sarteschi LM. Lo studio del varicocele con color Doppler. *G Ital Ultrasonologia* 1993; 4: 43–9.
18. Behre HM, Nashan D, Nieschlag E. Objective measurement of testicular volume by ultrasonography: evaluation of the technique and comparison with orchidometer estimates. *Int J Androl* 1989; 12(6): 395–403.
19. Karaman B, Koplay M, Ozturk E, et al. Retroaortic left renal vein: multidetector computed tomography angiography findings and its clinical importance. *Acta Radiol* 2007; 48(3): 355–60.
20. Lakhani P, Papanicolaou N, Ramchandani P, Torigian DA. Asymmetric spermatic cord vessel enhancement and enlargement on contrast-enhanced MDCT as indicators of ipsilateral scrotal pathology. *Eur J Radiol* 2010; 75(2): e92–6.
21. Varma MK, Ho VB, Haggerty M, et al. MR venography as a diagnostic tool in the assessment of recurrent varicocele in an adolescent. *Pediatr Radiol* 1998; 28(8): 636–7.
22. von Heijne A. Recurrent varicocele: demonstration by 3D phase-contrast MR angiography. *Acta Radiol* 1997; 38(6): 1020–2.
23. Palomo A. Radical cure of varicocele by a new technique: preliminary report. *J Urol* 1949; 61(3): 604–7.
24. Hirsch IH, Abdel-Meguid TA, Gomella LG. Postsurgical outcomes assessment following varicocele ligation: laparoscopic versus subinguinal approach. *Urology* 1998; 51(5): 810–15.
25. Cayan S, Shavakhabov S, Kadioglu A. Treatment of palpable varicocele in infertile men: a meta-analysis to define the best technique. *J Androl* 2009; 30(1): 33–40.
26. Chan PT, Wright EJ, Goldstein M. Incidence and postoperative outcomes of accidental ligation of the testicular artery during microsurgical varicocelectomy. *J Urol* 2005; 173(2): 482–4.

27. Marmar JL, Kim Y. Subinguinal microsurgical varicocelectomy: a technical critique and statistical analysis of semen and pregnancy data. *J Urol* 1994; 152(4): 1127–32.
28. Kuroiwa T, Hasuo K, Yasumori K, et al. Transcatheter embolization of testicular vein for varicocele testis. *Acta Radiol* 1991; 32(4): 311–14.
29. Bechara CF, Weakley SM, Kougias P, et al. Percutaneous treatment of varicocele with microcoil embolization: comparison of treatment outcome with laparoscopic varicocelectomy. *Vascular* 2009; 17(Suppl 3): S129–36.
30. Sze DY, Kao JS, Frisoli JK, et al. Persistent and recurrent postsurgical varicoceles: venographic anatomy and treatment with n-butyl cyanoacrylate embolization. *J Vasc Interv Radiol* 2008; 19(4): 539–45.
31. Iaccarino V, Venetucci P. Interventional radiology of male varicocele: current status. *Cardiovasc Intervent Radiol* 2012; 35(6): 1263–80.
32. Tauber R, Johnsen N. Antegrade scrotal sclerotherapy for the treatment of varicocele: technique and late results. *J Urol* 1994; 151(2): 386–90.
33. Colpi GM, Carmignani L, Nerva F, et al. Surgical treatment of varicocele by a subinguinal approach combined with antegrade intraoperative sclerotherapy of venous vessels. *BJU Int* 2006; 97(1): 142–5.

CASE

# 23 Prostate artery embolization for benign prostate hypertrophy

**Aidan Shaw and Irfan Ahmed**

**Expert commentary** Tarun Sabharwal

## Case history

A 72-year-old man with a known diagnosis of benign prostatic hyperplasia (BPH) returned to his urologist with worsening lower urinary tract symptoms whilst on a 5α-reductase inhibitor. He had a significant past medical history including myocardial infarctions and coronary stents. On examination, the prostate was grossly enlarged and had smooth margins. The International Prostate Symptom Score (IPSS) was 28 with a quality of life score of 6.

**Learning point** The International Prostate Symptom Score

The IPSS is used to assess lower urinary tract symptoms in men. The first seven questions are based on the American Urological Association seven-item symptom score (AUA-7) [1]. The questions refer to the following urinary tract symptoms: incomplete emptying, frequency, intermittency, urgency, weak stream, straining, and nocturia. The answers are assigned points from 0 to 5, with 5 being the most severe. Therefore patient's scores can range from 0 to 35 (asymptomatic to severely symptomatic). Symptoms are then categorized (see Table 23.1).

Question 8 refers to quality of life and was added by the World Health Organization when IPSS was adopted by the International Consensus Committee as an international questionnaire for evaluating prostatic symptoms. Unlike the previous questions, this question ranges from 0 to 6, with 0 being delightful and 6 being terrible. Although it does not globally assess the patient's symptoms, it acts as a good starter for doctor–patient conversation.

**Table 23.1** International Prostate Symptom Score

| Score | Correlation |
|---|---|
| 0–7 | Mildly symptomatic |
| 8–19 | Moderately symptomatic |
| 20–35 | Severely symptomatic |

The patient's prostate specific antigen (PSA) was elevated and measured 12μg/L. Prostate biopsies did not demonstrate any evidence of malignancy. An MRI scan demonstrated that the prostate was grossly enlarged with a volume of 300ml and no radiological evidence of malignancy.

**Clinical tip** Prostate-specific antigen

PSA is a protein produced by normal prostate cells. Elevation of PSA is thought to be due to disruption in the prostate cellular architecture. PSA is not specific to prostate cancer but to prostate tissue, and elevation of PSA can be due to a number of different prostate diseases as well as prostate cancer. The most common causes of PSA elevation are BPH and prostatitis. Other causes include urinary retention, catheter placement, prostate biopsy, and prostate examination. Prostate artery embolization has recently been shown to cause a sharp increase in PSA following the procedure, which then resolves after a month [2].

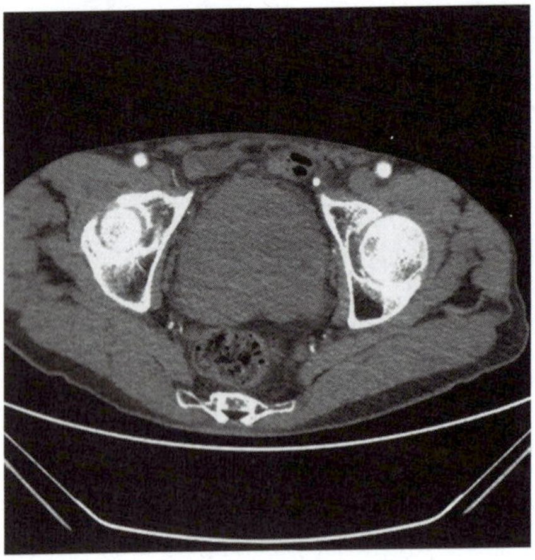

**Figure 23.1** CTA of the pelvis demonstrating a grossly enlarged prostate gland

Given the patient's anaesthetic risk, the patient was referred to interventional radiology for consideration of prostate artery embolization (PAE). Following consultation, a computed tomography angiogram (CTA) of the abdomen and pelvis was ordered for further evaluation of the prostatic arterial supply (Figure 23.1). The prostate arteries were identified to arise from the internal pudendal artery on the right side and the obturator artery on the left, with no stenotic or occlusive iliac atherosclerotic lesion identified.

**Expert comment** Computed tomography angiography (CTA)

CTA of the abdomen and pelvis is recommended prior to prostate artery embolization as it allows accurate assessment of any arterial atherosclerotic disease which may preclude embolization of the prostate artery (e.g. iliac occlusion or stenosis). It also allows visualization of the prostate arteries and pre-operative planning as there is anatomical variation in the origin of the prostatic artery on each side as well as from individual to individual. This reduces contrast dose and the time required to perform the procedure. The prostate arteries are very small and can be difficult to visualize. To assist with this, the patient is given two puffs of sublingual glyceryl trinitrate (GTN) on the CT table prior to the scan. The CT protocol for PAE is as follows:

- 120ml contrast
- rate 3.5–5ml/sec
- bolus triggering in the abdominal aorta
- 30ml saline given at the same rate before and after the injection of contrast
- two puffs sublingual GTN at the time of CTA.

After informed consent had been obtained, the patient was given pre-operative doses of cefuroxime 750mg IV and diclofenac 100mg PR. A retrograde puncture of the right common femoral artery was performed using local anaesthetic and ultrasound guidance and a 4Fr sheath was sited. The right internal iliac artery was successfully cannulated with a cobra catheter and an angiogram confirmed that the right prostate artery originated from the right internal pudendal artery. This was successfully cannulated with a microcatheter and an angiogram was performed to confirm the right prostatic arterial supply as well as to identify any aberrant arterial supply to the rectum, penis, or bladder (Figure 23.2). The artery was embolized to stasis using a 2ml syringe filled with polyvinyl alcohol (PVA) particles (initially PVA 100 and then PVA 200).

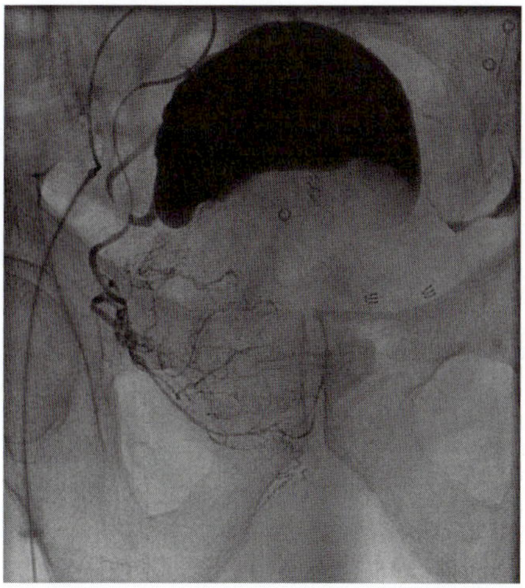

**Figure 23.2** DSA in the postero-anterior view demonstrating successful cannulation of the right prostate artery

> **Expert comment** Prostate arterial angiography
>
> Once the internal iliac artery is cannulated, the best projection for identification of the prostate artery and all the accessory branches is ipsilateral angulation of 350° and caudal-cranial angulation of 100°. A pump injection is performed using 6ml of contrast at a rate of 4ml/sec. Once the prostate artery is cannulated, ipsilateral oblique and postero-anterior views are obtained to identify collateral vessels and confirm parenchymal supply. Again, this is performed with an injection pump connected directly to the microcatheter using 4ml of contrast at a rate of 2ml/sec and a pressure of 300psi.

> **Expert comment** Preparing the PVA
>
> PVA 100 and PVA 200 are used for PAE and only a few millilitres are required to complete the embolization. Separate pots are used for the PVA 100 and PVA 200. The embolic agent is prepared by mixing a 'pinch' of PVA with 20ml of IV contrast and 20ml of saline. The embolization is then performed using a 2ml syringe.

The contralateral internal iliac artery and prostate artery were then cannulated and embolized using the same technique (Figure 23.3). The puncture site was then compressed manually. The patient was discharged later that day with no abdominal pain. He was prescibed ibuprofen 400mg three times daiy and cephalexin 500mg twice daily for seven days.

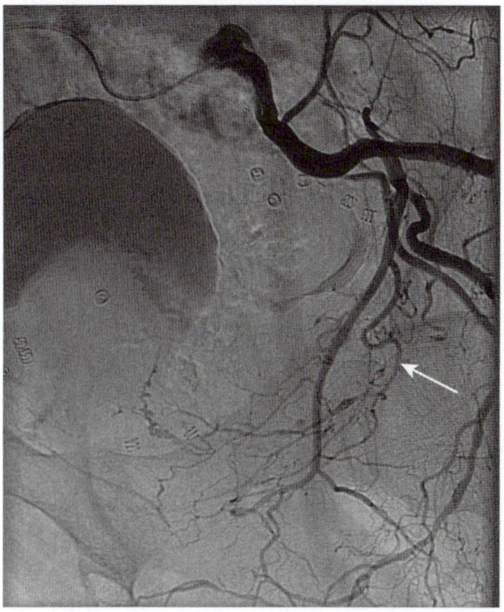

**Figure 23.3** DSA of the left internal iliac artery with 350° ipsilateral angulation and 100° caudal-cranial angulation demonstrating the prostate artery (arrow) originating from the left obturator artery

One month later the patient was well and the IPSS had fallen from 28 to 14. A follow-up CT two months later demonstrated that the volume of the prostate gland had significantly reduced and there was low attenuation in both lobes of the prostate gland in keeping with post-embolization change (Figure 23.4)

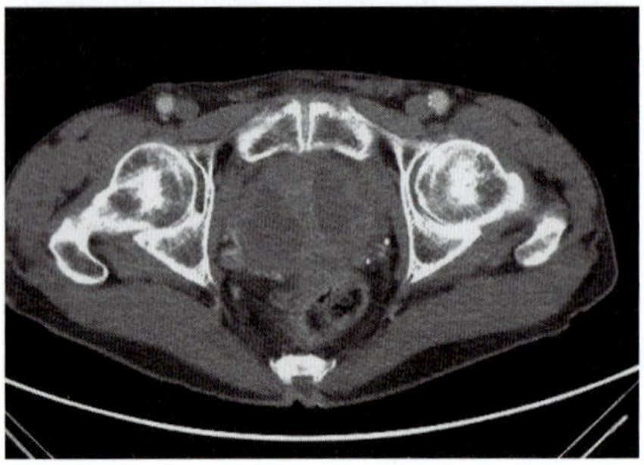

**Figure 23.4** Follow-up CT demonstrating significant volume reduction of the prostate with low attenuation in both lobes consistent with post-embolization change.

**Evidence base** Prostate artery embolization

Portugal

- PAE performed since 2010.
- Short- and medium-term results of a study including 255 patients have recently been published [3]. Technical success was defined as a completed PAE on at least one side, and clinical success was defined as improving symptoms (IPSS) and quality of life:
  - Technical success rate of 98%
  - Clinical success rate of 81% at one monthand 72% at three months with only one major complication.
- Concluded PAE is a safe and effective procedure with low morbidity and no sexual dysfunction [3,4].

Brazil

- PAE performed since 2010.
- A prospective study of patients with acute urinary retention due to BPH has been performed. Clinical and urodynamic parameters improved significantly following PAE. Ten out of eleven patients urinated spontaneously following Foley catheter removal at a mean of 12 days following PAE [2,5].
- Outcomes of unilateral versus bilateral embolization were also compared. The clinical outcome is better if bilateral embolization is achieved (75%); however, 50% of patients still achieved a good clinical outcome despite only unilateral success.

United Kingdom

- University Hospital Southampton was the first hospital in the UK to perform PAE. Twenty patients with BPH were treated.
  - The results were presented at the British Society of Interventional Radiology Meeting 2013.
  - IPSS decreased by 51% at one month, and was sustained at 46% at six months
  - Persistent improvements were found in IPSS, quality of life scores, and flow rates at one, six, and twelve months with no significant complications.
- The UK-ROPE (Registry of Prostate Embolization) trial has been launched in the UK in which 100 patients will be recruited from multiple centres across the UK

## Discussion

As the prostate gland enlarges in BPH, it starts to compress and obstruct the urethra, causing lower urinary tract symptoms (hesitancy, urgency, frequency, poor stream, and incomplete emptying). Once obstruction becomes complete it causes acute urinary retention. Indeed, over half the patients who present with a histological diagnosis of BPH have moderate to severe lower urinary tract symptoms (LUTS).

Patients presenting with mild or moderate LUTS can initially be managed with a trial of lifestyle modifications and oral medication (alpha blockers and 5α-reductase inhibitors). First-line treatment with alpha-blockers and 5α-reductase inhibitors as monotherapies or in combination have both proved effective in controlling LUTS with BPH [6,7].

If conservative management fails and LUTS are severe, surgical management will be offered. A number of different surgical options are available depending on the patient and the size of the prostate. All modern treatments favour conservation of the prostate and minimally invasive endosopic procedures rather than open prostatectomy. In addition to transurethral resection of the prostate (TURP), newer surgical options include holmium laser ablation of the prostate (HoLAP), microwave or radiofrequency ablation, and transurethral electrovaporization of the prostate (TUEVP).

TURP is associated with significant risk of morbidity (18%) and mortality (0.23%). It is regarded as the gold standard of surgery and is often successful. Patients usually stay overnight and are discharged the following day. However, the procedure has significant risks:

- significant blood loss requiring blood transfusion and prolonged hospital stay
- clot retention requiring bladder washouts
- urethral strictures
- 70% risk of retrograde ejaculation
- nerve injury resulting in impotence
- transurethral resection (TUR) syndrome (a rare but potentially life-threatening condition where hypotonic irrigation fluid is absorbed, causing severe electrolyte imbalance with neurological and cardiovascular manifestations).

## A final word from the expert

PAE has been performed for many years for intractable haematuria and has recently come to the forefront as a novel treatment for BPH. There are many advantages of PAE over surgical treatment options. The procedure takes around one to two hours and therefore can be performed as a daycase with the patient discharged later the same day provided that he is well. PAE can be performed on any size of prostate and does not involve urethral manipulation, therefore avoiding the risk of urethral strictures. Severe coorbidities that increase the anaesthetic risk are not a contraindication to the procedure. Patients can be converted to an open procedure following volume reduction. The only major complaint following PAE is retropubic pain and urethral burning, which are well managed on oral non-steroidal anti-inflammatory drugs. The main risk of the procedure is non-target embolization; however, only one patient worldwide has required surgical repair of the bladder following focal ischaemia. The procedure preserves the bladder neck and avoids nerve injury. This makes PAE particularly appealing to young male patients who are keen to preserve sexual function, as the risks of retrograde ejaculation and potential impotence are avoided.

The current results for PAE have shown the procedure to a safe, effective, and minimally invasive treatment option for BPH. More studies and follow-up are required to investigate the long-term outcomes, but given the results so far the procedure continues to have an exciting future.

## References

1. Barry MJ, Fowler FJ Jr, O'Leary MP, et al. The American Urological Association symptom index for benign prostatic hyperplasia. *J Urol* 1992;148(5): 1549–57, 1564.
2. Antunes AA, Carnevale FC, da Motta Leal Filho JM, et al. Clinical, laboratorial, and urodynamic findings of prostatic artery embolization for the treatment of urinary retention related to benign prostatic hyperplasia. A prospective single-center pilot study. *Cardiovasc Intervent Radiol* 2013; 36(4): 978–86.
3. Pisco JM, Rio Tinto H, Campos Pinheiro L, et al. Embolisation of prostatic arteries as treatment of moderate to severe lower urinary symptoms (LUTS) secondary to benign hyperplasia: results of short- and mid-term follow-up. *Eur Radiol* 2013; 23(9): 2561–72.
4. Pisco J, Campos Pinheiro L, Bilhim T, et al. Prostatic arterial embolization for benign prostatic hyperplasia: short- and intermediate-term results. *Radiology* 2013; 266(2): 668–77.
5. Carnevale FC, da Motta-Leal-Filho JM, Antunes AA, et al. Quality of life and clinical symptom improvement support prostatic artery embolization for patients with acute urinary retention caused by benign prostatic hyperplasia. *J Vasc Interv Radiol* 2013; 24(4): 535–42.
6. Greco KA, McVary KT. The role of combination medical therapy in benign prostatic hyperplasia. *Int J Impot Re* S 2008; 20(Suppl 3): S33–43.
7. Logan YT, Belgeri MT. Monotherapy versus combination drug therapy for the treatment of benign prostatic hyperplasia. *Am J Geriatr Pharmacother* 2005; 3(2): 103–14.

SECTION 4

# Non-vascular procedures and interventional oncology

CASE

# 24 Lung tumour radiofrequency ablation: what are the success factors?

Victoria St Noble

Expert commentary Nicos Fotiadis

## Case history

A 37-year-old female was referred with a past medical history of a testosterone-secreting adrenocortical carcinoma, resected 14 years previously. This recurred 5 years later within the adrenalectomy bed, prompting removal of the residual tumour along with unilateral nephrectomy, splenectomy, and distal pancreatectomy. Shortly afterwards, she was found to have several small lung metastases, two of which were treated by metastatectomy. A further five pulmonary metastases followed, which have been stable in number and slow-growing. The patient planned to become pregnant, and a decision to treat the metastatic disease radically before she conceived was made at a multidisciplinary meeting.

She was referred to the interventional radiology department for radiofrequency ablation (RFA) of the pulmonary metastases. She was asymptomatic at this time with no respiratory compromise or chest pain. Her biochemistry was normal with no evidence of hypersecretory state.

Staging chest CT showed a total of five lung lesions, with a size range from 7 to 21mm, located in four different lobes (Figures 24.1 and 24.2). There was no thoracic lymphadenopathy or evidence of metastatic disease elsewhere in the body.

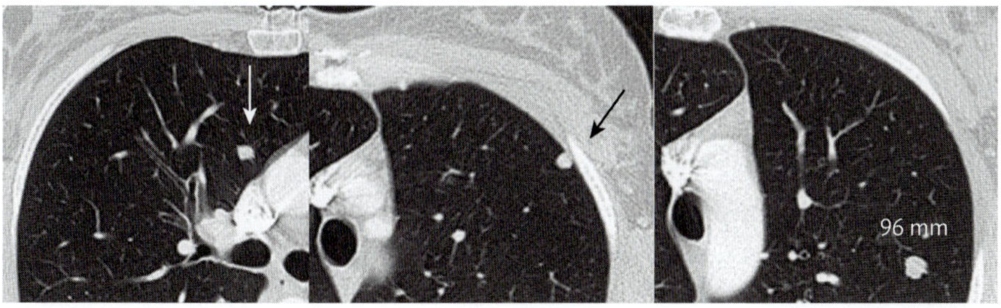


**Figure 24.1** Axial CT lung reconstructions showing a right upper lobe (left image) and two left upper lobe (middle and right image) metastases.

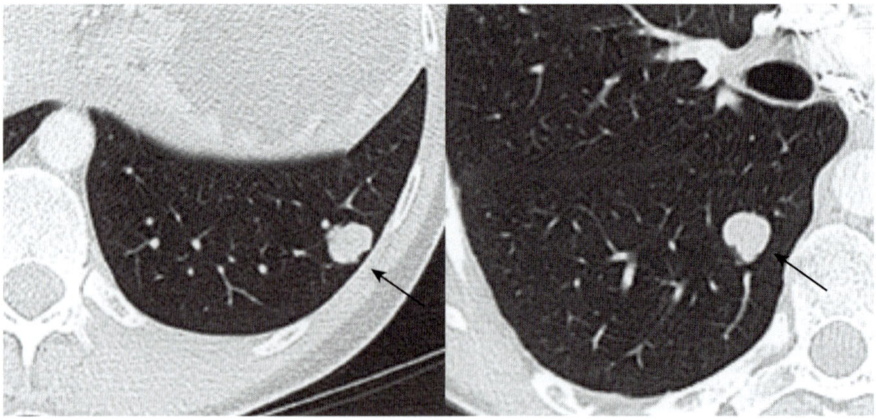

**Figure 24.2** Axial CT lung reconstructions showing left lower lobe (left image) and right lower lobe (right image) metastases.

**Learning point**

- Patients should be carefully selected for RFA by a multidisciplinary team, usually including a thoracic surgeon, an oncologist, and a radiologist. Pre-procedural work-up should include cross-sectional imaging of the chest, appropriate staging investigations, and biopsy of the lesion.
- The consensus opinion on size cut-off of lesions for RFA is 5cm. Lesions between 3 and 5cm should be considered with relative caution because of the higher incidence of recurrence. Nodules should be more than 1cm from the trachea, main bronchi, oesophagus, and central vessels in order to reduce the risk of complications. While some authors advocate treating patients with up to six lesions per hemithorax, the generally accepted upper limit is five nodules per lung [1,2].
- Patients with a life expectancy of less than a year and an Eastern Cooperative Oncology Group (ECOG) performance status >2 are not deemed good candidates for RFA. No minimum requisite pulmonary function parameters have been defined. The sole absolute contraindication for RFA is irreversible coagulopathy. Anticoagulation or antiplatelet agents should be stopped at least seven days prior to the procedure; warfarin should be discontinued five days before the procedure and recommenced 24 hours after [3].

The two larger lesions at the base of the left and right lower lobes were treated in the initial session. The procedure was performed with the patient in a prone position under conscious sedation administered by a consultant anaesthetist.

**Learning point** Anaesthetic considerations

- Anaesthetic options during lung ablation include conscious sedation by IV fentanyl, epidural anaesthesia, and general anaesthetic (GA), together with local anaesthetic infiltrated down to the pleura.
- Conscious sedation is used preferentially where possible. GA may become necessary where longer ablation times are needed, such as for larger lesions or several lesions in the same session. GA may also be preferred for lesions at the pleural surface, which are more prone to pain; alternatively, higher doses of IV fentanyl–midazolam or intercostal blocks may be used.
- Non-opiod oral analgesia is usually sufficient for post-procedural pain control [4].

The lesion in the left lower lobe was deemed to be too close to the parietal pleura and the diaphragm, and therefore an artificial pneumothorax was produced using a 21G IV needle. The needle was advanced towards the tumour in an axial plane with the intention of injecting $CO_2$ into the pleural cavity. This was unnecessary as the needle caused a small pneumothorax as soon as it was advanced into the pleural cavity (Figures 24.3 and 24.4).

A 3cm multi-tined expandable electrode (Leveen; Boston Scientific, Natick, MA, USA) was inserted in the lesion, which was displaced from the diaphragm and the parietal pleura. After successful ablation of the left lesion the small pneumothorax was aspirated with a three-way tap and a 20ml Luer-lock syringe. A tiny residual pneumothorax persisted. Since the patient was comfortable and asymptomatic, the 1.8cm right lower lobe lesion was subsequently ablated in a standard way. There were no associated complications. The patient was discharged the next day with no visible pneumothorax on chest X-ray (CXR).

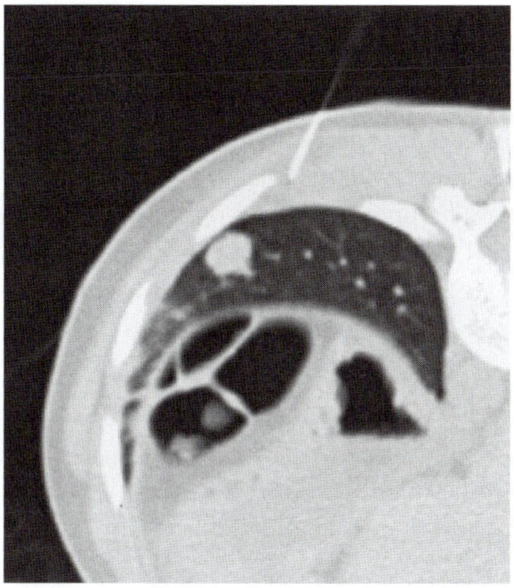

**Figure 24.3** Axial CT slice in the prone position showing advancement of a 21G needle towards the left lower lobe subpleural deposit.

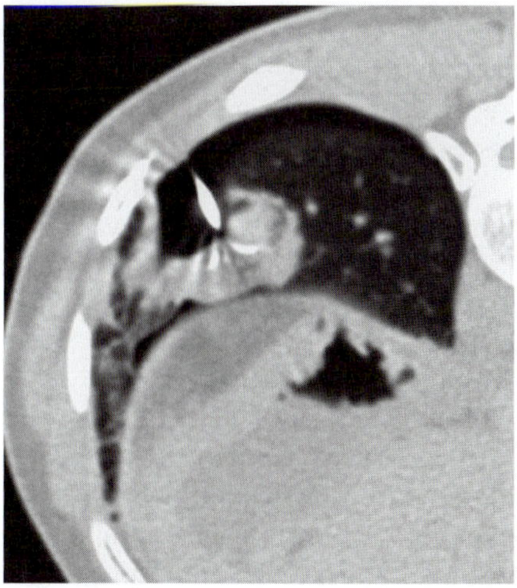

**Figure 24.4** Advancement of the needle results in a shallow pneumothorax and the RF probe is safely inserted in the lesion.

**Clinical tip**

A second metallic needle used in a tandem approach to perform an artificial pneumothorax should be removed prior to the ablation to prevent the current passing back along the tandem needle, therefore avoiding skin burns.

**Learning point** Creation of an artificial pneumothorax for subpleural pulmonary lesions

- Creation of an artificial pneumothorax has the advantage of separating peripheral lung nodules from the innervated parietal pleura, which may negate the use of GA.
- A multi-tined electrode, once sited within a peripheral lung lesion with the tines expanded, can be used to displace the tumour away from the parietal pleura. In a case review of seven patients by Hiraki et al. [5], this alone resulted in pain relief in one patient; in the remaining six patients pain relief was achieved by subsequent introduction of $CO_2$ into the pleural space, with no reported complications.
- Potential risks of this technique include inducing an air leak, necessitating pleural drain insertion, and potential tearing of the pulmonary parenchyma or pleura. It also has limited application in patients with known pleural adhesions [6].

Two weeks later the two left upper lobe lesions were ablated under conscious sedation and local anaesthesia. The procedure was complicated by a small haemopneumothorax (<10%) and lobar pulmonary haemorrhage. The patient remained stable and asymptomatic during the procedure, and a decision was made not to drain the pneumothorax. A seven-day course of antibiotics (amoxicillin and clavulanic acid) was started immediately after the procedure to prevent superadded infection. The patient's Hb remained unaltered at around 12g/dl and there was no need for transfusion.

The pneumothorax remained stable in the CXR taken four hours post-procedure and slowly improved in sequential CXRs during a three-day hospitalization. The parenchymal haemorrhage dramatically improved.

**Learning point** Complications of RFA

- Pneumothorax is the most common complication of lung ablation and occurs in up to 60% of RFA sessions [2], requiring chest-drain insertion in approximately 14% of cases [7]. Small intra-procedural pneumothoraces can be treated by insertion of a small needle catheter. Intractable pneumothorax due to bronchopleural fistula is a rare occurrence (0.6%) [8].
- Pulmonary haemorrhage following lung RFA is infrequent and usually self-limiting. The overall rate of pulmonary haemorrhage with or without haemoptysis has an estimated frequency of 1–6%. In a series of 164 patients undergoing lung RFA, there was one death secondary to massive pulmonary haemorrhage [9,10].
- Other infrequent complications include reactive pleural effusion, subcutaneous emphysema, infection, and pulmonary abscess [11].

Six weeks after the second RFA session a PET–CT scan was performed to evaluate the treatment response. There was no evidence of activity in any of the four treated lesions; however, there was marked inflammatory thickening of the left parietal pleural and multiple active lymph nodes in the mediastinum. The mediastinal nodes were interpreted as inflammatory and a decision to continue with RFA of the fifth right upper lobe lesion was made.

This was ablated under conscious sedation with a straight Cool-tip RFA probe (Covidien Healthcare, Boulder, CO, USA) with a 3cm active component. At the time it was considered that a straight needle could be more safely placed in close proximity to the superior vena cava and the ascending aorta (Figure 24.5). The procedure was uncomplicated and the patient was discharged the next day.

**Expert comment**

Aggressive management of pneumothorax with aspiration with or without drainage during the procedure significantly decreases the morbidity of the procedure and the in-hospital stay.

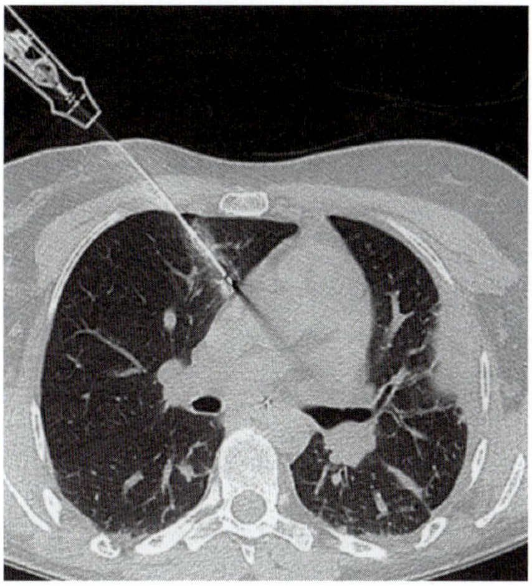

**Figure 24.5** Straight Cool-tip RFA electrode within the right upper lobe lesion. The subpleural shadowing in the left upper lobe corresponds to limited post-ablation pulmonary haemorrhage.

**Clinical tip**

A straight RF probe could be technically easier to place in hilar lesions and lesions closer to mediastinal structures.

**Learning points** Follow-up imaging post-RFA

- To date there are no universally agreed imaging criteria for follow-up of lesions post lung ablation. The generally accepted approach is to make assessments based on lesion size, geometry, and enhancement at follow-up CT imaging performed at 1, 3, 6, 12, 18, and 24 months, supplemented by FDG-PET CT. Size comparisons should take into account that the initial 'post-ablation mass' should be larger than the original tumour. The ablation zone should progressively shrink, as early as 2–3 weeks following treatment.
- Prolonged follow-up is necessary, as recurrences have been reported up to two years after treatment. Cavitation is described in up to 30% of treated lesions, most frequently when the lesion is in contact with a segmental airway. Cyst and cavity formation have also been described as indicators of response [2,12].

**Evidence base** The role of PET–CT in follow-up of lung ablation

- FDG-PET-CT has become a useful tool for the detection of incomplete treatment after lung lesion RFA.
- A recent retrospective five-year study, which followed 68 patients (94 pulmonary lesions), showed a number of different uptake patterns at ablation sites in PET–CT scans. Rim uptake was shown to be a favourable indicator relating to normal post-ablation inflammatory change. Conversely, discretely increased focal activity along the periphery of an ablation cavity was found to be a bad indicator [13]. The appearance of FDG uptake in mediastinal lymph nodes or at the site of the needle path used for RF ablation may occur and should not be considered as pathological.
- The optimal timing of initial follow-up PET imaging after ablation is still being evaluated. In a recent prospective study of 34 lung lesions (including five primary lung cancers) [14], the authors concluded that PET–CT at three months after RFA may be the most appropriate time for the initial study in order to limit false-positive results from inflammatory uptake.

The patient had another PET–CT scan three months after the final ablation session which showed no evidence of activity in any of the five treated lesions and decreased activity and size of the mediastinal nodes.

Twenty months after the initial ablation session the patient delivered a healthy baby girl. Forty days postpartum she had a CT of the chest, which showed a 1.9cm local recurrence at the site of the right upper lobe lesion. All the other lesions appeared completely ablated. A subsequent PET–CT confirmed the right upper lobe lesion as the only area of active disease (Figure 24.6).

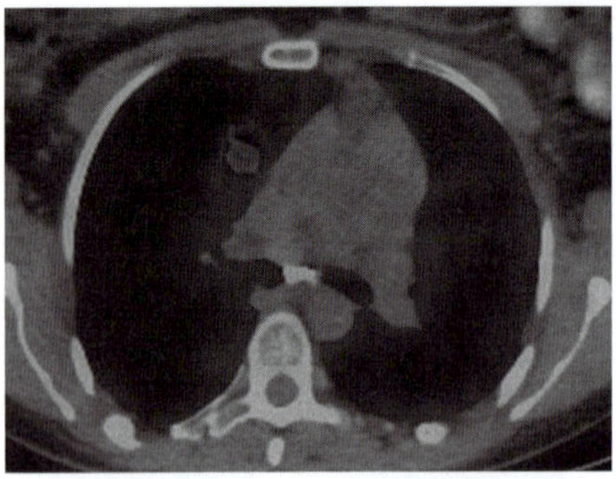

**Figure 24.6** Fusion PET–CT image showing FDG uptake in the previously ablated right upper lobe lesion.

The left upper lobe lesion was treated under GA with microwave ablation, as it is assumed that microwave will be less affected by the heat sink effect of the large mediastinal vessels. The procedure was uncomplicated and technically successful. However, subsequent PET–CT showed evidence of residual disease. The patient underwent a sublobar resection of the right upper lobe metastasis.

**Learning point** Heat sink effect

The efficacy of RFA is limited if there are large vessels adjacent to the tumour, as a result of the 'heat sink effect', whereby the circulating blood causes dissipation of the thermal energy. While larger vessels have the advantage of protecting themselves from substantial injury, the heat sink effect reduces the rate of perivascular tissue death. In the context of liver tumours, Lu et al. [15] found that a vessel size >3mm contiguous with a treated lesion has a strong correlation with incomplete tumour destruction by RFA. Therefore when treating tumours in close proximity to large vessels, one may consider more aggressive ablation strategies.

**Expert comment**

Ablation of tumours <3mm from large vessels or the pericardium is associated with increased risk of recurrence. Microwave ablation has a theoretical advantage for the management of those lesions since it is less affected by the heat sink effect, but this is not proven.

## Discussion

This case highlights some of the technical challenges and frequent complications of lung tumour RFA. As a minimally invasive technique, RFA is an attractive alternative to surgery for patients with small early-stage lung cancers or a limited number of metastases. Current evidence suggests that the outcome of pulmonary RFA is comparable with that of surgery, and more favourable than that of external beam radiotherapy. Two advantages of RFA compared with surgery are its lower procedural mortality rate (0.2% vs 1%) and the ability to perform repeated procedures [7].

The immediate technical feasibility of RFA shows good success rates in the literature, with a 98% success rate quoted in the RAPTURE study [16].

**Evidence base** RAPTURE study [16]

- Prospective multicentre trial of 183 tumours.
- Included a mixture of non-small-cell lung cancer (NSCLC) and metastases.
- Complete response lasting one year in 75 out of 85 assessable patients (88%).
- No differences in response between NSCLC and metastases. Overall survival was 70% at one year and 48% at two years for NSCLC, and 89% at one year and 66% at two years for colorectal metastases.
- Failure in only one patient was due to inability to transfix the lesion because of its small size.

A recent retrospective review of 46 studies, encompassing 1584 patients with a mixture of NSCLC and metastases, reported a mean overall survival of 59% following RFA treatment over a mean follow-up period of 18 months [7].

The pattern of recurrence following RFA occurs most commonly at the ablation margins.

Tumour size appears to be the most significant factor in predicting local recurrence; with tumour progression rates significantly lower in tumours <3cm in diameter. A retrospective review of 153 patients (189 lung ablations) revealed a median time to progression of 45 months for tumours of diameter 3cm or less, with one-, three-, and five-year survival rates of 83%, 57%, and 47%, respectively. This compared favourably with a median time to progression of 12 months for lesions >3cm, with one-, three-, and five-year survival rates of 45%, 25%, and 25%, respectively [17]. This mirrors findings of previous studies, and is due to the fact that complete coagulative necrosis of lesions >3cm in diameter is less likely. Some authors suggest that tumours of diameter 3–5 cm should be treated with six overlapping ablations in order to overcome this [18]. Achieving an adequate post-ablation margin, as demonstrated by ground-glass opacification on CT imaging, is crucial for ensuring successful tumour treatment. In a retrospective review, Anderson et al. [19] found that a minimum post-ablation ground-glass margin of 5mm significantly reduces the chance of tumour recurrence. Other factors associated with incomplete ablation include large vessel contact less than 3mm from the tumour and central location of the lesion [20].

**Evidence base** Beland et al. [12]

- Retrospective review of 79 RFA sessions on NSCLC.
- Recurrence in 34 (43%) at follow-up imaging, most often locally at the ablation margins (mean follow up 17 months, range 1–72 months), with intra-pulmonary recurrence elsewhere in the lungs and nodal recurrence making up the remainder.
- Increased tumour size and stage of the disease were associated with recurrence.

## A final word from the expert

As clearly illustrated in this case, patient selection is the key factor for successful lung ablation. Small metastatic lesions with favourable tumour biology are the ideal lesions for treatment with RFA. Five or more small (<3cm) lesions can be completely ablated in patients with no or well-controlled extra-pulmonary disease.

Bilateral treatment in one session should only be attempted in fit, young patients with no complications from the initial ablation.

Stage T1a primary lung cancer in poor surgical candidates could be successfully treated with RFA provided that an adequate ablation margin around the tumour is secured. A minimum of 5mm of ground-glass opacity around the treated tumour at the completion of the ablation minimizes the risk of recurrence".

## References


1. De Baere T. Lung tumour radiofrequency ablation. Where do we stand? *Cardiovasc Intervent Radiol* 2011; 34:241–51.
2. Bargellini I, Bozzi E, Cioni R, et al. Radiofrequency ablation of lung tumours. *Insights Imaging* 2011; 2(5): 567–76.
3. Pereira P, Salvatore M. Standards of practice: guidelines for thermal ablation of primary and secondary lung tumors. *Cardiovasc Intervent Radiol* 2012; 35(2): 247–54.
4. Hoffmann RT, Jakobs TF, Lubienski A, et al. Percutaneous radiofrequency ablation of pulmonary tumors. Is there a difference between treatment under general anaesthesia and under conscious sedation? *Eur J Radiol* 2006; 59:168–74.

5. Hiraki T, Gobara H, Shibamoto K, et al. Technique for creation of artificial pneumothorax for pain relief during radiofrequency ablation of peripheral lung tumours: report of seven cases. *J Vasc Interv Radiol* 2011; 22: 503–6.
6. Lee EW, Suh RD, Zeidler MR, et al. Radiofrequency ablation of subpleural lung malignancy: reduced pain using an artificially created pneumothorax. *Cardiovasc Intervent Radiol* 2009; 32(4): 833–6.
7. Chan VO, McDermott S, Malone DE, et al. Percutaneous radiofrequency ablation of lung tumors. Evaluation of the literature using evidence-based techniques. *J Thorac Imaging* 2011; 26(1): 18–26.
8. Sakurai J, Hiraki T, Mukai T, et al. Intractable pneumothorax due to bronchopleural fistula after radiofrequency ablation of lung tumors. *J Vasc Interv Radiol* 2007; 18: 141–5.
9. Dillon P, Sato K. Radiofrequency ablation of pulmonary neoplasm compicated by pulmonary haemorrhage. *Semin Intervent Radiol* 2011; 28(2): 175–8.
10. Nour-Eldin NE, Naguib NN, Mack M, et al. Pulmonary hemorrhage complicating radiofrequency ablation, from mild hemoptysis to life-threatening pattern. *Eur Radiol* 2011; 21(1): 197–204.
11. *NICE Guidelines: Interventional Procedure Overview of Percutaneous Radiofrequency Ablation for Primary or Secondary Lung Cancers* (London: NICE); 2010.
12. Beland M, Wasser E, Mayo-Smith W, Dupuy D. Primary non-small cell lung cancer: review of frequency, location, and time of recurrence after radiofrequency ablation. *Radiology* 2010; 254(1): 301–7.
13. Singnurkar A, Solomon SB, Gönen M, et al. $^{18}$F-FDG PET-CT for the prediction and detection of local recurrence after radiofrequency ablation of malignant lung lesions. *J Nucl Med* 2010; 51: 1833–40.
14. Deandreis D, Leboulleux S, Dromain C, et al. Role of FDG PET-CT and chest CT in the follow-up of lung lesions treated with radiofrequency ablation. *Radiology* 2011; 258: 270–6.
15. Lu DS, Raman S, Limanond P, et al. Influence of large peri-tumoral vessels on outcome of radiofrequency ablation of liver tumours. *J Vasc Interv Radiol* 2003; 14: 1267–74.
16. Lencioni R, Crocetti L, Cioni R, et al. Response to radiofrequency ablation of pulmonary tumours: a prospective, intention-to-treat, multicentre clinical trial (the RAPTURE study). *Lancet Oncol* 2008; 9(7): 621–8.
17. Simon CJ, Dupuy DE, DiPetrillo TA, et al. Pulmonary radiofrequency ablation: long-term safety and efficacy in 153 patients. *Radiology* 2007; 243(1): 268–75.
18. Steinke K, Glenn D, King J, Morris DL. Percutaneous pulmonary radiofrequency ablation: difficulty achieving complete ablations in big lung lesions. *Br J Radiol* 2003; 76: 742–5.
19. Anderson EW, Lees WR, Gillams AR. Early indicators of treatment success after percutaneous radiofrequency of pulmonary lesions. *Cardiovasc Intervent Radiol* 2009; 32:478–83.
20. Gillams AR, Lees WR. Radiofrequency ablation of lung metastases: factors influencing success. *Eur Radiol* 2008;18: 672–7.

CASE

# 25 Tracheobronchial stenting: covered versus uncovered

**Riccardo Inchingolo**

**Expert commentary** Tarun Sabharwal

## Case history

A 67-year-old patient presented with progressive dyspnoea and chest pain. A chest X-ray (CXR) showed a partial collapse of the left lung with an enlarged left hilum. The patient then underwent a CT scan which showed the presence of a left hilar mass (Figure 25.1a) involving the left lower bronchus and causing distal atelectasis of the left lower lobe, left-side pleural effusion, multiple enlarged lymph nodes throughout the mediastinal level, and multiple osteolytic bone lesions. Underlying CT signs of centrilobular emphysema, mostly located in the upper lobes, were evident. These results raised suspicion of a metastatic bronchogenic lung cancer (T3, N3, M1). A biopsy performed during bronchoscopy confirmed the diagnosis. The histological examination revealed non-small-cell lung cancer (squamous cellular carcinoma).

The patient's baseline symptomatology was severe with progressive dyspnoea and left chest pain. Physical examination revealed slightly reduced hypomotility of the left hemithorax. Blood gas analysis revealed severe hypoxaemia without hypercapnia and an almost acid–base balance: $Fio_2 = 0.21$, $Pao_2 = 62.8$mmHg, $Paco_2 = 36.8$mmHg, pH 7.424, and $[HCO_3^-] = 24.4$mmol/L. The patient then underwent lung function tests which showed severe obstructive respiratory deficit ($FEV_1/VC = 43\%$, $FEV_1/FVC = 42\%$, $FEV_1 = 1.03$L (44% of expected value), TLC = 6.43L (98% of the expected value), and DLco/VA = 2.87mL/min/mmHg/L (65% of the expected value)) and a bronchoreversibility test with 400µg of salbutamol ($FEV_1/VC = 45\%$, $FEV_1/FVC = 43\%$, $FEV_1 = 1.07$L (46% of the expected value)) which confirmed the clinical hypothesis of chronic obstructive pulmonary disease with a predominantly emphysematous pattern, as indicated by the CT scan.

> **Learning point**
>
> Malignant tracheobronchial obstructive disease can be caused by either a locoregional primary tumour or a metastatic tumour. Lung cancer is one of the leading causes of cancer death; most newly diagnosed lung cancers are already in an advanced stage. More than 50% of these patients will have involvement of the central airways [1]. This can be due to bulky endobronchial disease or extrinsic compression of the airways by either the tumour itself or lymphadenopathy. Obstruction of the central airways (trachea and main bronchi) can cause symptoms such as dyspnoea, cough, and haemoptysis, and when significant (>50% obstruction) cannot be tolerated for any length of time [2].

In a multidisciplinary meeting between interventional radiologists, thoracic surgeons, and oncologists, it was considered that the patient was considered

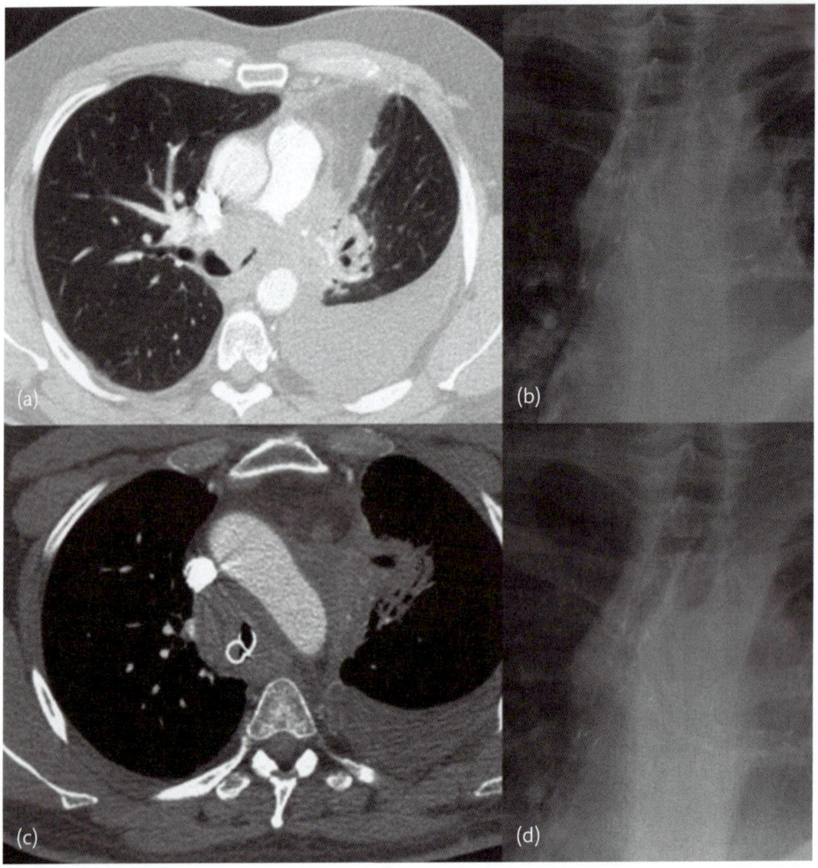


**Figure 25.1** (a) Central non-small-cell lung cancer with severe stenosis of the left main bronchus and carinal involvement. (b) A kissing stent procedure was performed. (c) The six-month CT follow-up showed tumour in-growth causing sub-occlusion of the upper right stent. (d) A further covered stent was inserted proximally to prevent complete occlusion.

**Clinical tip**

Pre-procedural imaging is vital for technical success. CT with multiplanar reconstruction is used to delineate the airway anatomy and diameter and to evaluate any further airway and/or parenchymal disease [3]. The stent size (length and diameter) and type (covered or uncovered) are selected on the basis of the CT findings and the type of obstruction (intrinsic or extrinsic) present.

**Expert opinion**

Although the use of flexible bronchoscopy and sedation in this the procedure has been reported to be safe and efficient, it is recommended that airway stenting is performed in theatre, under general anesthesia, using rigid bronchoscopy and fluoroscopy. We believe that this not only ensures the safety of the patient but also improves the accuracy of stent placement because of the combination of bronchoscopy and fluoroscopy [4].

non-operable and suitable for palliative treatment. Chemotherapy with four to six cycles of gemcitabine and a platinum analogue (cisplatin) was chosen for systemic therapy, with urgent tracheobronchial stenting as a palliative treatment to reduce his dyspnoea. Pre-procedural laboratory examinations included baseline complete blood count, platelets, and clotting profile.

Based on the pre-procedural imaging, it was decided to use a kissing stent procedure with an overlapping covered self-expanding metallic stent (SEMS) on the left side and an uncovered SEMS on the right. The procedure was performed in theatre under general anaesthesia. A thoracic surgeon used a rigid bronchoscope to gain access to the airway and to visualize the exact proximal margins of the lesion. Subsequently, the interventional radiologist advanced a standard 5Fr multipurpose catheter over a hydrophilic wire, under fluoroscopic guidance, to the level of obstruction. The hydrophilic wire was then used to cross the level of obstruction and then exchanged for a Stiff wire through the catheter. A further Stiff wire was positioned in the right bronchus. The stents used were a covered SEMS for the left side and two uncovered overlapping SEMSs for the right side. The stents were advanced over the wire and deployed under fluoroscopic guidance.

**Learning point** Stent types

- Silicone (e.g. Montgomery T-tube, Dumon, Dynamic):
  - advantages—cheap, removable, minimal granulation
  - disadvantages—need general anesthesia and rigid bronchoscopy, small lumen, interfere with mucociliary clearance, migrates.
- Uncovered SEMS (e.g. Niti-S, Gianturco Z, Ultraflex):
  - advantages—can use flexible bronchoscopy, large lumen, less migration, less ciliary interference
  - disadvantages—difficult to remove, tumour in-growth, radial force can cause necrosis and fistula formation, can collapse if external compression force is high.
- Covered SEMS (e.g. Niti-S, Ultraflex, Wallstent):
  - advantages—can use flexible bronchoscopy, can be used to treat fistulas, no tumour in-growth, large lumen, easier to remove than uncovered SEMS, less ciliary interference
  - disadvantages—may block bronchus, granulation tissue can form at ends, can collapse if the external compression force is high.

The post procedural CXR obtained 36 hours after the procedure showed satisfactory deployment of the stents (Figure 25.1b). Spirometry performed a week later showed increased $FEV_1$ (1.25L, 54% of expected value) and the patient no longer complained of rest dyspnoea.

The six-month follow-up CT scan (Figure 25.1c) revealed progression of the disease, with tumour in-growth in the upper right SEMS. Although the patient did not complain of rest dyspnoea and spirometry showed only a slightly reduced $FEV_1$, a decision was taken at the multidisciplinary meeting to deploy a new covered SEMS within the existing right stent to prevent future total occlusion. The procedure was successful, as confirmed by the post-procedural CXR (Figure 25.1d) and lung function tests with indices of obstruction almost the same as those obtained after placement of the first stent. The patient died three months later as a result of disease progression and multiple brain metastases, but had no further symptoms of severe dyspnoea.

An example of a similar procedure (right main bronchus stenting) is shown in Figure 25.2.

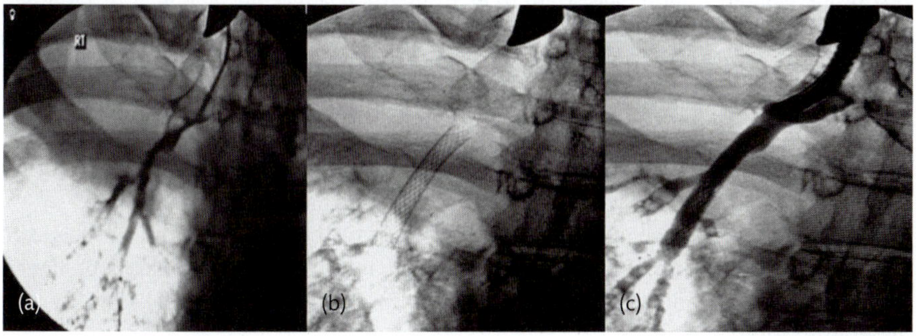


**Figure 25.2** Transcatheter pre-stenting right bronchogram showing (a) severe right bronchus stenosis and (b) stent deployment. (c) Post-deployment bronchogram showing an open airway.

## Discussion

Tracheobronchial stenting is an established palliative treatment for the management of patients with severe airway obstructive disease caused by non-operable malignant pathology, both loco-regional primary cancer and metastatic cancer [5]. Stenting can be utilized to alleviate acute respiratory insufficiency and therefore serve as a bridge to further adjunctive chemotherapy and/or radiotherapy. It is the main method for producing immediate symptomatic relief by treating extrinsic compressions.

Two large groups of stents are used for airway stenting: silicone and nitinol self-expandable (SEMS). SEMS can be either covered or uncovered, while silicone stents can be straight or Y-shaped. Each category has different advantages, disadvantages, and indications. The advantage of silicone stents is that they can easily be repositioned or removed and thus are suitable for benign lesions [6]. However, they have high migration and re-occlusion rates (20% and 15%, respectively), with decreased mucociliary clearance and higher rates of bacterial colonization. Moreover, because of their non-flexible and cumbersome design, their positioning usually necessitates general anaesthesia and rigid bronchoscopy, and reduced patient tolerance and an inability to place them into smaller-calibre airways has been reported [7].

SEMS are very flexible and conform to the airway anatomy more easily, resulting in improved tolerance, and their thin strut technology allows their deployment in bronchi of much smaller calibre than is possible with plastic stents. Uncovered SEMS are associated with a superior mucociliary clearance, low sputum retention, and low migration rates [8,9]. However, the patency of uncovered SEMs is compromised by the possibility of tumour or granulation tissue in-growth, which also results in difficult removal. Dedicated tracheobronchial covered SEMS have been developed to prevent tumour in-growth, facilitate removal, and successfully manage fistulas. However, these stents have an increased migration rate and lower mucociliary clearance compared with the uncovered type. In addition, airway obstruction can occur as a result of incorrect placement or migration [10]. Uncovered stents are used in cases of extrinsic obstruction in order to achieve a satisfactory grip on the respiratory mucosa and avoid migration, while covered stents are reserved for cases of intrinsic lesions and fistulas.

In our case, SEMS deployment was considered to be the approriate treatment because of the malignant nature of the stricture. A kissing stent procedure was performed and multiple stent were inserted; this decision was made because of the presence of a central bronchogenic tumour less than 2cm from the carina and evidence of enlarged mediastinal lymph nodes. In cases of lesions close to the bifurcation, a further contralateral stent is necessary to prevent occlusion of the main contralateral bronchus [11].

Left bronchus stenting was performed using two overlapping covered stents because an intrinsic lesion, eroding the mucosa, compromised the bronchus. However, the right-side stenting was performed using two uncovered stent in order to obtain a satisfactory grip on the non-diseased mucosa.

Another important consideration is the length of the stent. It should exceed the length of the lesion and, if possible, its proximal and distal ends should be deployed on normal mucosa adjacent to the lesion in order to provide adequate stability and avoid migration.

This technique has a high technical success rate (up to 91.8%), with low migration and occlusion rates (2.6% and 6.5%, repectively). [11].

Various peri- and post-procedural complications following tracheobronchial stent insertion have been reported: stent fracture or collapse, occlusion, migration, stent intolerance, infection, and haemoptysis. All of them are amenable to further minimal invasive management.

In the case of occlusion, as we experienced in our case, a new stent insertion should be considered, depending on the patient's life expectancy. Other complications, such as fracture and migration, can be managed with stent removal. In the past, biopsy forceps were used to remove expandable metallic stents [12,13] with potential risk of mucosal bleeding. Modern removal techniques are much easier to perform, because SEMS are manufactured with a hook-like device. To remove these stents, a hooked wire is introduced into the sheath. When the hook grasps the stent drawstring, the wire is withdrawn to obtain proximal stent collapse. The sheath, hook wire, and stent are then pulled out of the airway.

**Expert comment**

In cases of very tight stenosis a balloon predilatation may be necessary in order to allow accurate the advancement of the appropriate stent over the wire deployment under fluoroscopic guidance.

## A final word from the expert

Minimally invasive palliative stenting, under bronchoscopic and fluoroscopic guidance, for the management of symptomatic malignant airway disease is a safe and effective procedure. Making the correct choice between uncovered and covered SEMS results in high technical success and low long-term complication rates. Rigid bronchoscope access is valuable for accurate stent positioning, taking biopsies, and allowing adequate suction of airways. If there is an immediate misplacement, the stent can be repositioned more easily.

## References


1. Luomanen RKJ, Watson WL. Autopsy findings. In WL Watson (ed), ed. *Lung Cancer: A Study of Five Thousand Memorial Hospital Cases* (St Louis, MO: CV Mosby); 1968: 504–10.
2. Ernst A, Feller-Kopman D, Becker HD, et al. Central airway obstruction. *Am J Respir Crit Care Med* 2004; 169: 1278–97.
3. Bolliger CT, Mathur PN, Beamis JF, et al: European Respiratory Society/American Thoracic Society. ERS/ATS statement on interventional pulmonology. *Eur Respir J* 2002; 19(2): 356–73.
4. Furukawa K, Ishida J, Yamaguchi G, et al. The role of airwaystent placement in the management of tracheobronchial stenosis caused by inoperable advanced lung cancer. *Surg Today* 2010; 40(4): 315–20.
5. Martinez-Ballarin JI, Diaz-Jimenez JP, Castro MJ, Moya JA. Silicone stents in the management of benign tracheobronchial stenoses: tolerance and early results in 63 patients. *Chest* 1996; 109(3): 626–9.
6. Rafanan AL, Mehta AC. Stenting of the tracheobronchial tree. *Radiol Clin North Am* 2000; 38(2): 395–408.
7. Rousseau H, Dahan M, Lauque D, et al. Self-expandable prostheses in the tracheobronchial tree. *Radiology* 1993; 188(1): 199–203.
8. Beer M, Wittenberg G, Sandstede J, et al. Treatment of inoperabile tracheobronchial obstructive lesions with the Palmaz stent. *Cardiovasc Intervent Radiol* 1999; 22(2): 109–13.
9. Shin JH, Song HY, Shim TS. Management of tracheobronchial strictures. *Cardiovasc Intervent Radiol* 2004; 27(4): 314–24.
10. Shitrit D, Kuchuk M, Zismanov V, et al. Bronchoscopic balloon dilatation of tracheobronchial stenosis: long-term follow-up. *Eur J Cardiothorac Surg* 2010; 38(2): 198–202.

11. Inchingolo R, Sabharwal T, Spiliopoulos S, et al. Tracheobronchial stenting for malignant airway disease: long-term outcomes from a single-centre study. *Am J Hosp Palliat Care* 2013; 30(7): 683–9.
12. Filler RM, Forte V, Chait P. Tracheobronchial stenting for the treatment of airway obstruction. *J Pediatr Surg* 1998; 33: 304–11.
13. Nicolai T, Huber RM, Reiter K, et al. Metal airway stent implantation in children: follow-up of seven children. *Pediatr Pulmonol* 2001; 31: 289–96.

CASE

# 26 Early-stage hepatocellular carcinoma: the percutaneous approach

**Venus Hedayati**

**Expert commentary** Praveen Peddu

## Case history

A 54-year-old woman was found on routine blood tests to have abnormal liver function tests. Ultrasound revealed a fatty liver and, following referral to the hepatologists, the patient was monitored for non-alcoholic fatty liver disease (NAFLD). The hepatitis screen was negative and her alcohol consumption was moderate. This was reflected in the serum biochemistry outlined in Table 26.1.

Given the slightly elevated AFP, further imaging was undertaken, first with ultrasound and then with CT, which demonstrated features of cirrhosis with nodular liver and a dominant nodule in segment 6 measuring 2.7cm without typical characteristics of hepatocellular carcinoma; no definite arterialization was identified (Figure 26.1a). MRI depicted the lesion more clearly (Figure 26.1b). Although the imaging features were atypical, given the background risk a provisional diagnosis of solitary HCC was made. Following discussion at the multidisciplinary meeting, the decision was made to perform hepatic arteriography and treat the lesion with transarterial chemoembolization (TACE).

On arteriography, the lesion did not demonstrate a significant increase in vascularity, and despite selective chemoembolization with doxorubicin and lipiodol (Figure 26.1c), the post-chemoembolization CT did not demonstrate any morphological change within lesion. Therefore following a review at the multidisciplinary meeting and discussion with the patient, the decision was made to biopsy the lesion and to perform simultaneous radiofrequency ablation (RFA) of the lesion and the biopsy tract (Figures 26.1d,e) in order to prevent seeding of hepatocellular tumour. Histology of the lesion demonstrated well-differentiated HCC (Figure 26.2), and successful ablation was confirmed on a six-week post-ablation CT which did not show any residual tumour. Having confirmed the diagnosis of HCC, the patient was entered into the liver transplant pathway with enhanced regular surveillance to ensure no drop-out from the waiting list.

**Table 26.1** Serum biochemistry at presentation

| | | |
|---|---|---|
| INR | 1.14 | (<1.4) |
| Alkaline phosphatase (ALP) | 169 | (30–130IU/L) |
| Aspartate aminotransferase (AST) | 114 | (10–50IU/L) |
| Bilirubin | 12 | (3–20μmol/L) |
| Gamma glutamyl transferase GGT) | 1640 | (1–55IU/L) |
| Alpha-fetoprotein (AFP) | 17 | (<7 kIU/L) |
| Haemoglobin (Hb) | 12 | (11.5–13.5g/dl) |

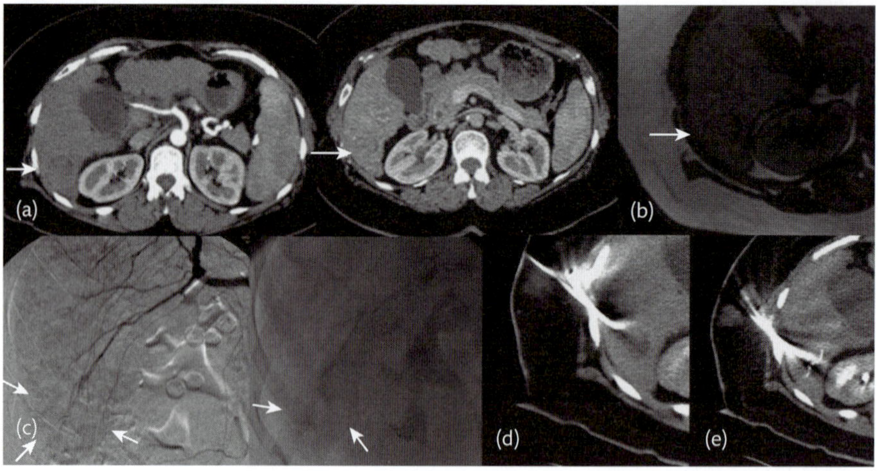


**Figure 26.1** (a) CT scan showing a nodular liver with splenomegaly. A rounded hypodensity, which did not enhance on arterial phase, is present in segment 6. (b) Non-contrast T1-weighted MRI image of the same lesion. (c) Selective angiography showss no significant increase in the vascularity of the tumour nodule in segment 6 (arrows). (d) A coaxial system was used to take a biopsy and (e) and perform radiofrequency ablation of the lesion and tract.

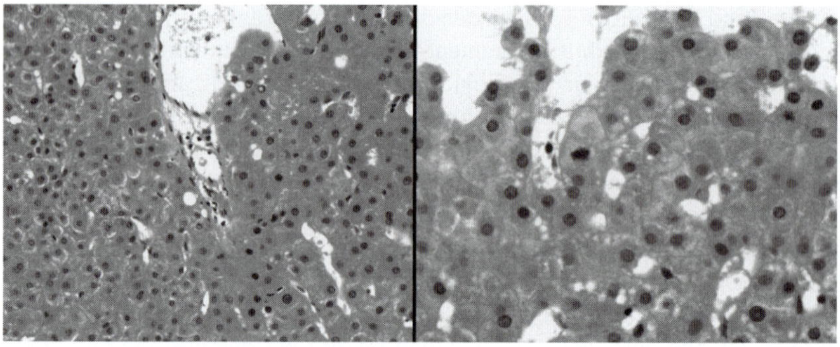

**Figure 26.2** Histology: H&E stained medium and high-power views of the lesion demonstrating variation in cell size and cytoplasmic volume, increased mitosis, and an unpaired arteriole, suggesting a well differentiated HCC

Courtesy of Dr A. Knisley, Consultant Histopathologist, King's College Hospital, London, UK.

**Expert comment**

A small number of patients with early-stage HCC do not have typical arterial enhancement and venous washout features on CT and MR. In this group the diagnosis is often influenced by their risk factors—serum AFP and severity of the background liver disease. In this case the patient had cirrhotic liver with significant background nodularity and a dominant nodule that could easily be identified on imaging. This, together with the mild elevation of AFP, tilted the clinico-radiological diagnosis more in favour of HCC. Hepatic angiography and chemoembolization with doxorubicin and lipiodol was chosen as the next step in clinico-radiological management as it is useful not only for characterizing atypical lesions but also for identifying other lesions which are not detected on axial imaging.

be treated 90% of the time with a recurrence rate of less than 1% [11]. Overall recurrence rate after ablation is not significantly different to that after resection, and is greater in lesions >3cm [4] Complications include intraperitoneal bleeding, pleural effusions or haemathoraces; RFA related mortality is up to 0.3%.

Transarterial embolization is used for BCLC stage B patients who have large or multifocal HCC but no signs of macrovascular invasion or extrahepatic spread. It may be combined with RFA, but is reserved for non-surgical candidates in whom RFA alone is not a treatment option. It results in tumour necrosis in approximately 50% of patients and improves survival [14]. It can be performed with or without chemotherapy agents depending on whether the patient can tolerate this. Conventional chemoembolization involves injection of the chemotherapeutic agent doxorubicin in combination with lipiodol into the lobar or segmental hepatic artery. Most centres have replaced conventional TACE with drug-eluting beads (DC Beads; Biocompatables, Farnham, UK). These allow slow release of the cytotoxic agent into the tumour, inflicting local ischaemia while reducing systemic concentrations [15]. Contraindications to treatment include extrahepatic tumour, Child–Pugh B or C liver disease, and macroscopic portal vein thrombus or poor portal flow for any other reason, as a potential complication is acute liver failure secondary to the procedure.

SIRT is another percutaneous approach which can be used if TACE fails but is generally reserved to extend the life of patients who are non-resectable or transplantable. The aim is to inject yttrium-90 microspheres bound to glass beads or resin which provide radiotherapy locally into the tumour circulation without the harmful effects of radiation necrosis to the remainder of the liver.

The treatment of advanced HCC with sorafenib, a once-daily oral multikinase and vascular endothelial growth factor receptor inhibitor, is outside the remit of this topic. It is used as a first-line treatment when other potentially more effective therapies, as discussed in this case, cannot be used.

In conclusion, the diagnosis and treatment of HCC requires a multidisciplinary approach. Radiologists play an integral role, from screening to diagnosis, and can provide a variety of treatments. According to the BCLC staging system, early HCC can be treated either with liver transplantation, resection, or percutaneous ablation. Asymptomatic patients with large-volume confined hepatic disease, no evidence of macrovascular invasion, and preserved liver function (Child–Pugh A) are treated with transarterial embolization with or without chemotherapy. Often patients are given a combination of treatments including TACE and RFA, which are used as a bridge to transplantation.

## References


1. Yoon SH, Lee JM, So YH, et al. Multiphasic MDCT enhancement pattern of hepatocellular carcinoma smaller than 3 cm in diameter: tumor size and cellular differentiation. *AJR Am J Roentgenol* 2009; 193(6): W482–9
2. Jang HJ, Kim TK, Burns PN, Wilson SR. Enhancement patterns of hepatocellular carcinoma at contrast-enhanced US: comparison with histologic differentiation. *Radiology* 2007; 244(3): 898–906.
3. Lu DS, Yu NC, Raman SS, et al. Radiofrequency ablation of hepatocellular carcinoma: treatment success as defined by histologic examination of the explanted liver. *Radiology* 2005; 234: 954–60.

4. Mazzaferro V, Battiston C, Perrone S, et al. Radiofrequency ablation of small hepatocellular carcinoma in cirrhotic patients awaiting liver transplantation: a prospective study. *Ann Surg* 2004; 240: 900–9.
5. Llovet JM, Schwartz M, Mazzaferro V. Resection and liver transplantation for hepatocellular carcinoma. *Semin Liver Dis* 2005; 25: 181–200.
6. Lu DS, Yu NC, Raman SS, et al. Percutaneous radiofrequency ablation of hepatocellular carcinoma as a bridge to liver transplantation. *Hepatology* 2005; 41: 1130–7.
7. Lesurtel M, Mullhaupt B, Pestalozzi BC, et al. Transarterial chemoembolization as a bridge to liver transplantation for hepatocellular carcinoma: an evidence-based analysis. *Am J Transplant* 2006; 6: 2644–50.
8. Otto G, Herber S, Heise M, et al. Response to transarterial chemoembolization as a biological selection criterion for liver transplantation in hepatocellular carcinoma. *Liver Transpl* 2006; 12: 1260–7.
9. Puneet P, Perera MT, Mirza DF. Current opinion on the role of resection and liver transplantation for hepatocellular cancer. *Indian J Gastroenterol* 2012; 31(3): 89–99.
10. Tinkle CL, Haas-Kogan D. Hepatocellular carcinoma: natural history, current management, and emerging tools. *Biologics* 2012; 6: 207–19.
11. Bruix J, Sherman M. Management of hepatocellular carcinoma: an update. *Hepatology* 2011; 53(3): 1020–2.
12. Pons F, Varela M, Llovet JM. Staging systems in hepatocellular carcinoma. *HPB (Oxford)* 2005; 7(1): 35–41.
13. Schwartz M, Roayaie S, Uva P. Treatment of HCC in patients awaiting liver transplantation. *Am J Transplant* 2007; 7(8): 1875–81.
14. Llovet JM, Bruix J. Systematic review of randomized trials for unresectable hepatocellular carcinoma: chemoembolization improves survival. *Hepatology* 2003; 37(2): 429–42.
15. Lammer J, Malagari K, Vogl T, et al. Prospective randomized study of doxorubicin-eluting-bead embolization in the treatment of hepatocellular carcinoma: results of the PRECISION V study. *Cardiovasc Intervent Radiol* 2010; 33(1): 41–52.

CASE

# 27 Small renal tumours: is radiofrequency ablation better than surgery?

**Miltiadis Krokidis**

**Expert commentary** Andy Adam

## Case history

A 64-year-old man presented to his GP with a three-month history of a productive cough that was resistant to common antibiotics. The GP requested a chest X-ray from the local hospital which showed an equivocal result. The radiologist suggested a chest CT scan to exclude the presence of a pulmonary mass. The CT revealed diffuse emphysema and interstitial lung disease but no pulmonary mass; however, some slices of the upper abdomen were included which showed the presence of a 29mm solid lesion and a 12cm simple cyst in the left kidney. The result was returned to the GP who referred the patient for an outpatient urological consultation. Prior to seeing the patient the urologist ordered a full blood count and a biochemical profile of the patient as well as a contrast CT scan of his abdomen in order to further delineate the incidental finding in the kidney. A CT scan was performed on an outpatient basis and showed a lesion that appeared solid in the non-contrast scan and significantly enhancing in the arterial and portal venous phase (Figure 27.1). The CT report was highly suggestive of renal cell carcinoma (RCC).

The case was discussed in the renal cancer multidisciplinary meeting and it was decided to treat the lesion with percutaneous radiofrequency ablation (RFA). The decision was made on the basis of the size of the lesion, the general condition of the patient, and local expertise.

**Learning point** CT characteristics of renal cell carcinomas

RCCs are often heterogeneous on unenhanced CT, with one or more low-density areas. Parenchymal calcification may be present, and the radiodensity of the mass is expected to be in the region of 20 Hounsfield units (HU). If the attenuation in the mass increases by more than 10HU after injection of contrast, the findings are highly suggestive of a solid lesion, and enhancement greater than 20HU is highly suggestive of malignancy.

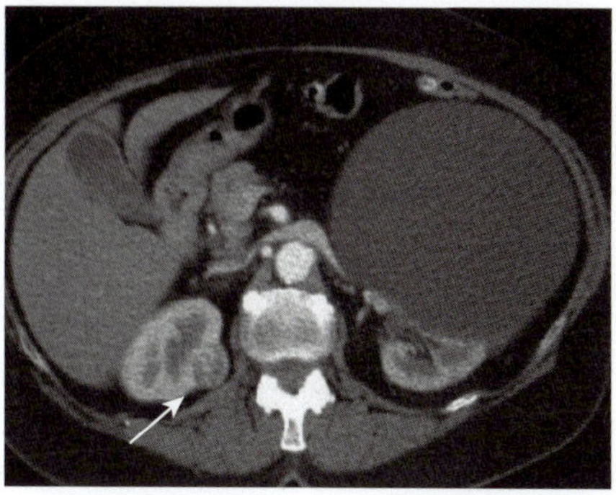

**Figure 27.1** CT with IV contrast showing an exophytic solid enhancing lesion in the right kidney (arrow). There is a large simple cyst in the left kidney.

**Evidence base** Radiofrequency ablation versus partial nephrectomy in patients with T1a RCC: comparable outcomes after five-year follow-up [1]

- Observational single-centre cohort study.
- Patients with a histologically confirmed solitary T1a RCC.
- Treated with either RFA or partial nephrectomy (PN).
- Overall survival, cancer-specific survival, local recurrence-free survival, overall disease-free survival, and metastasis-free survival were compared.
- Each group included 37 patients according to the selection criteria.
- Median follow-up time was 6.5 years for the RFA group and 6.1 years for the PN group.
- Five-year overall survival and cancer-specific survival were 97.2% (RFA) versus 100% (PN), $p = 0.31$.
- Disease-free survival was 89.2% (RFA) versus 89.2% (PN), $p = 0.78$.
- Local recurrence-free survival was 91.7% (RFA) versus 94.6% (PN), $p = 0.96$.
- Metastasis-free survival was 97.2% (RFA) versus 91.8% (PN), $p = 0.35$.
- The conclusion of the study was that, in selected patients, RFA is an effective minimally invasive treatment for RCC with long-term outcomes comparable with those for PN.

**Expert comment**

Outpatient consultations are an important part of the management of patients prior to image-guided tumour ablation. The proposed treatment should be put into context relative to alternative options, such as radiotherapy and surgery. During these consultations, the procedure is carefully explained to the patient, ideally with the help of diagrams or other images. The possible complications are outlined, as well as pre- and post-procedure care and follow-up arrangements. It is particularly important to explain that there may be a need for repeat treatment if there is local recurrence.

**Learning point** Histological classification of renal cell carcinoma

According to theWorld Health Organization, there are three major histological RCC types: clear cell RCC (80–90%), papillary RCC (10–15%), and chromophobe RCC (4–5%) [2]. Papillary RCC can be further divided into two subtypes, type 1 and type 2; the latter has a worse prognosis [3].

The patient was referred by the urology consultant to the Interventional radiology oncological outpatient clinic. The risks and benefits of the procedure were explained and consent was obtained.

The procedure was scheduled for the following week. The day before the procedure the patient was admitted and a full blood count and biochemical analysis were ordered. The interventional radiologist who had countersigned the consent form visited the patient again. The patient was kept nil by mouth from midnight. Premedication with pethidine 100mg IM and metoclopramide 10mg IV was administered an hour before the procedure.

The patient was transferred to the CT scanner and positioned prone on the CT table with his head towards the CT gantry. A radio-opaque body marker grid was applied in the skin projection of the left kidney and a topographic CT scan was performed (Figure 27.2a). The skin was then marked with a radio-opaque single marker and local anaesthesia was applied (20ml lidocaine 1%) (Figure 27.2b).

The procedure was performed under conscious sedation using midazolam 6mg and fentanyl 100µg administered intravenously. Initially,a CT-guided biopsy with an 18G cutting needle tray system was performed in the lesion (Figure 27.3a). A 22G spinal needle was then inserted in the lesion and 2.2ml of ethanol were injected prior to RFA (Figure 27.3b). The RFA system used was the Cool-tip RF System (Covidien, Boulder, CO; formerly Tyco Healthcare Valleylab). A single 17G electrode 15cm long was used (Figure 27.3c).

**Learning point** Characteristics of the Cool-Tip RFA system

The Cool-tip RF System consists of internally cooled electrodes connected to a generator which produces a 480kHz alternating current with a maximum power output of 200W. The energy output is adjusted based on the impedance of the tissue which is monitored continuously. The electrodes are internally cooled with saline to enhance the homogenous heating of the adjacent tissue and to reduce charring and vaporization. They are straight and monopolar and may be single or a cluster of three.

During needle placement two-dimensional reconstructions were obtained along the plane of insertion in order to make an accurate determination of the position of the needle tip relative to the tumour and adjacent tissues (Figure 27.3d). The

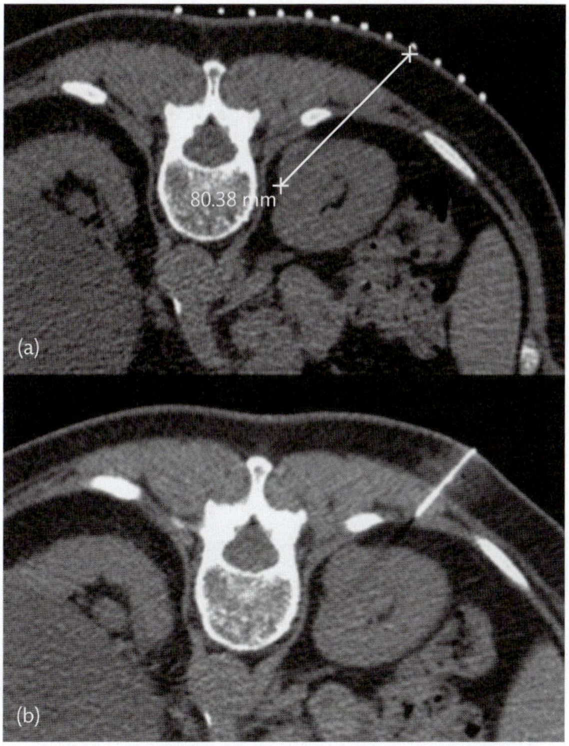


Figure 27.2 (a) A radio-opaque grid was used to plan the needle-insertion angle. (b) Local anaesthesia was administered.

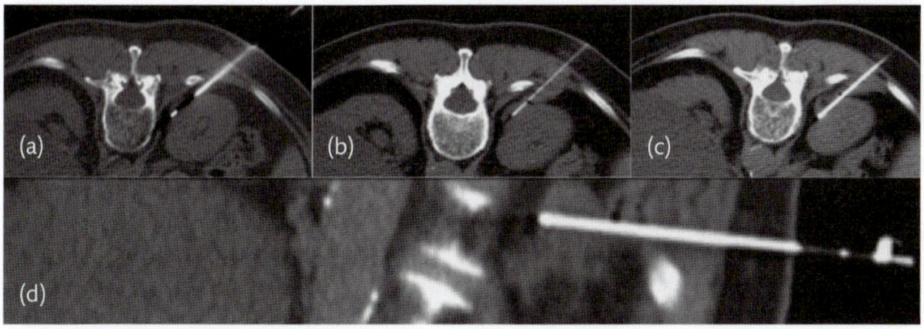


Figure 27.3 (a) A core biopsy was taken with a 16G needle. (b) Ethanol was injected prior to RFA. (c) A single RFA electrode was used. (d) Sagittal reconstruction of the CT image confirms that the electrode is in the centre of the lesion.

generator was operated in the impedance-control mode and the cycle of ablation lasted for 12 minutes. A CT scan performed at the end of the ablation process showed cavitation of the tumour area and no evidence of significant bleeding (Figure 27.4). The time required for the overall procedure was 40 minutes. At the end of the procedure the patient was transferred to the radiology recovery area and monitored haemodynamically for four hours. When he was fully awake he was transferred to the ward. A CT carried out the following morning demonstrated an area of coagulation, with no evidence of residual tumour. The patient was discharged an hour later. Follow-up scans performed every six months for the next three years showed no evidence of residual tumour (Figure 27.5).

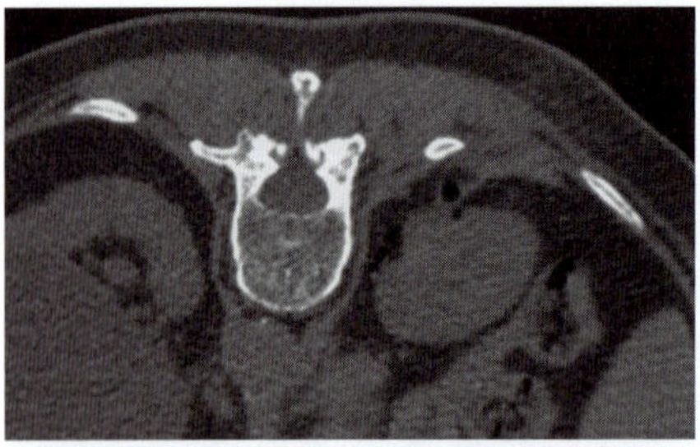

**Figure 27.4** Non-enhanced scan post-procedure shows cavitation of the tumour and no significant bleeding.

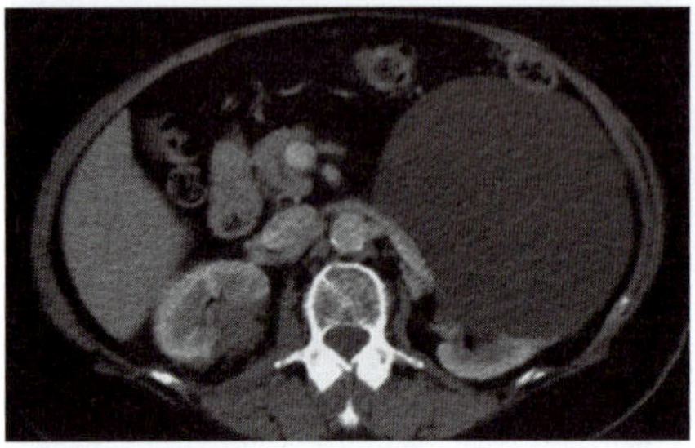

**Figure 27.5** Follow-up CT scan showing satisfactory treatment of the lesion.

**Learning point** Detection of residual tumour and tumour recurrence

For most of the groups performing RFA the detection of residual tumour is based on CT findings of persistent evidence of enhancement (10–15HU) of the lesion in the first three months post-RFA. The management of such patients consists of a new RFA treatment if there are no comorbidities. If MRI is used for follow-up, any qualitative increase in the signal intensity of the treated lesion post-contrast should be considered as residual disease. Repeat biopsy is not usually part of the management.

If the first scan shows complete response, but enhancement is detected in the follow-up scan, recurrence of the tumour should be considered. In such cases discussion in a multidisciplinary meeting is suggested in view of possible further treatment with RFA.

**Learning point** Definition of oncological outcomes

The oncological outcomes of the treatment of RCC are usually evaluated according to the recommendations of the American Urological Association Guideline Panel [4].

- Recurrence-free survival (RFS) refers to the proportion of patients withoutdisease recurrence in the ablation zone.
- Metastasis-free survival (MFS) refers to the proportion of patients without RCC anywhere in their body other than the treated kidney.
- Disease-free survival (DFS) refers to the proportion of patients with no disease at the last follow-up including both locally recurrent disease and evidence of metastases.
- Cancer-specific survival (CSS) is the proportion of patients who have not died from RCC.
- Overall survival (OS) is the proportion of patients who have not died of any cause.

## Discussion

Historically, surgical oncology followed the guidance of its founder, William Stewart Halstead, aiming for wide en bloc resection of the organ and the tumour that the organ contained. Surgical oncology has evolved towards an organ-sparing approach, aiming to excise the tumour but not the whole organ. Therefore minimally invasive in situ needle-guided treatments have been introduced and developed in the last 15 years, offering tumour treatment based on the destruction of tumour cells.

RFA is a thermal ablation method based on the interaction between high frequency rapidly alternating current and tissue. The alternating current causes water molecules in the biological tissue to vibrate, and the vibration is transmitted to adjacent molecules. The kinetic energy is transformed into thermal energy, leading to hyperthermia and coagulation necrosis of the biological tissue.

RFA has been the most diffuse ablative technique used and there is current evidence that shows that local control of RCC is effective with optimal long-term results.

**Evidence base** Long-term oncologic outcomes after radiofrequency ablation for T1 renal cell carcinoma [5]

- Retrospective review of 185 patients with sporadic T1 RCC.
- All patients with a histologically confirmed lesions.
- All patients were treated with RFA.
- Disease-specific survival and overall survival were calculated and stratified by tumour stage.
- Median tumour size was 3cm (range 2.1–3.9cm).
- The tumour stage was T1a in 143 cases and T1b in 42 cases.
- Twenty-four patients (13%) were re-treated for residual disease and there were 12 local recurrences.
- Median time to recurrence was 2.5 years.
- Tumour stage was the only significant predictor of disease-specific survival on multivariate analysis.
- Five patients developed metachronous renal tumors (2.7%). Four patients developed extra-renal metastases (2.2%), three of whom died of metastatic RCC (1.6%).
- The conclusion is that RFA results in durable local control and low recurrence risk for T1a RCC in poor surgical candidates.
- A higher stage correlates with a decreased disease-free survival.

The main advantage of RFA is the preservation of renal function, which may be at risk even with the most accurate PN procedure.

**Learning point** Factors influencing the loss of renal function after partial nephrectomy

PN is now considered to be the standard treatment for small renal masses [6]. The factor influencing the outcome of PN in terms of loss of renal function is warm ischaemia time (WIT). The exact period of accepted WIT is not known; however, the majority of the studies suggest 40 minutes as a cut-off [7–13].

The study by Pouliot et al. [14] included 182 patients where laparoscopic PN had been performed for tumours of median size 26mm. The baseline glomerular filtration rate (GFR) was 82ml/min/173m$^2$ and the median patient age was 62 years. Median loss of renal function occurred in 14%, and occurred predominantly if WIT was >30min. Other factors that were associated with loss of renal function were the endophytic location of the tumour, post-operative GFR, operative time, and blood loss.

RFA appears to offer very satisfactory long-term results, particularly in patients with only a single functioning kidney.

**Evidence base** Percutaneous radiofrequency ablation of small renal tumours in patients with a single functioning kidney: long-term results [15]

- Single-centre prospective study.
- Patients with a single functioning kidney and a tumour<3.5cm treated with RFA over a 7.5-year period were included.
- Nineteen patients were studied.
- Primary endpoints were technical success and tumour recurrence rate.
- Secondary endpoints were the deterioration of renal function and overall survival rate.
- The mean follow-up time was 56.1 months (range 36–102 months).
- The primary technical success was 100%.
- There was no significant difference between baseline GFR and GFR at 3, 12, and 24 months post-procedure.
- Recurrence was detected in four lesions (17%) and an additional RFA session was performed.
- None of the patients developed renal failure during their lifetime

In experienced hands, the effect of the RFA may also be enhanced by using ethanol, with optimal results.

**Evidence base** Combined percutaneous radiofrequency ablation and ethanol injection of renal tumours: midterm results [16]

- Single-centre prospective study.
- Twenty-seven consecutive patients with 28 renal tumours (mean diameter 2.87cm) were treated with ae combination of percutaneous RFA and ethanol ablation.
- Absolute ethanol (0.5–3ml; mean 1.7ml) was injected into the tumour immediately before RFA treatment.
- The mean follow-up period was 18.6 months (range 3–56 months).
- Twenty-seven of the 28 tumours were completely ablated following either one (21/27) or two (6/27) treatment sessions.
- No evidence of local recurrence or metastatic disease was seen during the follow-up period.
- Renal function was preserved in all patients

According to the current evidence, RFA appears to offer very satisfactory oncological outcomes in the treatment of small renal tumours. However, it is not clear whether or not RFA is better than surgery because there very limited direct comparison of the two methods has been reported in the literature, and none has been in the form of prospective randomized trials.

In 2007 Stern et al. [17] published a retrospective review of 77 patients who were treated for T1a renal masses in a single centre over an eight-year period. Thirty patients were treated with open PN, seven with laparoscopic PN, 26 with percutaneous RFA, and 14 with laparoscopic RFA. The mean follow-up for the RFA and PN groups was 30 months (range 18–42 months) and 47 months (range 24–93 months), respectively ($p < 0.001$), and the mean tumour size was 2.41cm and 2.43cm, respectively ($p = 0.45$). In the RFA group incomplete ablation occurred in one case and local recurrence in two cases. There were also two recurrences in the PN group. The three-year recurrence-free survival rate was 93.4% for the RFA group and 95.8% for the group who underwent partial nephrectomy, with no significant difference between the two groups ($p = 0.67$). Complications were also comparable between the two groups: one patient who underwent PN developed a hernia and two others developed prolonged ileus; one patient in the RFA group developed an obstruction

**Table 27.1 Comparative studies of RFA and PN**

| | | | | | |
|---|---|---|---|---|---|
| **Study** | Sung et al [18] | Olweny et al. [1] | Takaki et al. [19] | Stern et al. [17] | Bird et al. [20] |
| **Patients** | 150 | 74 | 115 | 77 | 69 |
| **Modalities** | Open PN (110) vs percutaneous RFA (40) | RFA (37) vs PN (37) for T1a RCC | RFA (51) vs radical (54) or partial (10) nephrectomy | Percutaneous (26) or laparoscopic (14) RFA vs open PN (30) or laparascopic PN (7) | Laparoscopic PN (33) vs laparoscopic RFA (36) |
| **Mean tumour size** | 24.4 ± 13.1mm (RFA) and 22.3 ± 10.2mm (PN) | 2.1cm (RFA) and 2.5cm (PN) | < 4 cm | 2.41cm (RFA) and 2.43cm (PN) | 2.8cm (RFA) and 3.1cm (PN) |
| **Type of study** | Retrospective single-centre study | Retrospective single-centre study | Retrospective single-centre study | Retrospective single-centre study | Retrospective single-centre study |
| **Conclusion** | RFA is superior to open PN with respect to the preservation of renal function with equivalent oncological outcomes | Comparable long-term oncological outcomes | Comparable with minor loss of renal function | Comparable oncological outcomes | No significant difference |

of the pelvi-ureteric junction, one developed pneumonia, and one developed an asymptomatic lower-pole hydrocalyx. The authors concluded that RFA for cT1a renal tumours has a comparable oncological outcome to PN.

In total five studies comparing RFA and PN are reported in the literature, and their results are summarized in Table 27.1.

## A final word from the expert

Percutaneous ablation is a useful alternative to surgery in carefully selected patients with small renal masses. This nephron-sparing technique produces satisfactory long-term oncological outcomes in patients with lesions up to 3cm in diameter. Its place in relation to partial nephrectomy has yet to be defined precisely. Ideally, this will be done through randomized comparative studies, although recruitment of patients may prove problematic and good registry data may make a significant contribution. In the meantime, percutaneous ablation seems particularly appropriate in patients with multiple tumours, chronic kidney disease, or tumours in solitary kidneys, and in those who are poor surgical candidates.

## References


1. Olweny EO, Park SK, Tan YK, et al. Radiofrequency ablation versus partial nephrectomy in patients with solitary clinical T1a renal cell carcinoma: comparable oncologic outcomes at a minimum of 5 years of follow-up. *Eur Urol* 2012; 61(6): 1156–61.
2. Eble JN, Sauter G, Epstein JI, et al. (eds). *Pathology and Genetics of Tumours of the Urinary System and Male Genital Organs. World Health Organization Classification of Tumours* (Lyon: IARC Press); 2004: 7.
3. Pignot G, Elie C, Conquy S, et al. Survival analysis of 130 patients with papillary renal cell carcinoma: prognostic utility of type 1 and type 2 subclassification. *Urology* 2007; 69: 230–5.
4. Campbell SC, Novick AC, Belldegrun A, et al. Guideline for management of the clinical T1 renal mass. *J Urol* 2009; 182: 1271–9.

5. Psutka SP, Feldman AS, McDougal WS, et al. Long-term oncologic outcomes after radiofrequency ablation for T1 renal cell carcinoma. *Eur Urol* 2013; 63(3): 486–92.
6. Ljungberg B, Hanbury DC, Kuczyk MA, et al. Renal cell carcinoma guideline. *Eur Urol* 2007; 51: 1502–10.
7. Thompson RH, Frank I, Lohse CM, et al. The impact of ischemia time during open nephron sparing surgery on solitary kidneys: a multi-institutional study. *J Urol* 2007; 177: 471–6.
8. Abouassaly R, Lane BR, Novick AC. Active surveillance of renal masses in elderly patients. *J Urol*. 2008; 180: 505–9.
9. Colombo JR Jr, Haber GP, Jelovsek JE, et al. Seven years after laparoscopic radical nephrectomy: oncologic and renal functional outcomes. *Urology* 2008; 71: 1149–54.
10. Foyil KV, Ames CD, Ferguson GG, et al. Long term changes in creatinine clearance after laparoscopic renal surgery. *J Am Coll Surg* 2008; 206: 511–15.
11. Godoy G, Ramanathan V, Kanofsky JA, et al. Effect of warm ischemia time during laparoscopic partial nephrectomy on early postoperative glomerular filtration rate. *J Urol* 2009; 181: 2438–45.
12. Becker F, Van Poppel H, Hakenberg OW, et al. Assessing the impact of ischaemia time during partial nephrectomy. *Eur Urol* 2009; 56: 625–35.
13. Desai MM, Gill IS, Ramani AP, et al. The impact of warm ischaemiaonrenal function after laparoscopic partial nephrectomy. *BJU Int* 2005; 95: 377–83.
14. Pouliot F, Pantuck A, Imbeault A, et al. Multivariate analysis of the factors involved in loss of renal differential function after laparoscopic partial nephrectomy: a role for warm ischemia time. *Can Urol Assoc J* 2011; 5(2): 89–95.
15. Krokidis M, Spiliopoulos S, Jarzabek M, et al. Percutaneous radiofrequency ablation of small renal tumours in patients with a single functioning kidney: long-term results. *Eur Radiol* 2013; 23(7): 1933–9.
16. Fotiadis NI, Sabharwal T, Morales JP, Hodgson DJ, et al. Combined percutaneous radiofrequency ablation and ethanol injection of renal tumours: midterm results. *Eur Urol* 2007; 52: 777–84.
17. Stern, JM, Svatek R, Park S, et al. Intermediate comparison of partial nephrectomy and radiofrequency ablation for clinical T1a renal tumours. *BJU Int* 2007; 100(2): 287–90.
18. Sung HH, Park BK, Kim CK, et al. Comparison of percutaneous radiofrequency ablation and open partial nephrectomy for the treatment of size- and location-matched renal masses. *Int J Hyperthermia* 2012; 28(3): 227–34.
19. Takaki H, Yamakado K, Soga N, et al. Midterm results of radiofrequency ablation versus nephrectomy for T1a renal cell carcinoma. *Jpn J Radiol* 2010; 28(6): 460–8.
20. Bird VG, Carey RI, Ayyathurai R, Bird VY. Management of renal masses with laparoscopic-guided radiofrequency ablation versus laparoscopic partial nephrectomy. *J Endourol* 2009; 23(1): 81–8.

CASE

# 28 Malignant biliary strictures: covered or uncovered stents?

Miltiadis Krokidis

Expert commentary Adam Hatzidakis

## Case history

An 87-year-old man presented with moderate melaena in the A&E department of a tertiary care centre. He was not significantly anaemic and he was transferred to a ward with a view to endoscopic examination the following day. His history included bilateral deep vein thrombosis (DVT), spinal stenosis with decompression five years previously, chronic kidney disease (CKD) stage 3 (baseline creatinine value 180µm/L) and hypertension. The endoscopic examination did not detect a bleeding source. The gastrointestinal bleeding was investigated further with a CT scan which revealed dilatation of the common bile duct (16mm) and pancreatic duct (12mm) and the presence of a 3.2cm diameter mass at the head of the pancreas (Figure 28.1).

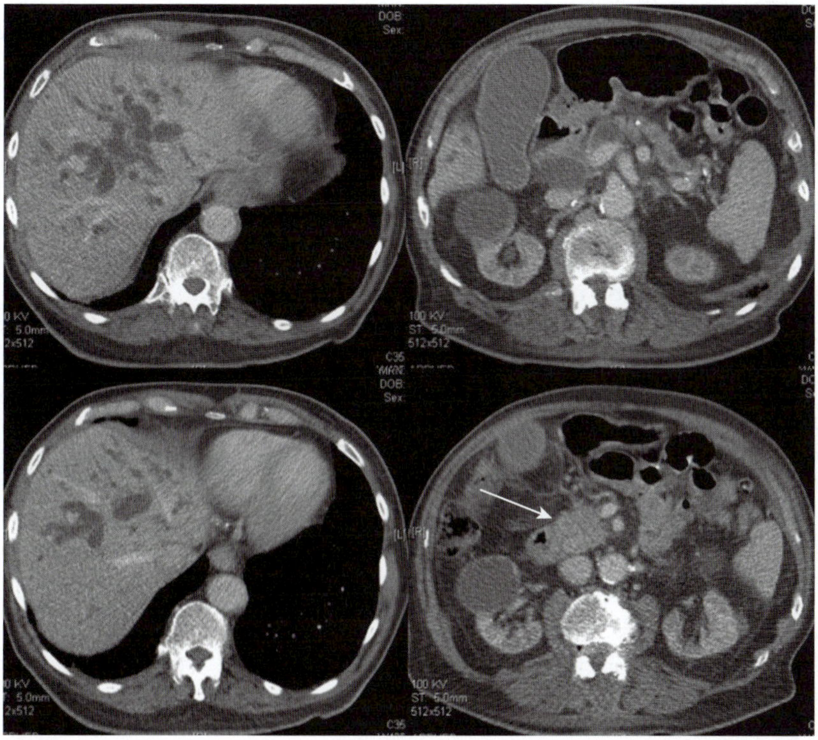

**Figure 28.1** CT with IV contrast showing a mass at the head of the pancreas (arrow). There is significant dilatation of the intra- and extra-hepatic ducts and the pancreatic duct.

**Learning point** CT protocol and characteristics of the of pancreatic adenocarcinoma

When there is suspicion of a tumour at the head of the pancreas a contrast CT scan is required. The timing of image acquisition is critical. The first image set should be acquired during the 'pancreatic phase' (approximately 40–50 seconds) and the second image set during the portal venous phase (90 seconds) [1]. Contrast injection should be performed at a rate of 4–5ml/sec, preferably with low osmolality contrast at an iodine dose of 1.5–2.0mg/kg, and thin slices should be obtained [2].

The lesion is frequently hypodense compared with the background parenchyma on IV contrast-enhanced imaging. It is important to obtain images when the enhancement of the background gland is maximal in order to reveal the attenuation difference between tumour and gland [3]. Secondary findings may include dilatation of the pancreatic duct and the common bile duct (CBD) when the lesion is located in the head of the pancreas.

The case was discussed in the regional hepatopancreatobiliary multidisciplinary meeting and it was decided to perform endoscopic ultrasound-guided fine-needle aspiration (FNA) and endoscopic stent insertion in the distal CBD. FNA confirmed the presence of a pancreatic adenocarcinoma, but endoscopic stent insertion was not feasible and a percutaneous approach was adopted.

The patient was transferred to the interventional radiology suite and ultrasound (US) confirmed the dilatation of the biliary tree. A left-side approach was decided. US-guided puncture of a left peripheral duct with a Chiba needle (Cook Medical) was performed and a cholangiogram was obtained (Figure 28.2a). A 0.021-inch guidewire was advanced within the central ducts and the needle was exchanged for a 6Fr dilator (NEFF set; Cook Medical) (Figure 28.2b). A 0.035-inch guidewire was then advanced in the common hepatic duct and an 8.5Fr external drain (Ultrathane; Cook Medical) was inserted in order to decompress the biliary tree. The patient was transferred to the ward and IV antibiotics were administered. Two days later a cholangiogram was performed and revealed the presence of multiple filling defects in the CBD due to the presence of multiple clots (Figure 28.3a). The external drain was exchanged over a wire to a 7Fr sheath (CheckFlo; Cook Medical), and the stricture in the lower CBD was crossed using a biliary manipulation catheter (BMC; Cordis Europe) and a hydrophilic guidewire (Glidewire, Terumo Europe). Because of the presence of blood clots an 8.5Fr internal–external drainage catheter was used (Figure 28.3b) and the patient was returned to the ward.

Two days later the patient was transferred back to the interventional radiology suite. A cholangiogram confirmed the decompression of the biliary tree and absence of clots (Figure 28.3c). The external drain was exchanged to a 7Fr sheath and a measuring pigtail catheter was inserted over a wire (Figure 28.4a). Contrast injection confirmed the distance from the cystic duct to the duodenum and a 10 × 100mm partially covered self-expandable metallic stent (Nitinella; ELLA-CS, Czech Republic) was deployed in the distal CBD (Figure 28.4b). A 5Fr access catheter was left in situ and the patient was checked two days later. The control cholangiogram confirmed satisfactory expansion of the stent (Figure 28.4c).

**Learning point** Biliary stents in malignant biliary strictures

Biliary stents are used in malignant disease for the palliative treatment of malignant jaundice. Plastic stents were initially used, but were rapidly replaced by self-expandable metallic stents. However, bare metallic stents tend to become occluded as a result of tumour in-growth, and therefore covered metallic stents have been developed and integrated into clinical practice.

**Expert comment**

The type of approach adopted for malignant biliary obstruction mainly depends on local expertise. In the majority of the tertiary care centres with experienced endoscopists and interventional radiologists the endoscopic approach should be tried first, and the percutaneous route will usually follow if the failed endoscopic attempt fails. The percutaneous approach is the first approach for patients with a Roux-en-Y loop or when severe oesophageal stenosis is present.

**Expert comment**

A staged approach with a couple of days interval between each stage may be necessary in some cases, particularly when sepsis or bleeding occurs. If a stent is inserted when blood clots are present it may become occluded; therefore clots should be removed from the bile tree before stent deployment.

**Evidence base** Plastic and metallic stents

A recently published meta-analysis included ten randomized trials and 785 patients, of whom 392 received a metal stent and 393 a plastic stent [4]. The results showed that metal stents were associated with significantly longer stent patency, fewer re-interventions, and longer patient survival times.

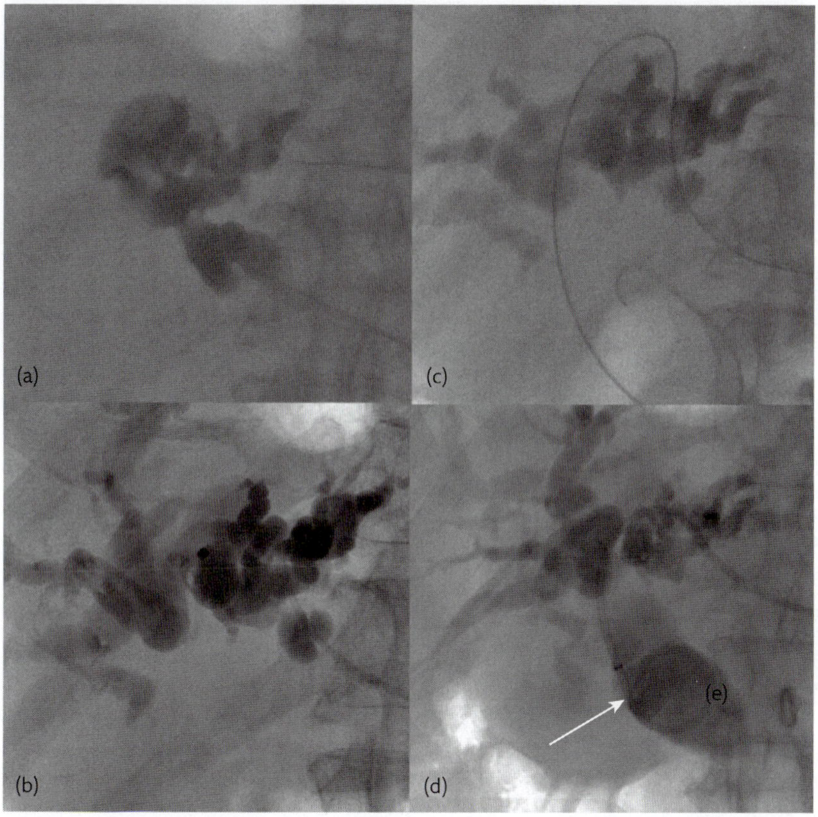


**Figure 28.2** (a) Cholangiogram performed from a left-side puncture confirms biliary duct dilatation. (b) This is followed by opacification of the rest of the biliary tree, and (c) a guidewire is advanced in the CBD. (d) An external drain (arrow) is advanced over the wire in the CBD.

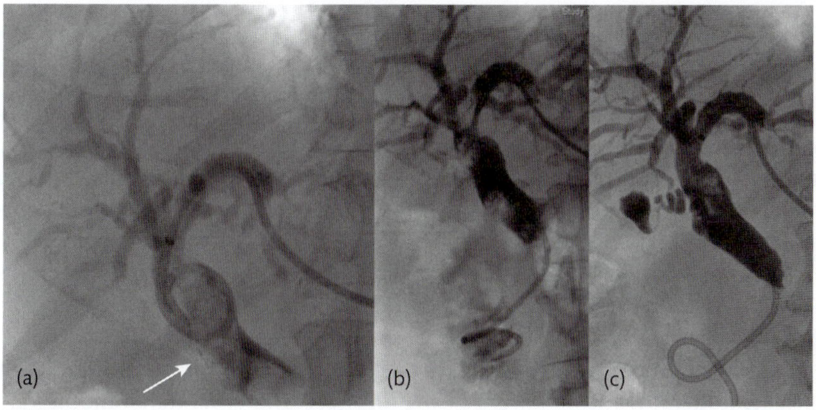


**Figure 28.3** (a) Cholangiogram through the external drain reveals the presence of filling defects due to clotted blood (arrow). (b) The external drain was internalized. (c) Two days later filling defects were significantly reduced.

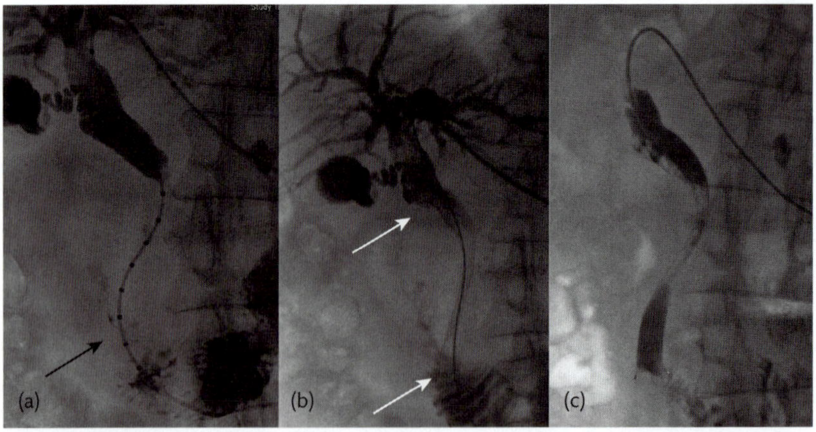


**Figure 28.4** (a) The drain was exchanged for a metric pigtail catheter (black arrow) in order to measure the distance from the cystic duct to the duodenum. (b) A covered stent was deployed in the stenotic area. (c) Cholangiogram obtained two days later confirming satisfactory stent expansion and contrast run-off towards the duodenum.

**Evidence base** Covering material for biliary stents

In attempts to reduce tumour in-growth several covering materials have been tested with various stents:

- Gore-Tex with biliary Gianturco-Rösch Z-stents [5]
- 0.015mm thick polyurethane with Wallstents [6–8]
- 0.015mm thick polyurethane with Strecker stents [9]
- 0.035mm thick polyurethane membrane with Gianturco-Rösch Z-stents and spiral Z-stents [10]
- 0.030mm thick polyurethane membrane with Niti-S stents [11]
- 0.040–0.050mm thick polyurethane with Wallstents [12]
- 0.050–0.060mm polyurethane membrane with diamond stents [13]
- 0.010mm expanded PTFE/FEP with nitinol stents [14–17]

## Discussion

In order to reduce tumour in-growth and re-intervention rate, with the aim of increasing the quality of life of oncological patients, covered stents with a large variety of designs and covering materials have been developed in the last two decades.

In the case described here a stent partially covered with silicone was used as a palliative measure for a patient with pancreatic cancer. The rationale of this approach is to obtain the longest possible patency period and avoid another episode of jaundice during the course of the patient's life that would interrupt chemotherapy and require a new procedure and potentially another stent. This is supported by two prospective randomized comparisons of covered and uncovered biliary stents in patients with pancreatic cancer and cholangiocarcinoma [18,19].

**Evidence base** Prospective multicentre clinical comparison of bare versus covered stents for patients with pancreatic adenocarcinoma and cholangiocarcinoma [18,19]

- Prospective single-arm two-centre studies.
- In the first study [18], 60 patients with Bismuth type I cholangiocarcinoma (36 men and 24 women, age range 46–78 years) were randomized.
- Technical success was 100% for both groups.
- Minor early complications were noticed in 13.3% of the bare-stent group and 10% of the patients of the covered-stent group.
- The mean follow-up period was 212 days (45–675 days). The 30-day mortality was zero for both groups. The median survival time was 180.5 days for the bare-stent group and 243.5 days for the covered-stent group. The mean patency rates were 166 days for the mesh stent and 227.3 days for the covered stent. Stent dysfunction occurred in nine patients in the bare-stent group after a mean period of 133.1 days, and forceps biopsy revealed tumour in-growth in 88.8% of these. Dysfunction also occurred in four patients in the covered-stent group after a mean period of 179.5 days due to tumour overgrowth in two patients and sludge in the other two. Tumour in-growth occurred exclusively in the mesh stent group. A cost analysis showed no difference in the overall costs for the two groups.
- In the second study [19], 80 patients with pancreatic adenocarcinoma (53 men and 27 women with an age range of 41–79 years, mean 62.7 years) were randomized into a bare-stent group and a covered-stent group.
- Technical success was 100% in both groups.
- Early complications were observed in 10% of the bare-stent group and 12.5% of the covered-stent group. Median follow-up time was 192 days (range 104–603 days). The 30-day mortality was zero for both groups. The median survival time was 203.2 days for the bare-stent group and 247 days for the covered-stent group which was not statistically significant. The mean primary patency was 166 days for the uncovered stents and 234 days for the covered stents ($p$ <0 .05). Dysfunction, which was due to tumour in-growth in 91.6% of cases, occurred in 12 patients in the bare-stent group after a mean period of 82.9 days. Dysfunction, occurred in four patients in the covered-stent group after a mean period of 126.5 days and was due to tumour overgrowth in two patients and sludge in the other two. A cost analysis showed no difference in the overall costs for the two groups.

As reported in previous studies [5,6], migration has always been a problem with covered stents. The use of anchoring fins in a partially covered stent with an uncovered portion decreases the rate of distal migration and therefore of dysfunction of the endoprosthesis.

Complications may occur when covered stents are used, particularly when the cystic duct is covered. In the case described here a measuring pigtail catheter was used to measure the exact distance from the cystic duct drainage point to the duodenum in order to avoid coverage of the cystic duct, which may lead to cholecystitis.

Covered stents may be able to prevent ingrowth, but they are unable to prevent overgrowth, i.e. growth of tumour at the proximal end of the stent. In order to prevent overgrowth an uncovered proximal extension can be integrated with the covered stent.

**Expert comment**

In cases of cholangiocarcinoma the cystic duct is probably infiltrated by tumour, and may be covered without problems. Similarly, in cases of pancreatic carcinoma the pancreatic duct can be covered without risk of pancreatitis.

## A final word from the expert

Covered stents are part of the management of patients with malignant biliary disease. However, their use should be restricted to patients where survival will be long enough to obtain a benefit, i.e. more than three months. Anatomical considerations are required in order to avoid obstructing the cystic or intrahepatic ducts, and an uncovered extension should be integrated in the design of future covered stents in order to reduce the rate of overgrowth.

## References


1. McNulty NJ, Francis IR, Platt JF, et al. Multi-detector row helical CT enhancement of the pancreas: effect of contrast-enhanced multiphasic imaging on enhancement of the pancreas, peripancreatic vasculature and pancreatic adenocarcinoma. *Radiology* 2001; 220: 97–102.
2. Tamm EP, Loyer EM, Faria S, et al. Staging of pancreatic cancer with multidetector CT in the setting of preoperative chemoradiation therapy. *Abdom Imaging* 2006; 31: 568–74.
3. Flether JG, Wiersema MJ, Farrell MA, et al. Pancreatic malignancy: value of arterial, pancreatic and hepatic phase imaging with multidetector row CT. *Radiology* 2003; 229: 81–90.
4. Hong WD, Chen XW, Wu WZ, et al. Metal versus plastic stents *for malignant biliary obstruction: an update meta-analysis. Clin Res Hepatol Gastroenterol* 2013; 37(5): 496–500.
5. Saito H, Sakurai Y, Takamura A, Horio K. Biliary endoprosthesis using Gore-Tex covered expandable metallic stents: preliminary clinical evaluation. *Nippon Igaku Hoshasen Gakkai Zasshi* 1994; 54: 180–2.
6. Thurnher SA, Lammer J, Thurnher MM, et L. Covered self-expanding transhepatic biliary stents: clinical pilot study. *Cardiovasc Intervent Radiol* 1996; 19: 10–14.
7. Rossi P, Bezzi M, Salvatori FM, et al. Clinical experience with covered Wallstents for biliary malignancies: 23-month follow-up. *Cardiovasc Intervent Radiol* 1997; 20: 441–7.
8. Hausegger KA, Thurnher S, Bodendorfer G, et al. Treatment of malignant biliary obstruction with polyurethane covered Wallstents. *AJR Am J Roentgenol* 1998; 170(2): 403–8.
9. Kanasaki S, Furukawa A, Kane T, Murata K. Polyurethane-covered nitinol Strecker stents as primary palliative treatment of malignant biliary obstruction. *Cardiovasc Intervent Radiol* 2000; 23: 114–20.
10. Miyayama S, Matsui O, Terayama T, et al. Covered Gianturco stents for malignant biliary obstruction: preliminary clinical evaluation. *J Vasc Interv Radiol* 1997; 8: 641–8.
11. Han YM, Jin GY, Lee S, Kwak HS, Chung GH. flared polyurethane-covered self expandable nitinol stent for malignant biliary obstruction. *J Vasc Interv Radiol* 2003; 14: 1291–1301.
12. Isayama H, Komatsu Y, Tsujino T, et al. Polyurethane-covered metal stent for management of distal malignant biliary obstruction. *Gastrointest Endosc* 2002; 55: 366–70.
13. Isayama H, Komatsu Y, Tsujino T, et al. A prospective randomized study of 'covered' versus 'uncovered' diamond stents for the management of distal malignant biliary obstruction. *Gut* 2004; 53: 729–34.
14. Bezzi M, Zolovkins A, Cantisani V, et al. New ePTFE/FEP-covered stent in the palliative treatment of malignant biliary obstruction. *J Vasc Interv Radiol* 2002; 13: 581–9.
15. Schoder M, Rossi P, Uflacker R, et al. Malignant biliary obstruction: treatment with ePTFE/FEP-covered endoprostheses-initial technical and clinical experiences in a multicenter trial. *Radiology*; 2002; 225: 35–42.
16. Hatzidakis A, Krokidis M, Kalbakis K, et al. ePTFE/FEP-covered metallic stents for palliation of malignant biliary disease: can tumor ingrowth be prevented? *Cardiovasc Intervent Radiol* 2007; 30: 950–8.
17. Fanelli F, Orgera G, Bezzi M, et al. Management of malignant biliary obstruction: technical and clinical results using an expanded polytetrafluoroethylene fluorinated ethylene propylene (ePTFE/FEP)-covered metallic stent after 6-year experience. *Eur Radiol* 2008; 18(5): 911–19.
18. Krokidis M, Fanelli F, Orgera G, et al. Percutaneous treatment of malignant jaundice due to extrahepatic cholangiocarcinoma: covered Viabil stent versus uncovered Wallstents. *Cardiovasc Intervent Radiol* 2010; 33(1): 97–106.
19. Krokidis M, Fanelli F, Orgera G, et al. Percutaneous palliation of pancreatic head cancer: randomized comparison of ePTFE/FEP-covered versus uncovered nitinol biliary stents. *Cardiovasc Intervent Radiol* 2011; 34(2): 352–61.

CASE

# 29 Vertebroplasty of the cervical spine

**Georgia Tsoumakidou**

**Expert commentary** Afshin Gangi

## Case history

A 13-year-old male patient presented with a three-month history of intractable pain in the neck. On clinical examination the patient presented no radiculopathy or neurological deficit. CT imaging revealed the presence of a well-defined expansile osteolytic lesion occupying the C6 vertebral body with cortical rupture towards the left transverse foramen (Figure 29.1a). The sagittal and coronal reformatted images demonstrated a pathologic compression fracture of the vertebral body (Figures 29.1b and 29.1c). There was no extension to the posterior spinal elements, intervertebral disk and paravertebral soft-tissue. The MR imaging confirmed the presence of a cystic lesion with multiple fluid-fluid levels on T2-weighted images and the absence of any solid enhancing elements. The diagnosis of primary aneurysmal spinal bone cyst (ABC) of C6 vertebral body was made.

**Learning point**

As defined by the World Health Organization, an aneurysmal bone cyst (ABC) is a benign tumour-like lesion. It is described as an expansile osteolytic lesion consisting of blood-filled spaces of variable size separated by connective tissue septa containing trabeculae or osteoid tissue and osteoclast giant cells. ABCs may:

- arise de novo (primary ABC)
- be caused by a reaction secondary to another bony lesion (23–32%) such as giant cell tumour, unicameral bone cyst, non-ossifying fibroma, fibrous dysplasia, chondroblastoma, or osteoblastoma (secondary ABC)
- arise in an area of previous trauma [1]

A multidisciplinary team consisting of an interventional radiologist, an oncologist and a spine surgeon decided that the best therapeutic option for the patient was percutaneous vertebroplasty of the ABC. The aim was to consolidate the cystic lesion, stabilize the fracture, and prevent any further vertebral body collapse. The surgical approach (tumour curettage and local spinal fusion) was not considered as the first therapeutic option because of its highly invasive character and associated risks (proximity to neurological and vascular structures).

The patient, accompanied by his parents, visited the treating interventional radiologist prior to the intervention to discuss the procedure, intended benefits, complications, and success rate. Written informed parental consent was waived.

A complete blood count, coagulation profile, and inflammatory marker (C-reactive protein) screen obtained the day before the intervention was normal. A single dose of prophylactic antibiotic cover (cefazolin 1g) was administered intravenously on the day of the intervention. The procedure was performed under general anaesthesia

**Learning point**

Patients with ABC usually present with pain, a mass, or a pathological fracture. Symptoms are usually present for several weeks to months before the diagnosis is made. Pathological fracture occurs in about 8% of ABCs, but the occurrence rate may be as high as 21% in ABCs with spinal involvement.

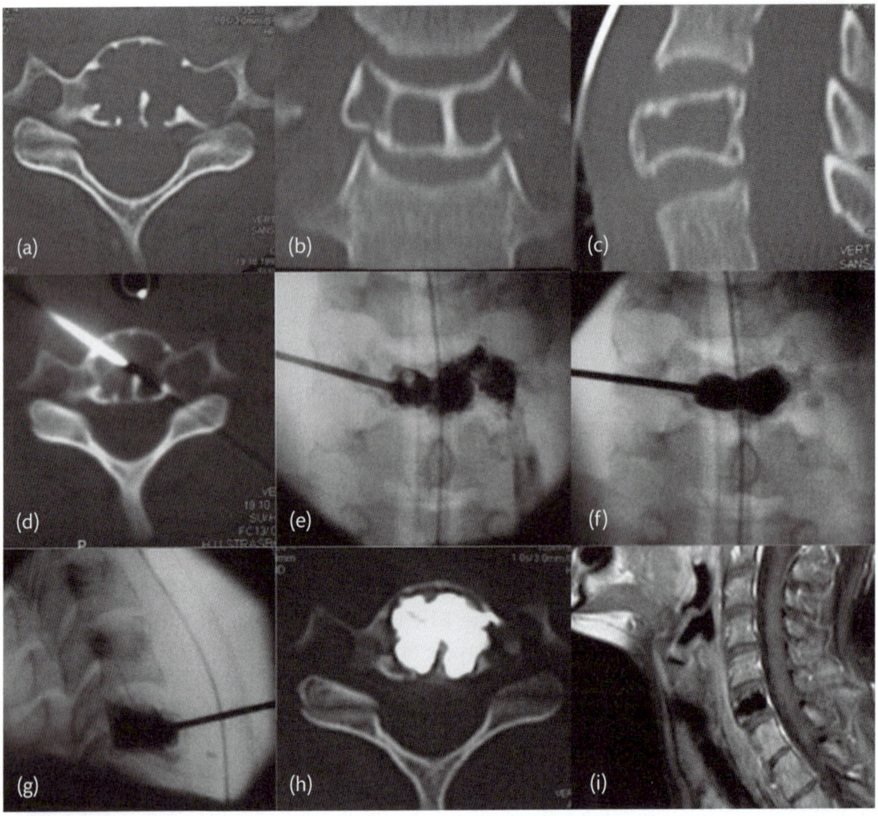


**Figure 29.1** (a) CT imaging showing a well-defined osteolytic lesion occupying the C6 vertebral body with a cortical rupture towards the left transverse foramen. (b,c) Sagittal and coronal reformatted images showing a pathological compression fracture of the vertebral body. (d) A 13G needle was placed on the vertebral body using an anterolateral approach. (e) The phlebogram showed a large drainage into the left internal jugular vein. (f,g,h) The cyst was completely filled with an injection of PMMA cement. (i) The three-year MR follow up shows absence of local recurrence, stability of the cement, and good preservation of the vertebral body height.

administered by the anaesthesiologist with continuous patient monitoring using ECG, pulse oximetry, and blood pressure.

Combined dual CT and fluoroscopic guidance was used. The patient was positioned supine on the CT table while the mobile C-arm was positioned in front of the CT gantry. A cushion was placed under his lower neck and upper thoracic spine to hyper-extend his neck.

After sterile draping, the carotid artery was palpated and the carotid sheath was pulled laterally and posteriorly so that the operator's fingers were in direct contact with the C6 vertebral body (while the carotid pulsations were felt behind the palpating fingers). A 13G needle was inserted just in front of the operator's fingers until bone contact was achieved. The needle trajectory was between the carotid sheath laterally, and the thyroid gland and the oesophagus medially. The needle was tapped into position under anteroposterior and lateral screening using a sterile medical hammer. A bone biopsy was then performed using a coaxial biopsy system (Figure 29.1d).

Once the needle was in position a few millilitres of contrast medium were injected to estimate the venous drainage of the ABC. The phlebogram showed a large drainage into the left internal jugular vein (Figure 29.1e).

**Expert comment**

Either the anterolateral or the posterior transpedicular approach can be used for cervical vertebroplasty below the C2 level. However, if the posterior transpedicular approach is used, the operator should always verify that the cervical pedicles are large enough and special care should be taken to avoid puncturing the vertebral artery

The cement was then prepared. A dedicated injection system with a connecting tube was used. The injection set allowed aspiration and direct injection of cement in a continuous flow, while the connecting tube increased the distance from the radiation source. The cement paste was injected under continuous lateral fluoroscopic control with intermittent anteroposterior screening. The lateral projection allowed early detection of any epidural leaks, while the anteroposterior projection detected any lateral leaks. The cement injection was stopped once the ABC was completely filled, as shown on the intermittent CT control. The stylet of the needle was reinserted under fluoroscopic guidance to inject the 1ml of cement remaining inside the needle lumen. The needle was then removed carefully under imaging to avoid leakage of cement along the pathway (Figures 29.1f,g,h). The patient was not removed from the operating table until the cement remaining in the mixing bowl had set. The total procedure time was 30 minutes.

Neurological evaluation following the procedure focused on the extremities. It was performed in the recovery room directly after the patient recovered from the general anaesthesia and two hours post-procedure. No neurological deficit was observed. A stiff cervical collar was not necessary. The patient was mobilized the same evening and discharged home the next day. He reported complete disappearance of pain immediately after the procedure and remained pain free at six- and twelve-month follow-up. No local recurrence was noted on long-term follow up (Figure 29.1i).

## Discussion

Percutaneous vertebroplasty (PV) is an image-guided therapeutic procedure which involves injection of radio-opaque cement into a painful partially collapsed vertebral body to splint it internally in an effort to relieve pain and provide stability [2,3].

PV was originally described by Galibert et al [4] in 1987 for the treatment of an aggressive vertebral haemangioma. Over the last decade, this technique has evolved to become a standard treatment for vertebral compression fractures (VCFs). Although PV is a fairly safe technique for fractures of the thoracic and lumbar level, it is considered technically challenging in the cervical spine because of the complex anatomy of this region.

Patients with cervical fractures requiring stabilization are usually cancer patients. Treatment options include surgical stabilization with or without associated radiotherapy and the use of external stiff cervical brace. Surgery in such patient populations carries a high risk of infection, a high complication rate and poor bone healing because of poor clinical conditions and the presence of comorbidities. The permanent use of an external brace significantly reduces the patient's quality of life.

**Learning point** Cervical percutaneous vertebroplasty

Indications are similar to those for PV at the lumbar and thoracic levels. Vertebral non-traumatic fractures at the cervical level are more often associated with the presence of a primary (haemangioma, ABC) or secondary (lytic bone metastasis, multiple myeloma) bone tumour [2,3]. Osteoporotic fractures of the cervical spine are rare.

Absolute contraindications include asymptomatic vertebral body tumours without impending fracture, presence of spinal cord compression, presence of osteomyelitis, discitis or active systemic infection, uncorrectable coagulopathy, and allergy to bone cement or opacification agents [2,3].

## Needle placement

The cervical level can be approached using fluoroscopic monitoring with or without CT guidance. In the anteroposterior approach adopted in this case the patient is placed in the supine position. The needle trajectory should be between the carotid sheath laterally and the thyroid gland and oesophagus medially (Figure 29.2).

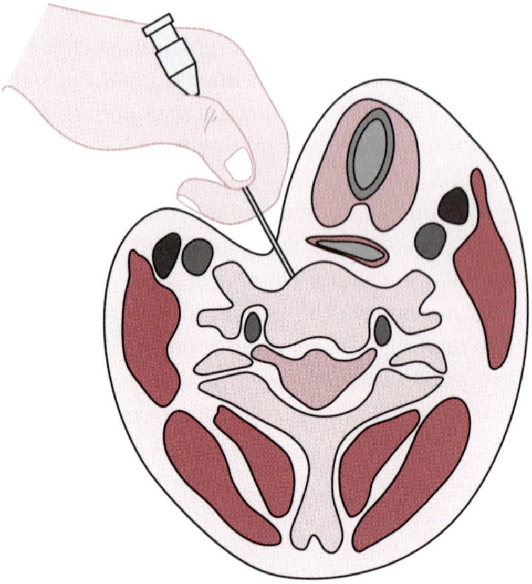

**Figure 29.2** The anterolateral approach can be used for cervical level vertebroplasty (below the C2 level). The operator's hands are placed just internal to the neurovascular sheath. The vessels are pushed laterally and the vertebroplasty needle is positioned in contact with the anterior vertebral wall. The needle trajectory is between the carotid sheath laterally and the thyroid gland and oesophagus medially.

A direct transoral approach should be used for C1 and C2 as this is the most direct route avoiding neural and vascular structures [5,6]. To prevent septic contamination of bone with oral bacteria, the tip of the bone trocar is protected with a thin sterile plastic bag (e.g. an ultrasound sterile probe cover) and the bag is perforated when the needle is in direct contact with the posterior oropharyngeal wall [2,3] (Figure 29.3)

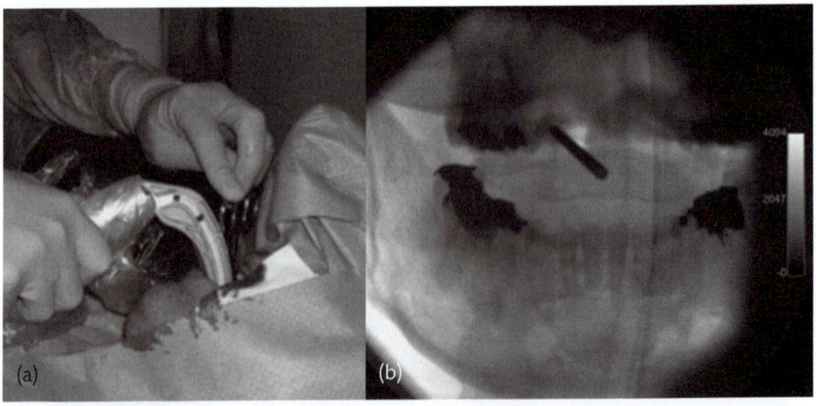


**Figure 29.3** (a,b) Transoral approach used for the C1 and C2 levels.

## Complications

Published data report the occurrence of complications in PV for osteoporotic fractures as <1% and for malignant disease as <10% [11]. Cement leakage is the most frequent complication reported and is usually asymptomatic [12]. Cement leakage rates are higher for malignant disease (incidence range 38–72.5%) than for osteoporotic vertebral fractures (incidence range 30–65%) [13]. Cortical destruction, the presence of a cortical soft tissue mass, highly vascularized lesions, and severe vertebral collapse are likely to increase the rate of complications.

Masala et al [8] report two cases (out of 62 cervical vertebroplasties) of non-symptomatic soft tissue cement leakage, and Guo et al. [7] reported asymptomatic cement leakages in 13% of patients undergoing PV of the upper cervical spine (C1–C3) [7].

Infection, puncture site bleeding, and allergic reaction to the cement are encountered less often [12]. Although post-vertebroplasty infection occurs in less than 1% of patients, strict asepsis should be maintained throughout the procedure.

**Evidence base**

A few data regarding the efficacy of PV at the cervical level have been reported in the literature [7–10]. Masala et al. [8] reported a significant reduction of pain 24 hours post-treatment (mean pre-treatment and 24-hour post-treatment visual analogue scale pain scores were 7.9 ± 1.7 and 1.5 ± 2, respectively) which was preserved at three months follow-up The results of Guo et al. [7] and Anselmetti et al. [1] were similar.

**Expert comment**

Complications reported after PV usually result from poor technique and poor patient selection.

- Injection of cement which is not sufficiently viscous, resulting in venous intravasation and bony extravasation.
- Injection at multiple levels (it is advisable not to treat more than five levels in one session), especially for patients with respiratory insufficiency. The prolonged prone position and possible fat embolism may result in a deterioration of respiratory function.
- Incorrect positioning of the needle tip (e.g. in a basivertebral vein or close to the posterior wall).
- Treatment of highly vascular lesions such as metastases from thyroid and renal cancer.
- Poor fluoroscopic image
- Cement with poor radio-opacity.

## A final word from the expert

The decision to treat patients should be made on a multidisciplinary basis. A detailed clinical examination in conjunction with the imaging findings must be carried out to determine the level(s) to be treated and rule out other causes of pain and neurological compromise. Cervical level vertebroplasty is more demanding than thoracic and lumbar level vertebroplasty, and should be performed by experienced operators.

## References


1. Martinez V, Sissons HA. Aneurysmal bone cyst: a review of 123 cases including primary lesions and those secondary to other bone pathology. *Cancer* 1988; 61: 2291–304
2. Gangi A, Guth S, Imbert JP, et al. Percutaneous vertebroplasty: history, technique and current perspectives. *Radiographics* 2003; 23: e10.
3. Gangi A, Sabharwal T, Irani F, et al. Quality assurance guidelines for percutaneous vertebroplasty. *Cardiovasc Intervent Radiol* 2006; 29: 173–8.
4. Galibert P, Deramond H, Rosat P, Le Gars D. [Preliminary note on the treatment of vertebral angioma by percutaneous acrylic vertebroplasty]. *Neurochirurgie* 1987; 33: 166–8 (in French).

5. Sachs DC, Inamasu J, Mendel EE, Guiot BH. Transoral vertebroplasty for renal cell metastasis involving the axis. *Spine (Phila Pa 1976)* 2006; 31: E925–8.
6. Martin JB, Gailloud P, Dietrich PY, et al. Direct transoral approach to C2 for percutaneous vertebroplasty. *AJNR Am J Neuroradiol* 2002; 23: 1619–20.
7. Guo WH, Meng MB, You X, et al. CT-guided percutaneous vertebroplasty of the upper cervical spine via a translateral approach. *Pain Physician* 2012; 15: E733–41.
8. Masala S, Anselmetti GC, Muto M, et al. Percutaneous vertebroplasty relieves pain in metastatic cervical fractures. *Clin Orthop Relat Res* 2011; 469: 715–22.
9. Zhang J, Hou M, Fei Z, et al. Clinical observation about percutaneous vertebroplasty for osteolytic metastatic carcinoma of cervical vertebra. *Zhongguo Xiu Fu Chong Jian Wai Ke Za Zhi* 2009; 23: 194–7.
10. Anselmetti GC, Manca A, Montemurro F, et al. Vertebroplasty using transoral approach in painful malignant involvement of the second cervical vertebra (C2): a single-institution series of 25 patients. *Pain Physician* 2012; 15: 35–42.
11. McGraw JK, Cardella J, Barr JD, et al. Society of Interventional Radiology quality improvement guidelines for percutaneous vertebroplasty. *J Vasc Interv Radiol* 2003; 14: S311–15.
12. Nussbaum DA, Gailloud P, Murphy K. A review of complications associated with vertebroplasty and kyphoplasty as reported to the Food and Drug Administration medical related web site. *J Vasc Interv Radiol* 2004; 15: 1185–92.
13. Laredo JD, Hamze B. Complications of percutaneous vertebroplasty and their prevention. *Skeletal Radiol* 2004; 33: 493–505.

CASE

# 30 Percutaneous neurolytic coeliac plexus block

**Angie Galea and Richard Guinness**

**Expert commentary** Anthony Watkinson

## Case history

A 53-year-old man was admitted to a medical ward with a history of weight loss, pruritus, and diarrhoea. On direct questioning he admitted to steatorrhea and dark urine. On examination there was a mass in the right upper quadrant. An ultrasound of his abdomen revealed a mass in the pancreatic head and a dilated common bile duct measuring 12mm down to the level of the pancreatic head. His CT demonstrated a poorly defined low-density lesion of diameter 19mm within the head of the pancreas. His liver function tests revealed an obstructive picture.

The patient underwent ERCP (endoscopic retrograde cholangiopancreatography), brushings were taken, and a plastic stent was inserted to relieve the obstruction. There was no evidence of malignancy on the brushings and pre-operative radiology suggested an operable tumour. At laparotomy there was a peri-ampullary mass that appeared to be infiltrating the portal vein which, if malignant, indicated inoperability. Therefore a palliative hepaticojejunostomy was performed. His post-operative recovery was uneventful and he was discharged home.

The patient returned four weeks later with increased epigastric pain, particularly after eating, as well as weight loss. He was on paracetamol 1g four times daily, tramadol 50mg four times daily, and amitriptyline 25mg daily. A CT scan showed a static appearance of the presumed pancreatic malignancy, but there was a new metastasis in the right lobe of the liver. Given the CT evidence of progression and the increasing need for analgesics the patient was offered a CT-guided coeliac plexus neurolysis.

Written consent was obtained and the patient was placed on continuous ECG, blood pressure, and oxygen saturation monitoring. He was encouraged to open his bowels just before the procedure. An IV cannula was inserted, and midazolam 2ml and fentanyl 50ml were administered intravenously. Further IV analgesia was titrated during the procedure. Entonox was set up and prepared for use later on in the procedure. The patient was positioned in a prone position and five parallel needles were taped to the skin at the level of T12–L2.

Five-millimetre CT scout images were acquired in held expiration with an angled gantry through the region of interest (Figure 30.1). The coeliac plexus was identified and the level was marked on the skin. Ten millilitres of 1% lidocaine was administered subcutaneously.

**Clinical tip**

Intense pain during alcohol injection stimulates sympathetic nerves that have both an inhibitory and an excitatory effect on the anal sphincter. This may lead to inappropriate relaxation of the sphincter and very rarely incontinence [1].

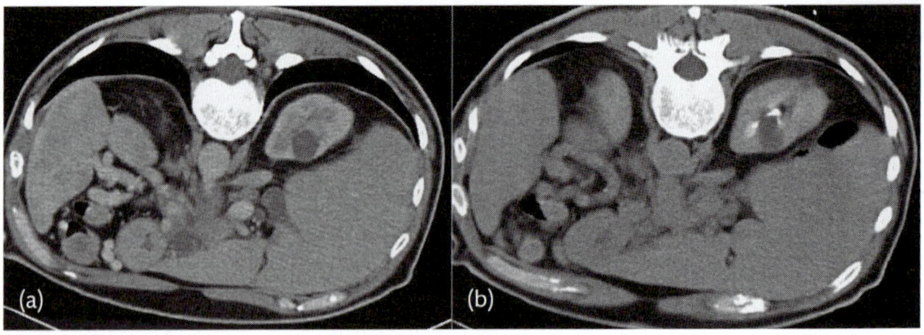


**Figure 30.1** (a) Image from a CT scan at the level of the coeliac artery acquired with a straight gantry. (b) Image at the same level obtained with an angled gantry. Note that the postero-inferior pleura can be avoided when this technique is used.

**Expert comment**

Avoid traversing the pleura with the needle as the injected alcohol can travel back along the track and cause intense pleuritic pain. Note that the inferior border of the pleura is curved so that the posterior pleura is at a lower level than the anterior border of the pleura. Therefore by angling the gantry by 5°–10° away from the patient's head (with the patient prone) you can avoid traversing the pleura and decrease the incidence of pleuritic pain post-procedure as well as the risk of pneumothorax.

Another valuable method of preventing pneumothorax is hydrodissection. Injecting 0.9% saline solution into the paravertebral extrapleural fat often creates a space wide enough for safe passage of the needle, thus avoiding transgression of the pleura.

Single CT slices were acquired by the radiologist whilst in the room using a foot pedal with a stop-and-shoot set-up (Figure 30.2). A safe needle route was planned avoiding the ribs, pleura, transverse processes, and renal cortex. A 15cm 20G Chiba needle (Cook, Bloomington, IN)was advanced into the left retrocrural space at a

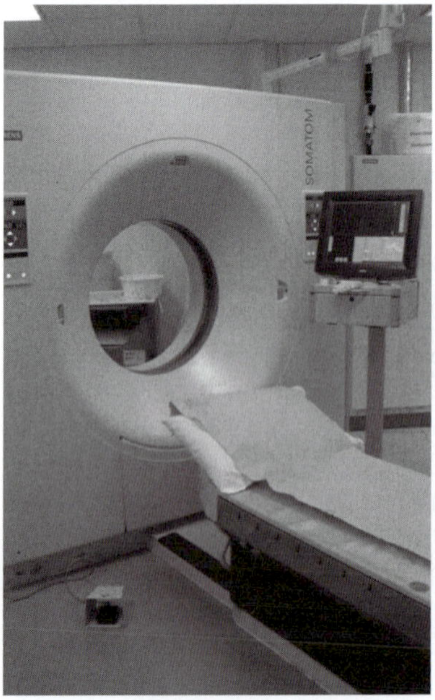


**Figure 30.2** CT suite showing the set-up of foot pedal and screen. The stop-and-shoot mechanism acquires two images 5mm apart that allow to assessment and correction of the needle-tip position

level between the coeliac axis and the superior mesenteric artery. A syringe was attached to the needle and negative pressure was applied to ensure that the tip was not in a blood vessel. The patient was warned that the alcohol injection was about to commence and a further 50ml of fentanyl IV was administered. The patient was asked to inhale some Entonox gas and, during held expiration, a mixture of 20ml absolute alcohol and 1ml iodinated contrast was injected without resistance into the retrocrural space (Figure 30.3). Correct placement of the needle tip was confirmed by observing the iodinated contrast material tracking over the anterior 180° of the aorta (Figure 30.4).

The procedure was repeated using a right retrocrural approach. There were no immediate complications and the patient was returned to the ward. He made an uneventful recovery and was discharged home.

**Expert comment**

Where possible, use a foot pedal in the CT suite in a similar set-up to the one shown in the image. This speeds up the procedure, resulting in better accuracy as the patient is less likely to move.

**Expert comment**

The alcohol injection is extremely painful and proper education pre-procedure is important. The patient should be fully analgized prior to injection, with Entonox used for breakthrough pain. Deep inspiration can lead to needle displacement, which usually leads to slight withdrawal of the needle rather than needle advancement".

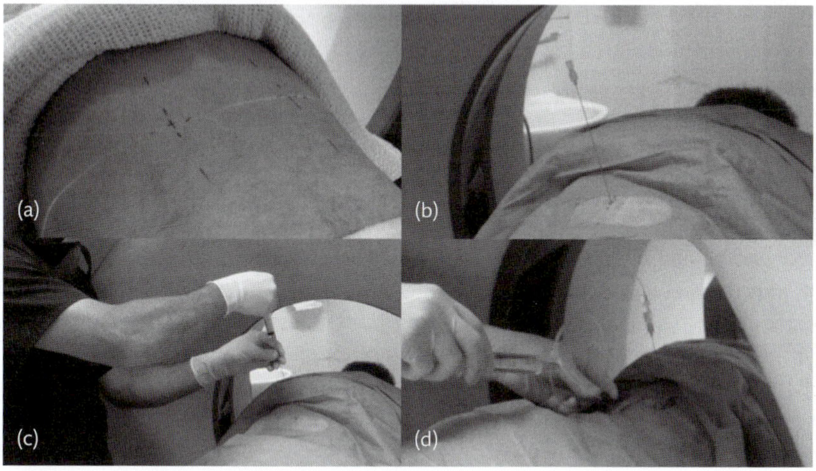


**Figure 30.3** (a) The CT laser is used to mark the level of entry, and needles (not shown here) are attached to the skin to mark the distance from the midline. Marking is performed in held expiration. (b) The Chiba needle is inserted into the retrocrural space using CT guidance. (c) The needle is inserted under aspiration to ensure that the needle tip is not intravascular. Correct needle placement is of paramount importance. (d) The solution of alcohol and contrast is injected.

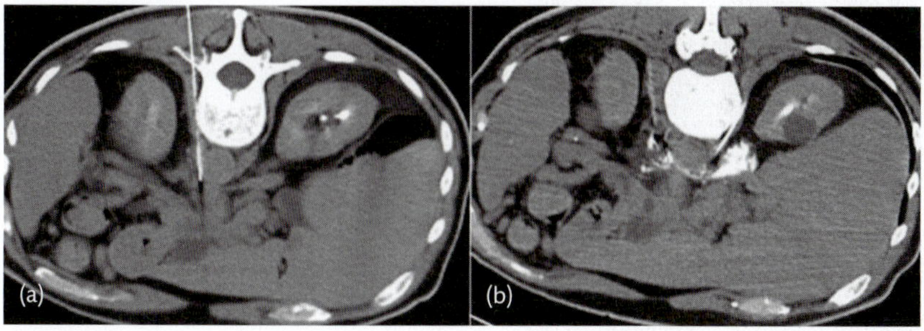


**Figure 30.4** (a) The needle is advanced into position with the tip lying just lateral to the aorta. (b) Right retrocrural approach: note that the iodinated contrast has coated the anterior aspect of the aorta, although, on the right, there is some spill into the retroperitoneal space, which is not ideal.

**Expert comment** Single versus bilateral injection techniques

If the initial injection (usually left) achieves 180° coverage around the anterior half of the aorta, a right-sided puncture is not necessary. If the needle tip is placed in the perivascular plane, good coverage can be achieved with one injection.

Post-procedure the patient reported a marked decrease in pain, a decrease in opiate use, and an improvement in his quality of life. This improvement persisted until his death four months later.

## Discussion

Coeliac plexus neurolysis is a palliative technique that has generally been used to control pain secondary to pancreatic cancer. Other indications that have been treated effectively with a coeliac plexus block include chronic pancreatitis, gastric cancer, oesophageal cancer, and colorectal cancer [2]

**Learning point**

The coeliac plexus is a network of presynaptic sympathetic nerve fibres derived from the greater (T5–T9), lesser (T10–T11), and least (T12) splanchnic nerves. The right ganglia are, on average, 0.6cm caudal to the coeliac artery, while the left are 0.9cm caudal to the coeliac artery [3]. On axial CT images the right and left ganglia demonstrate a multilobulated configuration that resembles the limbs of the adrenal gland. The coeliac plexus supplies the sympathetic and visceral sensory afferent fibres to the foregut structures. Pancreatic pain is mediated by sympathetic visceral fibres relaying via the coeliac plexus to the splanchnic nerves.

Coeliac plexus neurolysis does not completely abolish pain; rather, it decreases pain and reduces opoid requirements and their related side effects [2]. The alcohol interrupts the pain pathway by extracting the cholesterol and phospholipids from neural cell membranes and precipitating lipoproteins and mucoproteins [4].

Pain at the time of alcohol injection is inevitable, and posterior abdominal pain post-procedure has been reported in up to 96% of patients [3}. If the pleura is transgressed, pleuritic and shoulder pain which can persist for up to 72 hours after the procedure may be reported [4].

**Evidence base**

**Efficacy**

Methods of assessment of pain relief are varied, making analysis of the literature difficult, if not impossible. The results of a meta-analysis evaluating 21 retrospective studies in 1145 patients concluded that adequate to excellent pain relief is achieved in 90% of patients at two weeks and three months [2]. In a prospective randomized study, Ischia et al. [5] evaluated pain relief in 61 patients with pancreatic cancer pain; 29 (48%) experienced complete pain relief after the neurolytic block. In another prospective multicentre study on 22 patients who were followed until death, a significant reduction in pain, opioid use, and gastrointestinal side effects was obtained for at least four weeks [6]. The efficacy reported in earlier studies is summarized in Table 30.1.

**Neurolysis versus conservative therapy**

In a randomized controlled study (RCT) comparing neurolysis with opioids alone, Wong et al. [7] showed a significant reduction in pain relief post-neurolysis, but failed to demonstrate a statistical difference in quality of life or survival. Similarly, in another RCT comparing patients treated with coeliac plexus block or videothorascopic splanchnicectomy versus systemic analgesic therapy, neurolysis provided superior pain relief and quality of life scores, but differences between the two groups in overall opioid consumption, frequency of opioid adverse effects, and overall survival did not reach statistical significance [8].

**Table 30.1 Efficacy of coeliac axis neurolysis for pain relief in patients with pancreatic cancer**

| Reference | No. of patients | Type of study | Pain relief (%) |
|---|---|---|---|
| Bridenbaugh et al. 1964 [9] | 25 | RO | 88 |
| Black et al. 1973 [10] | 18 | RO | 70 |
| Hegedüs 1979 [11] | 38 | RO | 44 |
| Leung et al. 1983[12] | 13 | RO | 85 |
| Orwitz 1983 [13] | 80 | RO | 85 |
| Ischia et al. 1992 [5] | 20 | RCT | 60 |

RO, retrospective observational; RCT, randomized controlled trial.

**Learning point**

The artery of Adamkiewicz supplies blood to the anterior spinal artery and is recognized by its characteristic hairpin bend. It has a variable origin, and a review of 544 cases showed that is more likely to arise from a left intercostal artery (up to 83.3%) and can arise anywhere between T7 and L3 [18]. The anterior spinal artery supplies the anterior spinal cord and courses along the anterior aspect of the spinal cord.

**Evidence base**

**Duration of pain relief**

Pain relief is quoted to last from a month and a year because nerve routes may regenerate after a year [14]. A meta-analysis of the literature looking at pain relief at the time of death was presented for 53 patients in six studies [2]. This merged data indicated that 73% and 92% had partial or complete relief, respectively, within three months of their demise. In another RCT, pain relief until death was achieved in 60–75% of patients [5].

**Survival benefit**

The literature data are controversial. In a study by Staats et al. [15] neurolysis, compared with medical management alone, not only reduced pain, elevated mood, and reduced interference of pain with activity, but was also associated with an increase in life expectancy. Furthermore, in a group of 34 patients with pain before laparotomy, survival was improved in those receiving chemical splanchnicectomy [16]. However, as already noted, two RCTs showed no statistical survival benefit [7,8].

**Complications**

The incidence of complications reported in the literature differs depending on the approach used: 30–50% of patients experience hypotension after coeliac plexus block due to splanchnic vasodilatation and loss of sympathetic tone; 25–60% of patients report diarrhoea due to loss of sympathetic tone which may last for up to two days [5,17]. Neurological complications, including paraplegia, have been reported in <1% and are attributed to direct injection of the alcohol into either the artery of Adamkiewicz or another feeder artery, or spasm and thrombosis of a feeder artery due to the presence of the agent external to the vessel [17].

**Learning point**

Coeliac plexus neurolysis guided by endoscopic ultrasound (EUS) was introduced by Wiersema and Wiersma in 1996 [19]. This approach is reported to have a lower rate of neurological complications as the endoscopic route targets the coeliac plexus from an anterior approach. However, it requires advanced operator skill, particularly when injecting the neurolytic solution, as all the anatomy is obscured and distorted following injection.

Recent reports of identification of the coeliac ganglia with EUS raise the possibility of directly targeting the coeliac ganglia in the near future [20]. One can assume that direct targeting will be superior to current techniques and much smaller injection volumes will be needed. Furthermore, dedicated radiofrequency ablation of the coeliac ganglia may be worth exploration given the recent success of ablation for renal denervation [21].

## References

1. Carlstedt A, Nordgren S, Fasth S, et al. Sympathetic nervous influence on the internal anal sphincter and rectum in man. *Int J Colorectal Dis* 1988; 3(2): 90–5.
2. Eisenberg E, Carr DB, Chalmers TC. Neurolytic celiac plexus block for treatment: a meta-analysis. *Anesth Analg* 1995; 80: 290–5.
3. Romanelli DF, Beckmann CF, Heiss W. Celiac safety plexus block: efficacy and of the anterior approach. *AJR Am J Roentgenol* 1993; 160(3): 497–500

4. Fugère F, Lewis G. Coeliac plexus block for chronic pain syndromes. *Can J Anaesth* 1993; 40: 954–63.
5. Ischia S, Ischia A, Polati E, Finco G. Three posterior percutaneous celiac plexus block techniques: a prospective, randomized study in 61 patients with pancreatic cancer pain. *Anesthesiology* 1992; 76: 534–40.
6. Mercadante S, Catala E, Arcuri E, Casuccio A. Celiac plexus block for pancreatic cancer pain: factors influencing pain, symptoms and quality of life. *J Pain Symptom Manage* 2003; 26(6): 1140–7.
7. Wong GY, Schroeder DR, Carns PE, et al. Effect of neurolytic celiac plexus block on pain relief, quality of life, and survival in patients with unresectable pancreatic cancer: a randomized controlled trial. *JAMA* 2004; 291(9): 1092–9.
8. Stefaniak T, Basinski A, Vingerhoets A, et al. A comparison of two invasive techniques in the management of intractable pain due to inoperable pancreatic cancer: neurolytic celiac plexus block and videothoracoscopic splanchnicectomy. *Eur J Surg Oncol* 2005; 31(7): 768–73.
9. Bridenbaugh LD, Moore DC, Campbell DD. Management of upper abdominal cancer pain. *JAMA* 1964; 190(10): 877–80.
10. Black A, Dwyer B. Coeliac plexus block. *Anaesth Intensive Care* 1973; 1(4): 315–18.
11. Hegedüs V. Relief of pancreatic pain by radiography-guided block. *AJR Am J Roentgenol* 1979; 133(6): 1101–3.
12. Leung JWC, Bowen-Wright M, Aveling W, et al. Coeliac plexus block for pain in pancreatic cancer and chronic pancreatitis. *Br J Surg* 1983; 70(12): 730–2.
13. Orwitz S KS. Celiac plexus block: an overview. *Mt Sinai J Med* 1983; 50: 486–90.
14. Giménez A, Martínez-Noguera A, Donoso L, et al. Percutaneous neurolysis of the celiac plexus via the anterior approach with sonographic guidance. *AJR Am J Roentgenol* 1993; 161(5): 1061–3.
15. Staats P, Hekmat H, Sauter P. Lillemoe K. The effects of alcohol celiac plexus block, pain, and mood on longevity in patients with unresectable pancreatic cancer: a double- blind, randomized, placebo-controlled study. *Pain Med* 2001; 2(1): 28–34.
16. Lillemoe KD, Cameron JL, Kaufman HS, et al. Chemical splanchnicectomy in patients with unresectable pancreatic cancer: a prospective randomized trial. *Ann Surg* 1993;217(5):447–55; discussion 456–7.
17. Davies DD. Incidence of major complications of neurolytic coeliac plexus block. *J R Soc Med* 1993; 86(5): 264–6.
18. Melissano G, Bertoglio L, Civelli V, et al. Demonstration of the Adamkiewicz artery by multidetector computed tomography angiography analysed with the open-source software OsiriX. *Eur J Vasc Endovasc Surg* 2009; 37(4): 395–400.
19. Wiersema MJ, Wiersema LM. Endosonography-guided celiac plexus neurolysis. *Gastrointest Endosc* 1996; 44(6): 656–62.
20. Levy MJ. New approaches, including targeting the ganglia. *Gastrointest Endosc* 2009; 69(2 Suppl): S166–71.
21. Penman ID. Coeliac plexus neurolysis: best practice and research. *Clin Gastroenterol* 2009; 23(5): 761–6.

CASE

# 31 Vertebral augmentation techniques and pain management: is there a role in metastatic disease?

**Gianluigi Orgera and Miltiadis Krokidis**

**Expert commentary** Michele Rossi

## Case history

A 64-year-old female with history of papillary thyroid carcinoma returned to the hospital because of pain in the lumbar region for two weeks that had become unbearable and was not controlled by oral anti-inflammatory agents. Her visual analogue score (VAS) for pain was >7 at the time of admission.

The primary thyroid cancer had been treated three years previously by total thyroidectomy; histology revealed a well-differentiated follicular type with lymph node involvement. Post-surgical radiotherapy was performed with 100mCi of iodine-131 every 3–9 months during the first two years and then once a year. Thyroxine treatment at suppressive doses was given between radiotherapy treatments.

A CT scan was performed and revealed a lytic lesion in the left anterior portion of the body of the L2 vertebra. The lesion was partially eroding the cortex but there was no epidural compression (Figure 31.1). Treatment with non-steroidal anti-inflammatory drugs, steroids, and opioids in combination with physiotherapy did not appear to offer satisfactory pain control for the patient, and therefore it was decided to treat her with percutaneous vertebral augmentation.

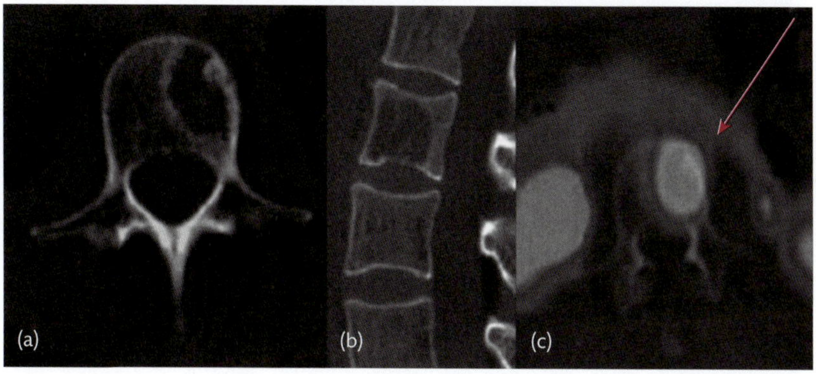


**Figure 31.1** (a) Axial and (b) sagittal reconstruction of the CT scan obtained before treatment showing a large osteolytic lesion at L2. (c) PET–CT scan shows high metabolic activity ($SUV_{max}$ = 15.50) before treatment.

**Evidence base**

The treatment of spinal metastases is extremely challenging because of the frequent severe pain that is the predominant symptom. This can be of three types: constant localized pain, radicular pain, and axial pain. Traditional pain management techniques involve a combination of pharmacology, radiotherapy, and surgical procedures. Axial pain is frequently associated with pathological vertebral body fracture and spinal instability secondary to destruction of its posterior portion. The standard options for management in these patients are medical therapy or surgical intervention [5].

**Learning point**

Following clinical assessment, a treatment strategy should be planned with the primary aim of providing palliative relief of symptoms, reducing analgesic adjuvant therapy and its side effects. The type, location, and extent of spinal metastases determine the optimal method of symptomatic management. Although metastases appear more frequently in the lumbar spinal region, thoracic metastases are generally more symptomatic because of the smaller calibre of the spinal canal in this area. Approximately 98% of spinal metastases are extradural, and 80% of these involve the posterior spinal elements (vertebral body and pedicles), often leading to instability, deformity, and pain [1,2].

Metastatic cancer is the most common tumour of the spine in about 10–30% of all cancer patients, with the most frequent primary sites being breast, lung, and prostate. Patients with spinal metastases have a median survival of 10 months, and effective palliation of symptoms is the principal clinical objective. Distant metastases, usually to the skeleton or lungs, occur in up to 20% of cases of primary thyroid carcinoma, and they represent the most frequent cause of thyroid-cancer-related death [3]. However, spinal metastases from thyroid cancer have the most favuorable prognosis of all tumours metastasizing to the spine [4].

**Learning point**

As the majority of these patients have a poor prognosis despite medium to long life expectancies, the aim of treatment is rapid symptomatic relief with consequent improvement in the quality of life. Conservative medical therapy may be ineffective, with inadequate pain relief because of insensitivity to ionizing radiation, resistance to chemotherapeutic agents, and tolerance to analgesic drugs. Inadequate pain relief may lead to immobility, which in turn increases the risk of venous thromboembolism, pressure sores, secondary respiratory problems, and depression [6].

**Evidence base** Is surgery an option?

Surgical spinal procedures are highly invasive and are generally unsuitable in this group of patients because of the high risk of complications and often the short life expectancy of this patient group. It is in this setting that recent technological advances combined with innovative interventional radiology techniques can now offer alternative less invasive treatment options for many patients with malignant vertebral body infiltration. Percutaneous vertebral augmentation procedures such as vertebroplasty, kyphoplasty, and skyphoplasty offer an attractive alternative with less soft tissue trauma, less blood loss, and the use of local anaesthesia, resulting in lower morbidity and mortality when compared with open spinal surgery.

**Learning point**

When selecting patients, a multidisciplinary approach is essential with input from the radiologist, spinal surgeon, and referring clinical specialist.

- Indications for percutaneous vertebral augmentation in patients with spinal metastases:
    - painful vertebral compression fracture or imminent vertebral compression fracture causing significant disability [6]
    - intense intractable pain t adjacent to vertebrae that have been diagnosed as fractured or osteolytic by recent imaging [7].
- Not indicated in:
    - asymptomatic vertebral compression fracture
    - pain that is responding to medical therapy.
- Absolutely contraindicated in:
    - local or systemic infection
    - uncorrectable coagulopathy
    - allergy to bone cement
    - tumour causing spinal cord compression.
- Relatively contraindicated in: [6,8,9]
    - lack of orthopaedic and neurosurgical support
    - complete or >70% vertebral collapse (as it is difficult to enter the vertebra)
    - patients with five or more metastases
    - vertebral fractures with posterior column involvement which increases the risk of cement extravasation
    - nerve root pain and/or radicular pain that is more severe than the axial pain (these patients often need adjunctive treatment with percutaneous vertebral augmentation and nerve root blocks to fully treat local pain).

The therapeutic strategy adopted was also based on the fact that the patient was unsuitable for surgery. A consensus for a combination of vertebroplasty and radiofrequency ablation (RFA) was obtained from the multidisciplinary team. The decision was based on the fact that there was no significant spinal cord compression or spinal instability.

After informed consent had been obtained, the vertebroplasty procedure was carried out in a daycase setting under local anaesthesia with 1% lidocaine combined with conscious sedation using midazolam 4mg and fentanyl 100µg). Clindamycin 600mg and Decadron 6mg were administered intravenously preoperatively. The procedure was performed in the prone position using CT-fluoroscopic guidance through a right transpedicular route. A 10G vertebroplasty needle was first advanced into the L2 body and then an 18G starburst array RFA needle was advanced coaxially. The lesion was ablated at 150W and a temperature of 100°C for five minutes. Following the ablation, PMMA cement mixed with barium (CementoRe set; Optimed, Ettlingen, Germany) was instilled under close imaging guidance until the anterior two-thirds of the vertebral body was filled and homogeneously distributed (Figure 31.2). After the procedure, the patient remained prone for 20 minutes to allow the cement to fully harden. There were no complications. A CT scan obtained immediately after the procedure demonstrated appropriate distribution of the cement (Figure 31.3a).

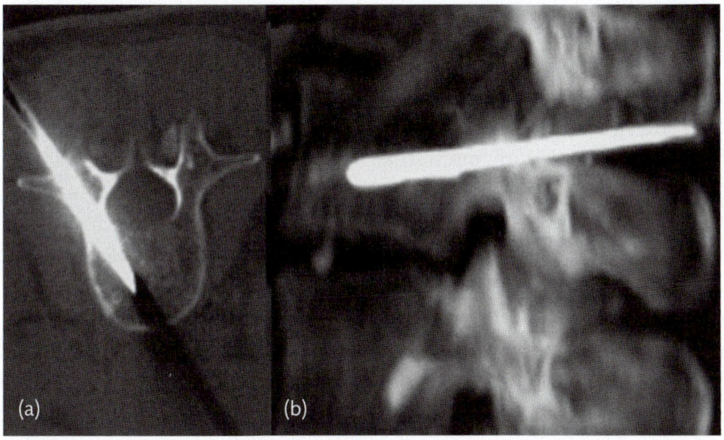


**Figure 31.2** Percutaneous vertebroplasty was performed under CT fluoroscopy immediately after thermal ablation via a transpedicular approach, (a) transverse and (b) sagital view of the needle.

Immediately after the procedure, the patient reported that her excruciating back pain had significantly improved, and the neurological evaluation reported that the VAS had dropped to 2.5. The patient was given seven-day cover with solumedrol and discharged home three hours after the procedure without any complaints. She continued to have radiometabolic therapy and the PET–CT was negative at one month (Figure 31.3b).

The procedure was defined as clinically successful with significant reduction of pain as demonstrated by the VAS score and the significant decrease in the amount of analgesia administered in the following weeks. At three months follow-up, the patient continued to report excellent pain control and resumed her normal daily activities.

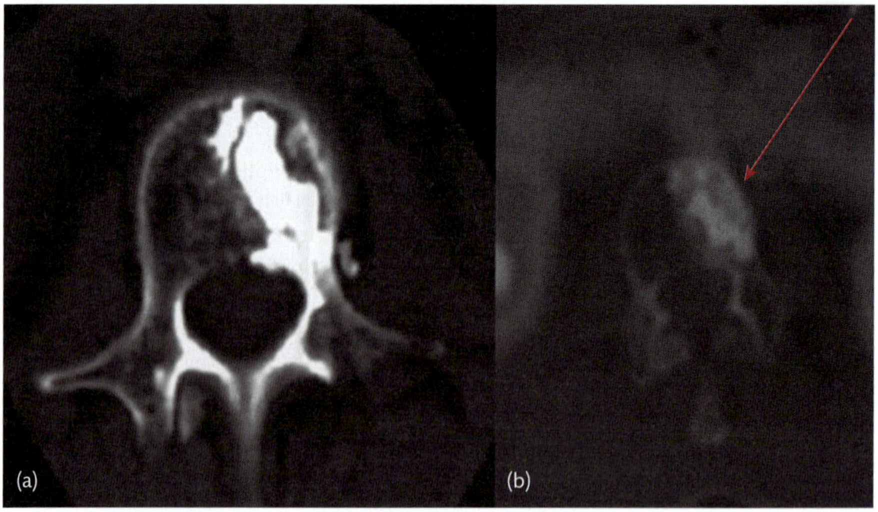

**Figure 31.3** (a) Control scan obtained immediately after the procedure shows a very good result, with a homogeneous filling of PMMA within the vertebral body without local complications. (b) PET–CT shows a consistent reduction of metabolic activity ($SUV_{max}$ = 3.00) at one month.

## Discussion

Percutaneous vertebral augmentation procedures were introduced 25 years ago by Harrington [10] in an intra-operative setting where 14 patients with metastatic spinal instability were treated with methylmethacrylate for anterior stabilization of the spine. Galibert et al. [11] wwre the first to describe the use of percutaneous acrylic cement injection for the treatment of an aggressive vertebral body haemangioma.

Currently, three vertebral augmentation procedures are licensed for clinical use: vertebroplasty, kyphoplasty, and skyphoplasty. Each of these requires a similar pre-procedural workup. Kyphoplasty provides restoration of vertebral body height with similar rates of analgesia to vertebroplasty, reducing the rate of cement leakage. However, it costs five to ten times times as much as vertebroplasty because of the equipment used and the requirement for general anaesthesia [7]. These two procedures provide similar pain control, so it is difficult to recommend kyphoplasty over vertebroplasty as the procedure of choice even if significant kyphosis is present. Skyphoplasty is the newest tool in the armamentarium of percutaneous vertebral augmentation procedures. It uses a stiff plastic tube that is deployed through a cannula and squashed into a popcorn-like shape to create the vertebral body cavity which is then filled with cement. The skyphoplasty device creates more pressure in a more predictable way than kyphoplasty. Another innovation is stentoplasty which uses a metallic stent as a scaffold that remains in situ after balloon deployment.

> **Learning point** Types of approach for percutaneous vertebral augmentation procedures
>
> A transpedicular approach is often used in the lumbar territory because of the broad-based pedicles. Costopedicular or paravertebral approaches are usually employed in the thoracic region as the pedicles have a narrow needle entry point. These approaches are also used in situations where there is significant tumour destruction of the pedicles.

Thermal ablation (RFA, microwave ablation, etc.) of spinal metastases can be carried out at the same time as percutaneous vertebral augmentation, with the two procedures acting synergistically to provide significant analgesia and increased vertebral stabilization within 24 hours of the procedure. There is also some evidence demonstrating that if RFA is carried out before percutaneous vertebral augmentation, the risk of cement extravasation is reduced [12]. Theories of its mechanism of action include destruction of sensory nerve fibres, reduction of the lesion size, and destruction of tumour cells producing nerve-stimulating factors. These combined procedures can give a patient stable and painless vertebra within 24 hours of admission with an unstable vertebra [13]. Cumulative analyses of literature data demonstrate that these patients have a significant reduction in pain, with minimal procedure-related morbidity, thus improving mobility, response to physiotherapy, and quality of life with minimal interference with adjuvant therapies and a reduction in analgesic-related side effects [14,15].

**Evidence base** Results and complications of percutaneous vertebroplasty from a multicentre trial—the European VErtebroplasty RESearch Team (EVEREST) [16]

- 4547 patients (3211 females and 1336 males, mean age 70.2 years).
- Percutaneous vertebroplasty (PV).
- 13,437 treated vertebrae.
- Procedures were performed using fluoroscopic guidance or combined CT-fluoroscopic guidance.
- 4004 out of 4547 (88.0%) patients reported significant pain relief within 48 hours.
- An average score of 8.3 ± 0.4 on the 11-point VAS dropped to 2.4 ± 0.4 in patients with metastatic disease.
- 430 osteoporotic patients (13%) were re-treated for a subsequent fracture.
- In 302 out of 430 patients (70.2%) a new fracture occurred in the contiguous vertebra.
- No major neurological complications were reported and the most frequent minor complication was venous leakage (20.5%).

## A final word from the expert

Vertebral metastatic disease has a huge negative impact on patient quality of life and survival. Palliative treatments (medical or radiotherapeutic and/or radiometabolic) are first-line treatments in diffuse disease. In vertebral metastases from thyroid cancer, a radical therapeutic attitude should be considered if clinically and technically indicated because of the good life expectancy of these patients.

Radiotherapy needs time to provide pain control and structural stabilization. In the specific case of thyroid metastases, radiometabolic therapy with iodine-131 in uptaking masses has good control of tumour growth. Moreover, samarium-153 has selective indications in bone methastases as it induces a peripheral osteoblastic reaction. Therefore it is effective at the edge of the mass and, potentially, controls pain. Both radiometabolic treatments can be combined with local thermal ablation as it induces an immediate tumour necrosis peripherally directed from the central site of the energy source. Thus, in theory, in this modality of action thermal ablation should favourably combine with and potentiate radiometabolic therapy with samarium-153.

The key to vertebral augmentation in these cases is cementoplasty. Techniques such as kyphoplasty, skyphoplasty, or even stentoplasty may have applications in metastatic disease, but their actual efficacy compared with standard vertebroplasty is unclear because of increased invasiveness, more pain, bilateral access, and higher costs. Moreover, cement diffusion within the osteolytic lesion after thermal ablation is usually is wide and quite homogeneous. Extravasation in the vertebral canal, root recesses, or root foramen can occur, but it can be carefully monitored by imaging and limited to an asymptomatic level. Therefore complications are rare. The low invasiveness of the procedure, which is always performed under local anaesthesia and mild sedation, often makes it possible to discharge the patient from hospital on the same day or the following day ('daycase surgery').

The ability of this combined procedure to provide rapid pain relief with little interference with other adjuvant therapies and minimal comorbidities should make it the first-line treatment in selected patients in centres that can offer it.

## References

1. Gokaslan ZL, York JE, Walsh GL, et al. Transthoracic vertebrectomy for metastatic spinal tumors. *J Neurosurg* 1998; 89(4): 599–609.
2. Jacobs WB, Perrin RG. Evaluation and treatment of spinal metastases: an overview. *Neurosurg Focus* 2001; 11(6): e10.
3. Benbassat CA, Mechlis-Frish S, Hirsch D. Clinicopathological characteristics and long-term outcome in patients with distant metastases from differentiated thyroid cancer. *World J Surg* 2006; 30:1088–95.
4. Hirabayashi H, Ebara S, Kinoshita T, et al. Clinical outcome and survival after palliative surgery for spinal metastases. *Cancer* 2003; 97: 476–84.
5. Georgy BA. Metastatic spinal lesions: state-of-the-art treatment options and future trends. *AJNR Am J Neuroradiol* 2008; 29(9): 1605–11.
6. Hamady M, Sheard S. Role of cementoplasty in the management of compression vertebral body fractures. *Postgrad Med J* 2009; 85(1004): 293–8.
7. Denaro L, Longo UG, Denaro V. Vertebroplasty and kyphoplasty: reasons for concern? *Orthop Clin North Am* 2009; 40 (4): 465–71.
8. Ofluoglu O. Minimally invasive management of spinal metastases. *Orthop Clin North Am* 2009; 40(1): 155–68.
9. Gangi A, Sabharwal T, Irani FG, et al. Quality assurance guidelines for percutaneous vertebroplasty. *Cardiovasc Intervent Radiol* 2006; 29(2): 173–8.
10. Harrington KD. The use of methylmethacrylate for vertebral-body replacement and anterior stabilization of pathological fracture-dislocations of the spine due to metastatic malignant disease. *J Bone Joint Surg Am* 1981; 63(1): 36–46.
11. Galibert P, Deramond H, Rosat P, Le Gars D. [Preliminary note on the treatment of vertebral angioma by percutaneous acrylic vertebroplasty]. *Neurochirurgie* 1987; 33(2): 166–8 (in French).
12. Chi JH, Gokaslan ZL. Vertebroplasty and kyphoplasty for spinal metastases. *Curr Opin Support Palliat Care* 2008; 2(1): 9–13.
13. Georgy BA. Percutaneous image-guided augmentation for spinal metastatic tumors. *Tech Vasc Interv Radiol* 2009; 12(1): 71–7.
14. Evans AJ, Jensen ME, Kip KE, et al. Vertebral compression fractures: pain reduction and improvement in functional mobility after percutaneous polymethylmethacrylate vertebroplasty retrospective report of 245 cases. *Radiology* 2003; 226(2): 366–72.
15. Barragan-Campos HM, Vallee JN, Lo D, et al. Percutaneous vertebroplasty for spinal metastases: complications. *Radiology* 2006; 238(1): 354–62.
16. Anselmetti GC, Marcia S, Saba L, et al. Percutaneous vertebroplasty: multi-centric results from EVEREST experience in large cohort of patients. *Eur J Radiol* 2012; 81(12): 4083–6.

# INDEX